General Administration in the Nursing Home

Second Edition

Wesley Wiley Rogers, B.A., M.R.E., N.H.A.

Program Director
Nursing Home Administration
McLennan Community College
Waco, Texas

Cahners Books

A Division of Cahners Publishing Company, Inc.
89 Franklin Street, Boston, Massachusetts 02110

Library of Congress Cataloging in Publication Data

Rogers, Wesley Wiley.
    General administration in the nursing home.

    Bibliography: p.
    Includes index.
    1. Nursing homes—Administration.   I. Title.
[DNLM: 1.   Hospital administration.   2.   Nursing
homes. WX150 R731g]
RA997.R55 1976   658'.91'36216   75–22325
ISBN 0–8436–0573–1
ISBN 0–8436–2055–2 student

Library of Congress Catalog Card Number: 75–22325

International Standard Book Number: 0-8436-0573-1
                                    0-8436-2055-2 (student)

Printed in the United States of America

Sci
R

Contents

Preface

Nursing home administration is changing so rapidly that it has become necessary to update and revise the former edition. Since the original work was published in 1971, a number of trends have developed within the nursing home industry that have required new legislation by government and new procedures by businessmen.

One change came about by reason of the most recent revision of the Social Security Act by Public Law 92-603, in which a common definition was given to those skilled nursing facilities contracting for either Medicaid or Medicare services. Recently, the Secretary of Health, Education, and Welfare published a new set of regulations in the *Congressional Register,* covering both the skilled nursing facilities, to conform to the law before cited and also a set of regulations for the intermediate facility.

They requested that all states set as a minimum standard the *Life Safety Code* (1967 edition) published by the National Fire Protection Association. When this code was imposed on nursing homes, there resulted sweeping changes in the various states. It was especially evident that many of the older nursing homes were subjected to repeated inspections and demands for greater fire protection.

Changes are developing in that comprehensive health planning has been imposed upon those facilities proposing to alter or increase their health delivery services to the public. New homes are much harder to get approved by the local governments and their health planning agencies. The effective efficient use of health care delivery systems can be seen as an aim of government in that the utilization review committee is now a common factor in the operation of both the Extended Care Facility of Medicare and the Skilled Nursing Facility of Medicaid.

A new breed of nursing home administrators is emerging. Formerly, the administrator was likely to be a family member operating a family business. Within the short span of time between the first publication of this book and the second edition, there developed a trend shifting the ownership of nursing homes from family ownership to chain ownership, that is, large corporate structures owning many nursing homes. In the change, administration has been converted to the hired administrator with stiff competition developing for those positions. Certainly, the licensed nursing home administrator has now found he has a marketable skill.

With change continuing at perhaps an ever-increasing pace within the nursing home industry, the former administrator is hard-pressed to keep up with the new breed of administrators. Indeed, any administrator who does not devote time daily to reading and digesting the increasing proliferation of printed materials coming to his desk in the form of regulations, laws, new business methods, etc., is likely to find himself out of the profession. Many administrators are finding increasing involvement with the fine work of such organizations as the American Health Care Association, the American Association for Homes for the Aged, or the American College of Nursing Home Administrators.

Finally, the administrator is suddenly faced with the problem that education in nursing home administration is becoming absolutely necessary if he is to keep his license a marketable product. Originally, the objective of most state licensing agencies for nursing home administrators was simply to get licensed most of the existing administrators at the time licensing was imposed. This trend has passed and in its wake much higher educational requirements are now imposed. The National Association of Boards of Examiners for Nursing Home Administrators, with membership drawn from 47 different states, has become a proponent of increased educational requirements for licensure. In fact, effective July 1, 1975, many state licensure boards are requiring an Associate Degree in Nursing Home Administration. This two-year degree requirement will later be increased to a baccalaureate level. Of course, these conditions can only be imposed on new candidates for licensure; however, any administrator at present licensed but not having a college degree in his profession will not compete in tomorrow's health-care industry. At first he will be passed by when he applies for choicer positions and later will find his applications for employment ignored altogether.

Notwithstanding the need for higher education, this text is directed to the beginning administrator or the licensed administrator who wishes a basic reference book in his work. The second edition may still be thought of as fulfilling the purpose of the orginal edition:

. . . the elements of the text are meant to define and explain the fundamental principles of nursing administration. It is a cataloguing and listing of these principles showing how they are applied to the nursing home. The evaluation and judgment of this material is left to the teacher and the student. Only occasionally has the material been evaluated. It was felt that one text could not adequately cover these vast resources needed. Therefore, the survey approach is intended.

The second edition has updated its materials to conform to changing concepts and new regulations. Some material has been added and other material expanded.

The original manuscript was intended as four manuals to be used as basic educational tools. In this edition, we have dropped this concept and simply numbered the chapters consecutively. The four "Books" of the previous edition are now Part One through Part Four.

We have eliminated the appendix section B because many of the definitions and principles may be found within the body of the text. The duplication was not necessary.

The author wishes to clarify the fact that he is a practicing nursing home administrator, that he is now entering his fourteenth year as the administrator of record of a Texas based nursing home, and that many of the concepts of the text have been proved at the Cedar Crest Nursing Home, Waco, Texas, which he owns with his wife, Janie. In addition, he now directs and teaches the Nursing Home Administration Program at McLennan Community College, Waco, Texas. This program leads to the degree of Associate in Applied Science in Long Term Health Care.

Acknowledgments for the

First Edition

This book is the result of a new and demanding need for education. It began when the author was requested to meet with a committee to plan and teach an adult education course to upgrade nursing home administration in McLennan County, Texas. The proposed course was to be offered through the Continuing Education Department of McLennan Community College, Waco, Texas. Dean James M. Summers' vision and inspiration was the dominant force in its development. The course or rather courses—the original course grew to five courses—was designed to meet the requirements of the Texas Board of Licensure for Nursing Home Administrators and the Texas Education Agency. The author's lecture outlines were later distributed to the 32 Junior Colleges in Texas approved to offer the licensure course.

The original committee was comprised of: Elmer Luckenback of the Lutheran Sunset Home, Clifton, Texas; Joseph P. McElligott, of the Regis Retirement Center, Waco, and the Central Texas Chapter of the Texas Nursing Home Association; Elmo Fischer of the Texas Association of Homes for the Aged; Theda Callaway of the Governor's Committee on Aging, Austin, Texas; Dean James M. Summers of McLennan Community College; Wesley W. Rogers, owner/administrator of Cedar Crest Nursing Home, Waco, Texas.

Sincere appreciation is extended to James P. Baker, Lufkin, Texas, President of the Texas Board of Licensure for Nursing Home Administrators; to E. M. Lawrence Jr., Executive Secretary; to Mrs. Wanda Morgan Iltis, Gonzales, Texas, Chairman of the Education Committee; and to members of the licensure board, Mrs. Johnnie M. Benson, Virgil N. Maxwell, Francis A. Flynn, J. W. Hornburg, Arthur B. Taylor, Dr. Wilfred G. Millington, and Dr. Phillip A. Gates.

Mrs. J. W. (Judy) Lohmann, Richardson, Texas, read the manuscript; undoubtedly it was my beloved and patient wife, Janie, who offered the greatest encouragement.

Acknowledgments for the Second Edition

The success of any book, especially when it has found acceptance through five printings, is more dependent upon the people who use it than on the writer. In this light, many have accepted and used this text for the improvement of nursing home administration.

Perhaps the best proponents of its use fall within the organization known as the National Association of Boards of Examiners for Nursing Home Administrators. Our sincere thanks are extended to E. M. Lawrence, Jr., Executive Secretary; to Ralph Marrinson, President; Dr. W. G. Millington, Vice President; Peg Freshman, Secretary; Jean Curtis, Treasurer; and Emanuel Bund, Legal Counsel.

We have worked with several state nursing home associations and have found help and encouragement. Our thanks also go to Rogers Wilson, Texas Nursing Home Association; Dr. Joe Rogers, Oklahoma Nursing Home Association; Ed Boudreaux, Louisiana Nursing Home Association; and Robert Russell, Florida Nursing Home Association.

Others have given encouragement and support, for which our thanks and appreciation are extended. Among these are Dr. Wilbur Ball, President, McLennan Community College; Robert K. Willis; Alvin Pollard; Dr. and Mrs. Lloyd DuBois, Dallas Baptist College; D. T. Hicks, Jr.; Lloyd Knect, Southwest Union College; and Dr. Robert Haacker, National Examination Service.

Several have indirectly influenced this text. These are: Mrs. F. L. Lohmann, Mrs. Mary Smith, R. D., Marshal Leazar, Dr. Cecil Edwards, Dr. C. C. Smith, and the Reverend Peter McLeod.

Undoubtedly, many others have encouraged me to continue our endeavor to improve nursing home administration. The strongest support comes from my family: from Janie who, as a licensed vocational nurse and a licensed nursing home administrator, has given me considerable insight into the medical aspect of the text; from Marcus, our son; and from our daughters, Debra, Cheryl, and Suzette.

PART ONE

Nursing Home

Administration

The nursing home administrator should know how to formulate goals. Some goals, called aims, are basic, primary, or general. Some goals, called objectives, are more specific.

The administrator will be familiar with the management process: planning, organizing, directing, controlling, and coordinating. Decision-making authority is invested in the administrator. He will establish policies of operation.

The administrator will be familiar with organizational structure. The governing board will be established; sole owner, partnership, corporation, or nonprofit organization. Departments will be determined by process of function, number, location, or service. The organization may be centralized in decision-making authority. He may use committees in decision making.

The administrator will delegate necessary authority by the use of written policies, job descriptions, directives, and instruction.

The administrator will establish patient-care policy administration by a patient-care policy committee, organized medical staff, or medical staff equivalent.

The administrator will develop systems of control to ensure quality patient care, functional control, financial management, and preventive maintenance. He may use consultation in social services, medical services, management, pharmacy, and nutrition.

The administrator will develop effective personnel administration. He will develop a manpower pool for recruitment, high standards of selection, and an adequate program of placement. He will develop personnel policies and abide with legal requirements: Fair Labor

Standards Act, Age Discrimination in Employment Act, and Equal Opportunity. He will work for good labor relations, using collective bargaining, arbitration, mediation, and conciliation to reach a labor agreement. It will be in accord with the Wagner Act, the National Labor Relations Act, the Taft-Hartley Act, and the Federal Mediation and Conciliation Board.

The administrator will be skilled in supervisory techniques. He will be skilled in planning and decision-making, using knowledge of methods, procedures, chance, risk, and statistical probability. He may use leadership by assignment, guiding, and inspiration; he will be familiar with laissez-faire, autocratic, democratic, and shared leadership.

The administrator may participate in Medicare or Medicaid.

The nursing home will secure a sound insurance program: fire insurance, bodily injury liability insurance, public liability insurance, malpractice insurance, automobile insurance, and unemployment insurance.

The administrator will be familiar with the law, legal contracts, the admission agreement, release of responsibility, written consent, statutes of limitations, the Uniform Commercial Code, and the Civil Rights Act.

The administrator will develop adequate training: orientation, on-the-job training, and in-service training.

The administrator will establish fair evaluation and recognition, performance ratings, promotion and transfer, and discipline.

Chapter *1*

Organization

The concept of organization of the nursing home will draw upon the business field for its principles and practices, because the nursing home is a business. While good patient care is the primary aim of the nursing home, business is the fundamental enterprise that allows the administrator to carry out this aim. Therefore, the study of general administration in the nursing home will include a study of how a business is organized, how employees are selected and supervised, business law, and insurance. Studies of labor, its problem, human relations, training, staff meetings, and group dynamics are but a few of the areas that will concern the administrator.

Our text will not follow the accepted pattern of a business manual, because we are concerned with the administrator of the nursing home. He will have certain immediate needs in his work which we shall deal with first. Fundamentally, the greatest need will be the organization of the nursing home.

The nursing home may be organized according to several patterns, i.e., centralized management, decentralized management, formal organization, informal organization, committees, etc. There is no definite rule, since the size, type, and ownership of a business usually determine its methods of operation. However, the type of management personnel may dictate the type of management of the home. Normally, the governing board is the owner of the nursing home and will select the administrator. The selection will be by a written agreement specifying the responsibility of the administrator.

The Sole Proprietorship

The sole proprietor is the individual owner. In many cases, the owner serves as his own administrator and is in a sense hiring himself. Thus he has a dual role: governing board and administrator. There are some advantages in this arrangement, and there are also several disadvantages. The nursing home operated by the sole proprietor usually gives more personalized care, is usually caught up in problem solving, often works directly with the employees, has a close relationship with the employees' and patients' families, tends to use an "open door" employee policy, and has tight control on the economic growth and stability of the business.

Usually, the sole proprietor got his start when a family enterprise was passed on to him. Originally, the majority of nursing homes were family businesses. By nature, the sole proprietorship is the easiest method of starting a business, and the individual with some savings, an ability to manage, and a concern for the aged can start a nursing home. However, it is becoming increasingly more difficult because of more rigid licensing laws. Because of the licensing law for nursing home administrators, he now must take specialized training if he is to serve as the administrator of record for the facility. Because of Comprehensive Health Care Planning, he may not be eligible for federal funds from Medicare or Medicaid, if he does not secure the approval of his local planning agency. He may find himself limited in capital, which could restrict his growth potential; banks and lending institutions are very cautious about underwriting a business that is built primarily by one person. The sole owner has unlimited liability, which may restrict his raising money for operation and expansion. In spite of this, nursing homes operated by the sole proprietor continue to comprise a large percentage of the nursing home industry. However, corporate or nonprofit organizations continue to gain in numbers.

The Partnership

Normally, there are two types of partnerships in the nursing home business: the general partnership and the limited partnership. All owners share equally in the management and liability of the operation in a general partnership. In the limited partnership, by contract and law, an agreement may be made in which the partnership restricts management responsibility for all but one partner. Secret partners are restricted by licensing and contractual agencies, which require affidavits of ownership. The partners constitute the governing board.

The Corporation

With the advent of Medicare and Medicaid, nursing homes have tended to grow larger. Recent trends have made the 100-bed home the nearly average size, with projected trends to increase this number upward. Limited in growth capital, the sole proprietor finds his only way to compete is to "go public" and incorporate. Of course, the stock may be owned by the individuals incorporating and may never be offered to the general public. In this condition it resembles single family ownership.

A more recent trend is the growth of "chain" nursing homes. They are referred to as chains simply because of the number controlled by one corporation. Some advantages of the corporate structure may be passed on to the consumer. The ease with which ownership may be shifted without disturbing the management of the corporate nursing home makes it an attractive investment. Because the size of the corporation may reach into the millions of dollars, some advantage in starting new enterprises may be noted. Because the corporate structure limits the liability of the individual owner to the shares he may own in the corporation, many sole owners have incorporated. Such factors as these have tended to bring many nursing homes into chain corporations.

Nonprofit Organization

The nonprofit corporation exists for charitable purposes. Actually, there is no such thing as a purely nonprofit business, since all business must make a profit to continue to exist. The question is merely who benefits from the profits of the corporation. Of course, trust funds may exist for dispensing certain funds.

The nonprofit corporation or voluntary organization, as it is sometimes called, is chartered by the Secretary of State of the state in which it exists. All activities of the business must function within the stated purpose of the charter. Like a regular stock corporation, it is limited to carrying on its business activities in compliance with corporation law.

The trend among voluntary organizations is to enter the nursing home field on a larger scale. The health care field has always appealed to charitable organizations as a vehicle of service. Admittedly, the voluntary organization may have several advantages, i.e., the raising of capital by subscription, a definite tax advantage, etc.

It may be noted that many states now have associations of nonprofit homes for their improvement and support, e.g., the American Association of Homes for the Aged.

The board of trustees or a board of directors will be designated by charter as the governing board having final authority.

The Board of Directors

The minimum requirement is that at least three persons must comprise a corporation. Normally, the administrator wishing to incorporate his business will secure the services of a corporation lawyer who will prepare the necessary articles of incorporation and file them with the Secretary of State of his state. The minimum articles of incorporation include the names of the corporation and the incorporators, the period of its duration, the purposes, and the value of the firm.

Once the incorporators have raised the necessary minimum amount specified as the value of the firm, they hold an organizational meeting to select officers and to pass the necessary resolutions empowering these to conduct business. Because all business conducted by the corporation must be according to state corporation law, no actions are valid without proper authorization. Thus resolutions should be passed for authorization to acquire property, to fix salaries, to pay the organizational expense, to deposit money or draw checks, and to conduct the business.

One rigid requirement of the corporation is the documentation of all meetings of the board of directors or the annual meeting of the stockholders. An attorney should guide the secretary in framing the format of the minutes of each meeting. Another requirement is an annual meeting at a specified time, preceded by a proper notice of this meeting. All actions of the corporation must be conducted within the stated purpose of the corporation. Thus, if a corporation clearly states that the purpose of the business is to conduct a nursing home, it may conduct no other type of business without a charter ammendment. The corporation attorney should always be available to review the actions of the corporation.

The Development of Management Theory

In our attempt to organize the nursing home as a management enterprise, we should look into the historical background of the development of management theory. Essentially, two theories, called scientific theory and functional theory, developed simultaneously. Like all theories, they had their origin in experience, in this case, that of Frederick Taylor and Henri Fayol.

Frederick Taylor, working for Bethlehem Steel during the latter part of the nineteenth century, began to apply scientific principles to management. He concerned himself with such factors as methods, training, equal division of work, wages, cooperation between workers, and time study.

Henri Fayol, a Frenchman, is credited with developing the functional approach to management. He began his studies in 1885 and systematically analyzed the functions of management. A function might be described as the natural or logical divisions of work. An example might be the economic factor concerning a business. Fayol found that work or business could be studied as to its technical aspect, its management relationships, its commercial and accounting functions, its problems of security, and its operational functions.

The development of this text covers, in general, the same points. It begins by studying the organizational or operational functions of the nursing home, the relationship of the administrator to his staff, something of the commercial aspects, and it progresses through governmental relationships. It studies other functions of the nursing home, such as the technological aspect and the human relations involved in its operation.

Refinements of management theory since the time of the initial studies by Fayol and Taylor have developed certain aspects of organizational management. Management can be typed, generally, according to three levels: top, middle, and operating. *Top management is considered to be the decision-making level and will include the administrator.* Middle management is any level of supervision between the top management level and the operating level. In the local nursing home the Director of Nurses will be considered middle management. The operating level, of course, includes the line worker. The charge nurse is considered the line manager.

The Principles of Organization

There are certain basic principles that govern the method used to establish an organization. When the administrator begins to define the relationship of authority and responsibility, he will adopt these principles. Essentially, it is *how* an organization is developed. What is the working relationship of one worker to another? How are the workers grouped together? How do you expand the organization? How does authority extend from the top management to the operating level?

The administrator may adopt a well-defined system of delegating authority and responsibility. There are definite relationships, definite written job descriptions, and accepted functional relationships. This would be called a formal organization and would apply "line" relationships to guide the "chain of command." *"Line" means a direct path of communication, authority, and responsibility between a subordinate and a superior.*

In contrast with the formal organization and operating within its framework is an informal organization. *Informal organization concerns the attitudes, emotions, likes, and dislikes of the employees.* It is a cohesive element that affects decisions, movement, progress, and success. It functions loosely in spite of management. It may, however, be a powerful tool when understood and integrated in the power structure. It should be noted that the smaller the nursing home, the more influential the informal organization becomes. It may be observed at work when the supervisor of nurses influences the laundry in the processing of laundry, or when the aide becomes a self-appointed foreman. A secretary may be more in charge of an office than the administrator and give direction to employees. Precisely for this reason the administrator will define his position, establish definite channels of communication for his authority, and supervise wisely within these channels. He may use informal organization for feedback reactions, evaluation, and judging the temper of his organization, but he should never allow it to run the nursing home for him.

Forming Departments

The administrator should learn the principles of organization concerned with departmentalization. *This is the act of grouping the functions and activities of the nursing home into departments.* This may be done in several ways. The process may dictate the type of organization formed. An example within the nursing home would be the laundry. Since clothing is processed by washing, drying, folding, etc., it naturally would be separated from other activities and called the laundry department, would be given a supervisor and workers, and be established in the chain of command. Such a working department may be referred to as a line department.

Departmentalization concerns the basis chosen to make departments. In the nursing home, there are several variations of this, but the most common is the first, second, and third shift of nursing. Each shift is essentially a department with its own charge nurse and its workers, called aides. The basis for departmentalization is the number

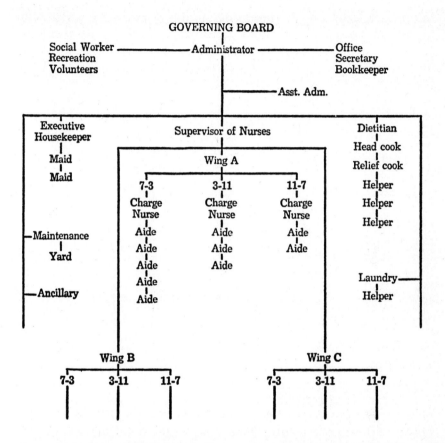

GOVERNING BOARD

Social Worker ———————— Administrator ———————— Office
Recreation   Secretary
Volunteers   Bookkeeper

———————— Asst. Adm.

Executive
Housekeeper   Supervisor of Nurses   Dietitian
                                                    Head cook
Maid   Wing A   Relief cook
Maid
                 7-3   3-11   11-7   Helper
                 Charge   Charge   Charge   Helper
                 Nurse   Nurse   Nurse   Helper
—Maintenance   Aide   Aide   Aide
                 Aide   Aide   Aide
Yard   Aide   Aide
                 Aide   Laundry——
—Ancillary   Aide   Helper

            Wing B   Wing C
       7-3   3-11   11-7   7-3   3-11   11-7

Organizational Chart of Small Nursing Home

or time of shift. It is also possible to departmentalize on the basis of territory. When you say, "upstairs," "West wing," or "First floor," you are giving examples of departmentalizing on the basis of territory. There is an additional way of departmentalizing which is applicable to the nursing home. This is by customer. This occurs when a portion of the facility is assigned to a certain level of care. For example, when one wing is an extended care facility, the customer is the Medicare patient.

Centralization and Decentralization

In the search for a method of grouping the workers, the services, or the activities of the nursing home, there are two other considerations: centralization and decentralization. Such consideration applies to the decision-making authority of the nursing home, but it also relates to the organizational and departmental structure of the organization.

The decision-making process, making use of the knowledge of methods, procedures, chance, risk, or statistical probability, includes the determining of policy establishing the organization and rendering judgment.

In the centralized concept, the management's decision-making authority is reserved for top management. In the decentralized organization, decision-making authority is delegated to a subordinate.

To grasp the importance of this differentiation in the nursing home organization, consider the administrator who personally directs every department supervisor. This is centralized management. On the other hand, the administrator may give some decision-making authority to the heads of departments. This is called decentralized decision making. The administrator who allows the department heads to hire and fire their particular workers illustrates decentralized management. Normally, only the large unit or a multi-unit practices decentralized management. It is not uncommon for the nursing home chain to decentralize its management; however, it may also adhere to centralized management. The statement, "I will have to check with the home office," denotes centralized authority.

Growth is affected to some degree by whichever concept the management may have of decentralization or centralization. With the centralized viewpoint, the administrator will extend the scale of the organization when he adds new departments. This will simply mean that more supervisors are responsible to the administrator. However, should he place an additional supervisor between himself and the line supervisor, he will diversify his authority further. Picture the aide, who is responsible to the supervising nurse, who in turn is responsible to the administrator.

Functional Relationships

The administrator will develop certain relationships with his employees and the work they perform in behalf of the patients. These are commonly known as line, staff, or functional relationships. These relationships are an integral part of the organizational pattern and are effective when utilized wisely by the administrator. The development of the functional relationships overlaps the line relationships. Normally, the functions of an organization follow those identified by Henri Tayol, i.e., technical, financial, security, etc. Today we refer to them as staff relationships.

Within the management of the nursing home, a number of staff relationships exist for the support of the administrator's direction of the nursing staff and deal with the service or advisory areas of organization. Staff relationships are said to exist when advice, counsel, or assistance is offered in support of the line organization. They are essentially functional relationships and carry neither authority nor right of discipline.

There are a number of roles that a staff relationship may play in the nursing home organization. The assistant administrator is a good example. Another is the consultant who counsels. The personnel manager may offer his services in selecting employees. It should be noted in identifying these positions that a conflict of terminology exists in the ideal staff position. The popular use of the term "staff" has been to identify the entire organization, e.g., calling a "staff meeting" or referring to the "supervisory staff." In business terminology, "staff" in organization means the supportive employee, not the "line" supervisor.

Another supportive role in administrative decision-making is the committee. The committee is a type of organization, but it is also a function relationship. The administrator may find a very practical use of the committee as a tool for making decisions, and rightly so, since it enlists a variety of talent and gains their support. It broadens the use of staff development as it utilizes a wider range of experience. Its function, however, is to support the administrator in making nursing home decisions. Some administrators find the committee system to be too slow, with a tendency to become rubber stamps for his decisions.

Patient Care Policy Administration

The nursing home administrator will discover he has achieved a place of professionalism in the health care community. He will also discover the need to utilize interprofessional cooperation in the development of patient-care policies. Normally, he may draw upon the professional disciplines of his own staff or go outside the home to obtain professional assistance. *The basic idea behind the development of policies for patient care is to draw upon the wide range of knowledge and experience of the medical and paramedical health care team.* It is, therefore, necessary to bring together a consensus of opinion as to the best way to meet the needs of the patients. The patient-care policy committee serves this purpose.

The customary method of administering patient-care policies is the one required by most licensing agencies or contractual agencies. For example, the Texas Department of Public Welfare, in contracting for medical assistance for Medicaid recipients, requires of the administrator:

> Written patient care policies shall be formulated with the advice of one or more physicians and one or more registered and/or licensed nurses.

Thus, if the administrator were to establish such a committee as a standard for participation in the welfare program, it would be composed of himself, a nurse, and a physician, and may include any other personnel he deems necessary, i.e., dietitian, therapist, pharmacist, dentist, social worker, etc. The normal function of the committee is to formulate policy; however, this should also include making such amendments as may be necessary, and a periodic review, perhaps annually, to bring them up to date.

A second method of administering patient-care policy is to develop an organized medical staff of the physicians practicing in the nursing home. Such an organization would be self-regulating and would develop policies for medical practice and attendance. It would approve policies concerning patient care. Such an organization may include physicians, paramedical personnel, and health advisory members. A medical director would be employed by the nursing home as the coordinator.

The first two methods will generally relate to the single nursing home; however, it is possible to go to the county medical society, or any community-wide medical group to obtain supervision of the patient-care policy planning. Such a device will be *equivalent to a medical staff* and will function within the several nursing homes cooperating in the project. In other words, several nursing homes join together to enlist the community medical society to develop patient-care policies applicable to the various cooperating nursing homes. It is possible for a chain operation to use this device for formulating patient-care policies.

The organized medical staff has the advantage of giving uniformity and discipline to the medical attendance expected within the home. It also enlists the medical practitioners' cooperation in handling the problems of patient-care policy planning.

Essentially, the administration of the patient-care policy is based on written policies. Policies are of a two-fold nature: general administrative policies and patient-care policies. Besides these two policies, we may go a step further and develop procedures which define step by step how a policy will be carried out. Methods are more specific and define a single step of a procedure. Thus, the administrator will have in the policies, procedures, and methods adequate tools in which to administer the home.

For the benefit of the administrator, we have included a sample manual of patient care. The administrator will notice some overlapping of other policies of the nursing home such as the personnel policy. In the final analysis, each administrator decides how to define the policies of his nursing home; indeed, some administrators will have only a single policy statement. Logically, a nurse will need three policies. When she is hired, she will be given the personnel policy. Then she may receive a copy of the patient-care manual because she is a nurse. finally, she would receive a copy of the administrative policies because she has supervisory responsibilities.

Patient Care Manual

"Grow old along with me; the best is yet to be."—Robert Browning.

The Objective. The primary objective is to restore and maintain each patient at his best functional level so as to encourage dignity, self-care, and independence.

Personnel shall pursue this objective through physicians' services, nursing services, restorative services, dietary services, patient activities, counseling, and guidance.

Discrimination Forbidden. Compliance is pledged with section 601 of Title VI of the Civil Rights Act of 1964, which stipulates: "No person in the United States shall, on the ground of race, color, or national origin, be excluded from participation in, be denied the benefits of, or be subjected to discrimination under any program or activity receiving Federal financial assistance." Substantial proof of such discrimination by any employee is grounds for dismissal.

Prerequisites of Good Nursing. Nursing is of a confidential and personal nature; therefore, only the management will deal with the families. Remember that the condition, treatment, medications, etc., of patients is considered privileged information. This means an employee cannot publish, gossip, or reveal information concerning patients except to those legally privileged to receive it. The charts are for the nurses, the physicians, and the management only. The medicine boxes are for management use only; therefore, it is best that medicine and treatments be discussed by the nursing supervisor and/or charge nurses with the patient and guardian/relatives. While employees are expected to be courteous and tactful in receiving relatives and visitors, they should avoid giving out privileged information both on the job and off the job.

Every nurse will receive a patient report before rendering service to the patients. Such reports will be given to the in-coming shift by the charge nurse of the shift going off duty. However, patient care still has priority, and will be done, if needed, during the report period.

Each nurses' aide will report on the conditions of the patients she attends regarding all matters which should be included in the shift report and the clinical charts.

Changes in patients' conditions, observations, and progress shall be recorded in the clinical charts.

All charting will be done by the charge nurse and/or ward clerk. The charge nurse will sign all charting concerning her actions. The 7:00 A.M. to 3:00 P.M. charts are recorded in blue ink. The 3:00 P.M. to 11:00 P.M. charts are recorded in green ink. The 11:00 P.M. to 7:00 A.M. charts are recorded in red ink.

Every incident, whether or not resulting in injury, and every allegation of mistreatment of patients by the nursing home staff shall be described in an Incident Report. The charge nurse must sign and file one copy with the administrator, and the other copy is placed in the clinical charts.

The charge nurse or supervising nurse will accompany all doctors making rounds of their patients and will assist in such a manner as would be prescribed by good nursing practices. She will be cooperative and efficient, and perform such tasks as requested by the doctor to assist in bedside procedures.

Medications are to be kept under lock at all times when not being prepared or administered. The charge nurse will keep all keys (medicine room, medicine cabinet, narcotic cabinet, re-frigerator, etc.) in her possession while on duty. Keys are to be surrendered to the in-coming shift's charge nurse.

No medications or treatments shall be given patients except on orders of a licensed physician prescribing to his patient.

There is an automatic stop-order for all controlled drugs such as narcotics, sedatives, and antibiotics, which must be adhered to unless the physician prescribes the specific number of doses and time to be given.

Patients shall not be allowed to have custody of any medications except at the time administered or as ordered by the physician.

The narcotic record is to be kept up to date.

The administration of medications and treatments shall be recorded on the clinical charts.

Personal Hygiene for Bed Patients.

Brush and comb hair daily.
Shampoo hair as needed.
Male residents will shave at least daily.
Male residents will have haircuts monthly.
Teeth are brushed twice daily.
Dentures are cleaned twice daily.
Provide containers for dentures at night.
Cut fingernails as needed.
Cut toenails as needed.
Change clothing daily, more often if needed.
Turn and rub bed patient every two hours.
Apply body lotions, powders, and deodorants.
Give complete bath every day.
Give partial bath after each incontinent episode.

Personal Hygiene for Ambulatory Patients.

Encourage residents to brush and comb hair daily.
Have hair shampooed as needed.
Male residents are to have a haircut every month.
Male residents will shave daily.
Encourage residents to brush teeth twice daily.
Clean all dentures twice daily.
Cut fingernails and toenails as needed.

Bathing and Linen Changing Schedule. The supervisor of nurses will correlate and post schedules.

Required Shift Duties. 7:00 A.M. to 3:00 P.M.

All medications will be administered by the charge nurse.

The charge nurse will check each patient.

The charge nurse will do all charting or use a ward clerk.

Aides will keep note pads and make notes for the charge nurse.

Early A.M. care will be given patients not attending the dining room.

Assistance will be given any patient needing help to the dining room.

All nurses will assist with breakfast.

Bathe and groom patients. Attend patients while bathing.

Serve nourishment and fluids at 10:00 A.M.

Provide water set-ups at the bedside tables.

Prepare patients for the noon meal. Offer assistance as needed.

Encourage activities and render assistance for organized recreation.

Check linen rooms, bathrooms, and utility rooms. Pick up, straighten, and clean as necessary.

Clean and store all nursing equipment not in use.

Make a final check of patients before shift is finished.

Aides will give notes and reports to charge nurse.

Charge nurse will give report to in-coming shift.

Required Shift Duties. 3:00 P.M. to 11:00 P.M.

All medications will be administered by the charge nurse.

The charge nurse will check each patient.

The charge nurse will do all the charting or use a ward clerk.

Aides will give notes and reports to charge nurse.

Serve fluid and nourishment at 3:00 P.M. and 7:00 P.M.

Prepare patients for the evening meal and assist them.

Encourage activities and render assistance in organized recreation.

Prepare and assist patients to bed.

Personal hygiene requirement for patients will be met.

Attend patients while bathing.

Check linen rooms, bathrooms, and utility rooms; pick up, straighten, and clean as necessary.

Clean and store all nursing equipment not in use.
Make a final check of patients before shift is finished.
Aides will give notes and reports to charge nurse.
Charge nurse will give report to in-coming-shift.

Required Shift Duties.   11:00 P.M. to 7:00 A.M.
All medication will be given by the charge nurse.
The nurse in charge will check each patient.
The charge nurse will do all charting.
Fulfill Personal Hygiene requirements.
Carry out assigned bathing requirement.
Offer water to bed patient during each turning period.
Place clean washcloth and towel in each patient's unit.
Place clean bed linens where needed.
Place disposal pads in each incontinent patient's unit.
Assist ambulatory patients in dressing (robes are permitted at breakfast).
Check linen rooms, showers, bathrooms, and utility room; pick up, straighten, and clean as necessary.
Clean and store nursing equipment not in use.
Make final check of patients before shift change.
Aides will give notes and reports to charge nurse.
Charge nurse will give report to in-coming shift.

The Nursing Home Staff

The recruitment, selection, and placement of the nursing home staff is perhaps the most important function of the administrator and his assistant. This function may be assigned to the administrative assistant or personnel director, but should be supervised carefully. *The nursing home's primary commodity is the service rendered by the employees.* Success is built on the best selection of personnel.

In order to recruit and keep an adequate staff for the nursing home, the administrator should first anticipate the staffing needs. Generally, there are several factors affecting needs. Because of the diversity of tasks, the requirements for performance, and the replacements owing to shifting personnel, job needs will vary. The administrator will anticipate these variations. Because of the variation in occupancy of the nursing home, and the variation in costs, personnel needs may change. The administrator will devise some system of anticipating employment needs which will be coupled with a method of authorizing staff positions.

The administrator will be aware of some other factors, psychological in nature, that affect the staffing pattern. For example, more aides are needed when a number of patients become critically ill, when seasonal changes affect the health of employee or patient, or when the bed capacity is increased. The normal course is for these aides to become accepted as a part of the normal staffing pattern even though they were temporarily added. The employees, including the supervisors, will accept them and expect them to remain, resisting the efforts of the administrator to return to a normal staffing pattern when special needs no longer prevail.

The development of the staffing pattern will be affected by requirements of the licensing agency which may specify a minimum staff. Contractual agencies such as Medicaid and Medicare will also specify certain minimums. The administrator will methodically list the staff from time to time, collect data concerning the staffing needs, analyze this in relation to the goals and objectives of the home, the costs of operation, or seasonal or emergency needs, and then make his personnel staffing decisions.

Locating Qualified Nursing Home Personnel

The personnel director will develop his sources of applicants for employment. Within the home there will come recommendations from the employees, the patients, and the relatives of patients. These are good sources that should not be overlooked. However, the relative of an employee may not be a good choice. In addition, the administrator will look at all recommendations objectively.

A number of external sources are available and should be cultivated. These would include employment agencies, educational institutions, professional organizations, labor unions, and social agencies. Of course, advertising through the local newspaper is an accepted pratice in business and should be used. During the summer, especially for vacation relief, there are many fine high school and college students who could be used to great advantage by the nursing home. Such student development is important. For a number of years, the Vice-President of the United States has sponsored campaigns to employ students during the summer. The local state employment offices usually coordinate this activity, serving as well as a source of referrals of the unemployed. An apprenticeship program through an educational institution may be another source. The administrator himself may locate an assistant-in-training through a local junior college.

Finally, we must consider the unsolicited applicants. While careful evaluation must be made of each of the applicants, the administrator will discover these usually come as a result of word-of-mouth referrals by friends, relatives of patients and employees, former patients, or business associates. An objective selection method will weed out those not suited for employment. The administrator who selects his applicants well can discover potential employees who will help him meet business objectives.

Methods of Employee Selection

Recruitment is finding applicants and selection is hiring suitable applicants. Selection of employees involves the techniques and methods of evaluating candidates as to the necessary qualifications for specific jobs. There are several basic factors that may be used in selecting employees from among those recruited.

It is the function of management to make selections. While the task may be delegated to a personnel manager or department supervisor, it will be a cooperative process among all levels of management with the final approval resting in the administrator. Usually, the administrator formulates the policies and objectives, and then the task of selection is delegated to an assistant. His policies must ensure that the standards used are ethical and legal. Each state has fair labor practices which should be adhered to in the selection of nursing home employees. While several laws apply, the two most important federal laws are the Fair Labor Standards Act of 1938 as amended in 1966 to include nursing homes and the Age Discrimination in Employment Act of 1968. Employment practices should not exclude the handicapped.

Interviewing the Applicant

Greeting the applicant cheerfully at the beginning of an interview will place him at ease, allowing a better appraisal. The more he talks, the more he will reveal about himself. Remember, the interviewer is selling the applicant on working in the nursing home, and it is just as possible to lose a potentially good employee as it is for him to lose the chance of getting a job. Normally, there would be a short preliminary interview. This is to determine if major obstacles are evident that would prevent employment. If the job opening were for a registered nurse and the applicant were a registered technician, this would constitute a major obstacle. If the nursing home carried no staff position of technician, it would benefit the nursing home and the applicant to terminate the interview. Of course, continue the interview if there may exist a probable need in the future for a technician.

In preparation for the interview, the personnel manager will have ready the necessary application forms, testing materials, and interview data. He will have formulated his interview plan.

Conducting the interview is a skill to be learned and developed. *The objective of the interview is to encourage the applicant to reveal as much information regarding his ability, attitudes, reliability, and potential for performance as possible.* Certainly, the person conducting the interview will have had study and practice in the techniques of interviewing. He will also keep in mind that his nursing home will be no better than the people he selects for employment. If he forms the wrong first impression of an applicant, he may never reach a true estimate of ability. And if he estimates an applicant's ability without adequate reasons, his evaluations will not ring true. He should be ever aware of how his applicant will rate when compared with the present staff, and whether he can discover a true picture of the past ability of the potential worker. The interview is designed to discover as much information as is possible within the alloted time. If there are unanswered questions, additional time will be needed.

At the conclusion of the interview, the personnel manager will begin immediately his investigation and appraisal. Time will be at a premium, because most unemployed persons are in need and will not delay very long waiting for the personnel manager to make a decision to hire. The background check of references, previous employment, and educational qualifications should be done thoroughly. He will request the prospective employee to submit to a physical examination to determine his fitness for the position.

In the employee interview, the following points are covered:

> Verification of the application data.
> Estimate of the applicant's appearance.
> A physical examination to determine fitness.
> An estimate of his attitudes.
> An estimate of his motives for work.
> Knowledge of past work experiences.
> Evaluation of the past work experiences.
> Forecast of potential work ability.
> Check of character references.
> Test of job skills.

Educational achievement.
Estimate of reliability.

A preliminary selection may be made by the personnel manager or the administrator. However, the final decision should be made after an appraisal by the department supervisor. The importance of cooperative effort in choosing employees cannot be stressed too greatly.

After the employee has been selected and employment requirements have been completed, he is given information about the nursing home, and its policies are discussed. Rules and regulations of the company are explained. The salary is agreed upon, deductions determined, and fringe benefits clarified. Some personnel managers make this a part of the interview; however, it should be noted that the discussion of benefits, salaries, deductions, etc., is normally a part of the final agreement.

After final evaluation of the interview, testing, and recommendations, and after agreement concerning salary is made, the personnel manager or the administrator will hire the applicant. This should be a formal act, such as stating the position and the salary. For example, the administrator might say, "Mr. B., we have carefully evaluated your qualifications and would like to offer you a position as ———— with your starting salary to be $————. Is this acceptable?"

If this is agreeable, the starting date and time schedule are set, orientation is scheduled, and any other requirements of the nursing home are met. Notes should be kept concerning all agreements or promises made to the new employee.

Placement of Employees

How an employee is placed on the job will often determine his effectiveness. It may determine whether the employee gets through the first day or week on the job without difficulty. A placement program follows set guidelines that have been determined in advance. Little will be taken for granted. The program should be thorough and complete. However, care will be taken to see that the employee is not overwhelmed by the presentation. This is especially true where the educational level of the employee is low.

Orientation

Orientation as a placement tool is an organized effort to acquaint the new employee with his job. Each person with whom the new worker is to have some association, will be properly introduced and given some time for comments. This should be done either formally or informally. In a formal situation, the administrator, nursing supervisor, department head, and staff personnel are brought together for the orientation period. This usually will be done when there are several persons in the orientation program. In contrast, the informal method of orientation indicates where the new employee meets and talks with the various supervisory personnel individually. Each person is given sufficient time for personally orienting the new employee as to the responsibility or authority exercised by each of them.

Orientation should be objective and not personal. At least one person will develop the plan for orientation and carry it through to conclusion. For example, the personnel director will develop a checklist that will include the functions and responsibilities of each person involved in the orientation of the new employee. He should ascertain that it is comprehensive and is accomplished according to the plan.

The supervisor's checklist will include those items of importance that are to be accomplished when the employee first reports. It will include specific activities to be done during the first day on the job. Some form of checkup should be planned at periodic times. A typical list may include:

> Introduction and welcome to the nursing home staff.
> Showing where personal items are stored.
> Location of washroom and rest room.
> Facilities for eating.
> Review of personnel policies.
> Use of the time clock.
> Introduction to work group.
> Tour of nursing home and place of work.
> Safety rules in the use of special equipment.
> Safety rules in the handling of patients.
> Parking rules.
> Briefing concerning department.
> Starting employee on his job.
> Initial performance check.
> Follow-up evaluation.
> Miscellaneous.

In discussing the employees job training, explain the requirements for training and the accomplishments expected. A copy of the training plan, including some curriculum, may be placed in the hands of the beginning employee during the orientation period. Even if he is to be given only on-the-job training, this should be well planned.

It should be noted that while this discussion focuses on the orientation of the new employee, orientation is part of the directing process when it is used to familiarize all employees with new methods, procedures, or policies.

Personnel Policy

Every employee in the nursing home should have the benefit of two sources of information concerning his job. The first is the personnel policy, and the second is a complete description of the job he is expected to do. The administrator is responsible for providing this information for each employee.

The personnel policy is general in nature, dealing with information concerning all employees. The job description is for the individual employee. It is developed cooperatively with the various levels of management. It may be the result of cooperation with the workers, their representatives, or negotiation between labor and management. Usually, personnel policies are developed cooperatively, while job descriptions are prepared by the supervisors.

The personnel policy will be brief and concise, yet thorough enough to anticipate all the needs of labor as related to management. It should include:

> The nursing home statement of objectives.
> Working hours, including over-time pay.
> Holidays, rest periods, and time off.
> Benefits such as insurance, employer liability, hospitalization, and pension plans.
> Sick leave, leave-of-absence, extended leave.
> Vacation and requirement for eligibility.
> Safety rules.
> The pay period and pay day.
> Rules of conduct, etiquette.
> Liability of the employees.
> Miscellaneous information.

The administrator will establish a definite means of informing the employees of the personnel policy and changes in it. There will be a need for a periodic review of policies by the supervisory staff and with the employees. At any time a change in policy is made, sufficient time to inform the employees will be given before the change becomes effective. All policies and policy changes should be in writing.

Personnel policy should be correlated with the written job descriptions. For example, the job description for the nurse's aide is nearly the same as patient-care policy and both are closely related to some of the items of personnel policy.

Principles of Job Analysis

Every job is analyzed before a proper job description is written. The amount of detail needed will depend upon several factors related to company personnel policy. Certainly, the size of the nursing home organization or its parent organization, the scalar length of the management, the organizational method, and the type of management will dictate the amount of detail written into a job description. This is not to say that any job analysis should be brief and less thorough, but that in the smaller nursing home there is a shorter communication span between worker and administrator and/or top management.

A detailed study includes several factors such as the physical motions involved in the specific aspects of the job, psychological considerations, and any unique methods. A general study or analysis may be preferred in the smaller nursing home. This will include the basic factors of the task as outlined below.

The "what?" factor is simply an explanation of the job. In simple terms, the various responsibilities and duties are itemized. These may be listed at random or in order of importance. Usually, the chronological order is best.

The "when?" factor lists the job in relation to time. This may be thought of as a duty schedule. However, close analysis of a specific job is not always practical; it may take longer to describe a task than to perform it. An example is scheduling the nurse's aide's time for giving bed baths. If the analysis were made of each step in bathing a patient, i.e., preparation, positioning, application of soap, rinsing, drying, repositioning, etc., such information would hardly serve as a duty schedule. If, however, this information were to evaluate the time for each type of patient, it would be useful in scheduling the number of bed baths to each aide, or valuable in training for efficiency.

The "where?" factor lists the place, or places, the job is to be accomplished. It may involve more than the specific location of the work to be done. The source of supply, the check-in and check-out station, distance traveled, elevator waiting time, communications, etc. will be considered in the analysis. One administrator discovered an approximately 15% loss of time by cleaning employees waiting for the elevator in a multistory nursing home that formerly had been a hotel. This affected efficiency greatly and required the hiring of additional help.

The "how?" factor lists the skills and techniques needed to accomplish the job. It may specify the educational requirements necessary for performance. It will also include a discussion of the tools and equipment needed as well as the skill required in their use. This will likely be the primary analysis, since it is fundamental to the entire job. Certainly, an analysis of a bookkeepers's job should not be carried further than to gather enough information to make a practical job description. Bookkeeping is too involved to make a minute listing of every detail. The analysis may, however, describe the system used, the machines and machine skills, and the techniques required. On the other hand, the housekeeper's position will be analyzed carefully, since there is the probability of wide variation in practice.

The "who?" factor lists the person or persons involved in the task. In the analysis, the management or administration will make the final decision as to who is assigned to a job. There are times when the analysis will include some of the function of related personnel. For the benefit of defining the functions of the nurse's aide, the administrator may show some of the responsibilities of the supervisor of nurses, the charge nurse, the medication nurse, the administrator, and the physician in order to avoid duplication and unauthorized nursing.

The "why?" factor is important in that it gives the reason for the job. Before the staff can be recruited for the opening of a nursing home, an analysis of job requirements must be made. When a change in the staffing pattern is made, the administrator should resurvey each job requirement. Periodically, the administrator will review the work of each person and weigh his efficiency. When a question arises concerning an individual employee and his performance, the job analysis will help the administrator in making a fair decision.

Writing the Job Description

The student of administration should practice the art of job description using the methods described under job analysis. While they are interrelated, the analysis is a scientific study of the task and the description is a written detail of how an individual should perform a given task. In other words, a job description tells an employee what he is hired to do and includes anything of significance related to the performance of the job. The job description will define the limit and the scope of the task to be performed.

The contents of the job description are:

The job title.
Classification of the job in relation to the staff.
A general description of the scope of the task.
Any limits placed on the task.
A list of the materials to be used.
The normal position and place the work will be done.
A discussion of the skills required.
The methods that are used.
The training necessary.
Optional information.

The job description may contain certain optional information: promotion opportunities, compensation, working hours, dress requirements, health safeguards, and safety requirements. There may be some unusual aspect of an individual job such as the handling of contaminated materials, subjecting the employee to adverse heat or cold, dealing with patients that are not responsible for what they do or say, etc.

If the student is actively engaged in nursing home work, he should describe his own position and then be given the responsibility of writing several other job descriptions. If the student is not active in the profession, he might visit a nursing home and observe, discuss employee qualifications with the management, and research from written materials the job details. We include below a job description for administrator.

TITLE: NURSING HOME ADMINISTRATOR

Classification. Administrator of record, having full supervisory responsibility for the management of the nursing home. He shall answer directly to the governing board for his actions and the actions of his subordinates.

General Description of Responsibilities. He shall supervise the employees, administer the patient-care policies, and manage the total operation of the home, including policies, financial matters, staffing, cooperation with state and local agencies, community relations, professional relations, and patient relations.

Personal Qualifications. He must be at least 18 years of age, hold a current state license as a nursing home administrator, meet the educational requirements of that license, be capable of making mature judgments, be of good physical and mental capabilities, and maintain a life style and character that reflects a genuine love and concern for the nursing home patient.

Working Conditions. The administrator shall work a minimum of forty hours per week, either in his office, in the nursing home proper, and/or within the community.

Skills Required. The administrator will develop and possess skills of supervision. He shall be responsible for procuring adequate, trained personnel, their supervision, their working assignments, their job descriptions, and a periodic review of performance. He shall further be able to organize, direct, and coordinate all phases of the administration.

Chapter *2*

Supervision and Supervisory Policies

Goals As Related to Supervision

The administrator, with the governing board, is responsible for formulating the purpose of the nursing home, which may be stated in general terms, such as "service to the infirm and aging." Goals are important and must be pursued actively and positively, otherwise energy must be expended to remedy the negative results. For instance, if there is failure to strive for good public relations, the nursing home may discover itself faced with the necessity of overcoming bad public relations; if the aim of supplying superior nursing care is ignored, the administrator may find himself trying to reverse a declining occupancy rate.

The broad, general goal of nursing home operation, in addition to service to the patient, includes ethical business practices, a favorable public image, and a good economic position. One may think also in terms of helping to benefit the social, spiritual, and psychological life of the patients. As fundamental as these objectives are to the success of the nursing home, however, the administrator will be quick to realize that he cannot become too idealistic; he also must be practical.

If the nursing home administrator were to say, "We aim to give good nursing service," it would be quite evident that his purpose was commendable, but the question, "How do you intend to do it?" would immediately arise. If he can then reply, "We intend to train our nursing personnel in the best nursing home techniques," he gives evidence of

28

being thoroughly practical: his constructive reaction to a specific need brings the overall goal of the nursing home closer to attainment.

Goals can be illusive and vague unless one can properly describe them in terms that are attainable. There are several aids to making identification: *a survey of needs, opinions of others, the interest of the workers, imagination, analysis, etc.* The administrator should first discuss needs with those related to the area in consideration, arouse their interest, and gain their opinion. By engaging them in the solution of problems, an objective may be established. A brainstorming conference or round-table discussion is sometimes used to spark ideas which the administrator then analyzes before deciding on a course of action. The consideration of practicality is a key factor in choosing a goal.

State a goal in its simplest terms. Be concise and to the point. This is the first step of planning. Usually, the administrator will formulate a specific goal, and will make it the first statement of a plan. While this may be done as a part of planning, discovering a goal is a separate step that should be done before anything else. Once this has been stated, the details of the plan will come quickly.

State a goal as it may relate to the organization. Goals relating to the nursing home as a whole are broad and general. Goals relating to the various departments will be more specific. Finally, goals relating to the line worker will be very specific. In fact, the more specific the goal, the more objective it will become. In addition, the larger the organization, the greater the need for the coordination of goals and objectives.

State any limitations and restrictions imposed on the goals and objectives. This may be a time limit, restriction of materials, or specific conditions.

State goals and objectives in terms of human behavior. They could more nearly be called behavioral objectives. The use of action verbs will focus on the human aspect of goal setting, since they describe a desired result. Verbs such as "train," "learn," "demonstrate," "recognize," "eliminate," etc., describe actions to be accomplished.

Examples of Types of Goals in Nursing Home Administration.

A learning goal: To learn the fundamentals of selecting the proper person to be employed on the staff of the nursing home.

A supervisory goal: To develop a job description.

A motivation goal: To formulate a plan of worker recognition to improve the quality of work in the nursing home.

A human-relations goal: To discover what causes absenteeism of the employees and make plans to eliminate it.

An improvement goal: To discover how creativity and imagination can be used to improve the quality of work being done in the nursing home.

A policy-making goal: To review the policy of the nursing home concerning the arrival of a new patient and to rewrite it in more specific terms.

An operational goal: To review the systems and facilities necessary for the preparation and serving of proper diets in the nursing home.

A health goal: To develop methods of sanitation that will ensure adequate hygiene in the nursing home environment.

An improvement goal: To review the importance of constantly maintaining and repairing the facility and to inaugurate a system of preventative maintenance.

Development of Supervisory Policy

Policies are guidelines that have been established by experience and decisions to serve certain needs, tasks, procedures, and functions. The personnel policy is only one of several that will be needed for the proper operation of the nursing home. The development of policies is the responsibility of the administrator. He will probably draw upon many sources of information, but his primary sources will be the requirements laid down by good nursing care practices, good management practices, the licensing agency, Medicaid, and Medicare. Under "Conditions of Participation for Extended Care Facilities," a delineation of policy is required in the following areas:

The personnel policy.
Policy for notification of changes in patient status.
Patient-care policy, including admission, transfer, discharge.
Nursing and medical-care policy covering physician services, nursing services, dietary services, restorative services, pharmaceutical services, diagnostic services, emergency care, dental services, social services, patient activities, clinical records, transfer agreement, and utilization review.

There follow examples of statements of policy for some of the cases mentioned above.

ADMISSION POLICY

A. Patients are admitted only upon the recommendation of a qualified physician, who will continue supervision of patient-care needs and furnish current orders for treatments, activities, and medications.

B. The patient shall have a physical examination prior to and within 14 days of admission.

C. Upon admission, the physician shall furnish current medical findings, diagnoses, rehabilitation potential, a medical history, plus a medical plan to include medications, treatments, diet, and activities.

D. The patient and his relative or guardian will have freedom of choice of physician, pharmacy, dentist, and other paramedical services.

E. The supervising nurse will develop a patient-care plan from medical findings, patient information, physician's orders, social data.

F. The Medicaid caseworker shall assist in the formulation of the social care plan.

G. The admission form shall be completed at the time of the patient's admission.

H. An admission agreement shall be completed and signed at the time of the patient's admission.

I. Patients will be given a copy of the nursing home operational policy.

CHANGE IN THE PATIENT'S STATUS

I. Change in the physical condition of the patient:
   A. Notify the physican. (The charge nurse shall first make necessary observations and record vital signs.)
   B. Notify the relative/guardian. (Charge nurse's responsibility.)
   C. If the change is significant to the degree that the Medicaid classification may change, the caseworker will be notified.
   D. If the change results in a change in the medication regimen (other than temporary), the caseworker will be notified for Medicaid patients, and the relative/guardian for private patients.

II. Change in billing:
   A. An increase in rates for private patients will be preceded by at least one week's notice.

B. Charges on the patient's account are to conform to prior agreements and shall conform to Medicaid standards for those patients receiving assistance.

III. Change in status may result in a change of residence.

    A. A prospective patient shall be fully informed that a change in status may result in a change of residence.

    B. Private patients will be asked to remove to another facility should the level of required care exceed that offered by the nursing home.

    C. Only when the care offered the patient is adjudged sufficient and adequate by the physician, will a patient be allowed to remain.

    D. Should the change of status of the Medicaid patient result in a change of classification, he will be required to move to a facility offering the required level of care. Sufficient time to move shall be granted.

TRANSFER POLICY

I. Transfer to a hospital:

    A. The physician will recommend and admit patients to the hospital. The charge nurse will call the hospital to alert it of the transfer.

    B. The relative/guardian will be notified immediately when hospitalization has been recommended.

    C. The choice of hospital is vested in the patient and/or his relative/guardian.

    D. The Medicaid caseworker will be notified when the patient is receiving medical assistance.

    E. The hospital chosen is recorded on the patient's cardex.

    F. The transfer form is completed and sent with the patient.

    G. The relative/guardian should accompany the patient. When such person is not available, administrative personnel will be assigned.

    H. Personal effects sent with the patient should include: sleeping apparel, dentures, toothbrush, personal items.

II. Transfer to another facility: same as transfer to the hospital except that all personal effects will be sent with the patient. Also, the patient/relative/guardian may select the facility and inform the physician, who then dismisses the patient.

DISCHARGE POLICY

I. Patients may be discharged under any of these conditions:
  A. The physician dismisses him.
  B. The relative/guardian who signed the patient into the nursing home signs the patient out.
  C. The patient signs a release of responsibility.
  D. At the request of the nursing home, when the admission agreement is not met or a change in the status of the patient places him beyond the level of care normally offered.
  E. By transfer to hospital and the patient's space in the nursing home is not reserved.

II. Prerequisites for discharge:
  A. The physician is notified.
  B. The guardian/relative is notified.
  C. The home receives notice as per admission agreement.
  D. The patient is competent to dismiss himself.

III. Procedures for discharge:
  A. Notify the physician and get his release.
  B. Notify the relative/guardian who signed the admission form.
  C. Notify the Medicaid caseworker in time for him to arrange predischarge consultation.
  D. Send caseworker notice of discharge within 48 hours after discharge.
  E. Help the patient pack his or her belongings.
  F. Close out petty cash, financial record, and return valuables stored in safe.
  G. Notify pharmacy, kitchen, laundry and other departments.
  H. Close patient register; get forwarding address.
  I. Assist patient to waiting transportation.

WHEN DEATH OCCURS

I. Nursing procedures:
  A. Record exact time of apparent death, i.e. when the vital signs of the patient cease.
  B. Notify the physician immediately. Normally, when death seems probable, the nurse will already have consulted with him. When apparent death occurs, he will be notified again.
  C. The body shall not be removed from the home without the authority of the attending physician, his alternate, or legal rep-

resentative having authority, e.g., coroner. Normally, the funeral home chosen by the relative/guardian is called and the body surrendered to the mortician. In some cases, the body may be transferred for an autopsy.
- D. Notify the relative/guardian if they are not present. As death approaches, give the family assistance, privacy, and consideration.
- E. When death has been pronounced by the physician, call the funeral home of the family's choice.
- F. Remove the nursing equipment.
- G. Cleanse the body.
- H. Dress the body, comb hair, groom.
- I. Freshen the bed, use clean linen as required.

II. When the ambulance comes:
- A. If the family has not arrived, delay calling, if possible.
- B. The ambulance attendant will request information for his records, i.e. exact name, physician, responsible person, etc.
- C. Secure receipt for the transfer of the body.

III. Closing of the records of a deceased patient:
- A. Record death in permanent register.
- B. Close and collect the clinical records.
- C. Notify the Medicaid worker.
- D. Close the financial record and make final billing.
- E. It is recommended that records be closed and stored within one week.
- F. Medications die with the patient. They are stored and released only to the appropriate representative of the Board of Pharmacy.
- G. Possessions are to be released to the authorized person, e.g., executor of estate.
- H. Information is to be considered privileged and confidential. The guardian/relative should release all press information.

The formulation of policy will be the largest single responsibility of the nursing home administrator. While middle management usually formulates policy in cooperation with the operating level, only top management can ensure that it is in complete accord with the objectives of the home. Some nursing home policy arises out of a need observed at the operating level and consequently is entirely practical in nature. In order to be enforceable, therefore, it must be useful to and compatible with all concerned.

Wordy, ambiguous statements do more harm than good. Terminology should be brief and exact. Some method of informing those affected should be adopted. The bulletin board is good, but the administrator should look with favor on placing a written copy of his policies in the hands of each person responsible. He may further ensure compliance by publicly informing those responsible. Word of mouth is subject to misinterpretation. The need for uniform interpretation and enforcement cannot be stressed too greatly.

The Procedure Manual

Procedure instructions are written for a wide variety of routine duties performed by the nursing staff or other personnel. The usual method is to write procedures for the different departments i.e., dietary procedures, nursing procedures, etc. The reader will note the statement of policy illustrated in this text entitled, "When Death Occurs." This is actually a procedure, since it is specific in nature and is written for the benefit of the nursing staff, especially the charge nurse.

The basic approach to writing procedures is the same as that for writing policy. The student may refer to the suggested method of job analysis as a starting point. Another approach is through the in-service training manual, in which case the same material serves both as a description of procedure and as the training curriculum. The student should note the section in the text concerning "On the Job Training," in which we have illustrated a basic procedure entitled, "Turning the Bed Patient." He will readily connect the training motive with accepted patient-care nursing procedures and recognize that they are interrelated.

Skills of Supervision

Every administrator needs certain supervisory skills. While all administrational functions will not demand every skill, nevertheless, each is important to the successful operation of the nursing home. *Normally, supervision requires five basic skills: planning, organizing, directing, controlling, and coordinating.* Each is a distinct function, and each can be learned with practice, study of techniques, and appraisal of effectiveness. Lack of these skills may be detected by difficulties in the management of the nursing home. The administrator as a planner is like the physician who investigates signs and symptoms to discover the source of illness of the patient. By careful analysis, he should be able to discover where supervision is failing. The requirement of supervisors to submit periodic performance ratings on those employees in their charge is but one of the various techniques of supervision.

Planning

Planning is a skill. It is not readily learned, since it is a part of the nature and working characteristics of the administrator. Some people plan and others do not. Others plan as they work. All methods have some merit, but the person who develops his plan first will have greater success. Planning essentially involves decision-making, which is the function of the administrator and the governing board. The more thorough he is in his approach to decisions, the better his chance of success. Since decision-making is often a matter of selecting the best course possible from several alternatives, many data may be needed. Their collection and assembling involves planning.

Planning is deciding general strategy. This is your goal.

Planning is setting limits. Any activity is limited as to time, place, money, personnel, materials, skills, etc.

Planning is deciding who shall be involved, and what their part of the plan will be.

Planning is deciding methods. This is listing the various activities in terms of chronological steps.

Planning is deciding on material requirements, specifications, availability, and procurement.

There is more likelihood of a project failing due to poor planning than through the failure of any other single skill of supervision. The administrator plans how he will organize, how he will direct, how he will control, and how he will coordinate; thus, if planning fails, all the other skills of supervision will go astray.

There is a normal sequence to planning: goal setting, data collection, establishing the plan. Thus, if the administrator will give proper perspective to each, goals, data, and plans, his administration will improve.

Directing

Directing is guiding the organization to accomplish its planned activities and functions. It, too, is a skill that involves many talents. The administrator must be able to communicate with his employees. He must gain their confidence and loyalty. He must inspire. He must be able to correct gently.

Directing may include training of an individual in order that he may fully understand the functions of his task. It may be necessary for the administrator to use counseling to make the employee aware of his responsibility, or it may be necessary to use discipline. Directing is achieving the motivation of the employees. The ultimate aim of directing is getting the job done.

Controlling

The administrator, to supervise properly, must maintain control of his nursing home and the various activities and functions that are happening within it. Measures of control have to be established. Evaluation techniques and methods of correction are necessary.

Controlling involves measuring the success of the nursing home against the objectives established by the administrator and governing board. Measurement of profit is readily made with the financial statement; however, unless there are established goals in other areas, the administrator will have little indication of his progress. He will find it useful to analyze absenteeism, employee turnover, occupancy, inventory, purchasing, etc. Actually, for purposes of control, the administrator will establish many methods of evaluation that he will constantly be reviewing.

Controlling always involves an established standard. It involves using feed-back data to establish deviation from the standard. Finally, it involves judgment in making corrections. Record keeping should be for the purpose of control.

When the administrator notes a problem, he will institute a corrective method. One example may be the inventory of the pantry. Since food staples are usually the object of employee pilfering, a cross-check of inventory against usage may discover discrepancies requiring additional control methods.

Employee evaluation based on performance ratings is a form of control. The standard is the working agreement. Performance ratings by supervisors note how well an employee achieved or deviated from the working agreement. The administrator may use this information to take corrective actions. Even discipline is a control measure. An employee may be summoned to the office of the administrator. He is told what the standard working agreement is for his job. He is advised how he has failed to meet this standard. Finally, the administrator exercises his judgment and decides what disciplinary action should be taken to correct the situation.

Coordinating

Coordinating is related to controlling, but there is a difference. *Coordinating is relating the many aspects of the operation to the goals of the administration.* It is placing each function in its proper perspective. A nursing home is a multifunctional organization. Each activity has its place and contributes to the whole operation. However, one activity out of harmony is likely to disrupt the entire home.

An excellent example of coordination is the scheduling of the flow of soiled linens from the nursing home to the laundry, to be processed and returned in time for their next use. The preparation of meals to coincide with the nursing activities is another. Scheduling of recreational activities must also be coordinated. Performance of housekeeping duties relates directly to patient care, rest periods, visiting periods, and eating.

It should be noted that coordination involves two or more distinct activities. It may involve two distinct aspects of a single activity. Perhaps the single best instrument of coordination is a calendar listing chronologically various activities. In addition, the magnitude of each task must be considered in their proper relation.

Leadership in Supervision

How does one supervise? There are certain techniques and methods that help an administrator to perfect his ability to supervise. They all have to do with the elements of leadership. In other words, the administrator becomes a leader for his employees to follow. The organization will function better, produce finer results, and inspire greater loyalty with good leadership. The output of an organization is dependent upon leadership. Poor leadership results in poor effort. Related problems, such as absenteeism or shoddy work habits, are overcome by good leadership. Good leadership is useful in avoiding accidents and incidents between employees.

Leadership may be divided into several categories and types according to the levels of management. Beginning with top management, which establishes the spirit and psychological incentive for employee loyalty, there follows the midmanagement level that correlates line management functions, and finally, there is the all important line supervisor who directs the actual work of the nursing home. At each and every level, the supervisor will need to become skilled in the various techniques of leadership. He is dealing with the motivation of his subordinates and their performance in order to attain the goals of the nursing home. He uses an organizational chart or the structure of group relationships for which he is responsible. He will take into consideration the mutual trust, respect, and cooperation he may generate between employees, and assist them in properly relating to the task. He may use democratic or autocratic means; however, there are other considerations of leadership.

The value of coercive leadership is doubtful. The use of fear tactics can be questioned. The employee who fears for his job will not make the best motivated employee. Too great an emphasis on rule and regulation will restrict fellowship as much as it would control response.

Leadership by assignment may have value. In this, the supervisor makes all the decisions, arbitrarily makes assignments, and controls by disciplinary measures. Some hospitals and nursing homes use this as a primary method because of the frequent change of assignment and personnel. It involves written instructions, but its success depends on how thoroughly the supervisor may explain the duties. It will need to be used with some consideration to the human relations involved. Since it tends to arouse suspicion of the supervisor as to his sincerity in representing management, steps should be taken to show as much consideration for the employee as possible.

Leadership by guiding is similiar to teaching. The leader is primarily concerned with the employee knowing his job. He is readily available to explain when the employee has a problem. He is personally interested in his subordinates and tends to make his supervision employee-centered. Personality differences are tolerated, while adjustments are made for the individual needs of employees.

Leadership that is inspiring is perhaps the finest leadership in supervision. The administrator will emphasize teamwork and group spirit. Good morale is important, and imagination and creativity are welcome. This type of leadership may lean toward democratic techniques which require counseling, discussion, and an interplay of ideas. Supervision need not be "easy" or "soft" when it is democratic. Discipline must be maintained due to the necessity of enforcing nursing home policies. The supervisor will be far more concerned with motivating for achievement of the nursing home goals. He will focus on group dynamics, ethics, achievement, reward, fair play. Teamwork is all important.

History has developed several unique concepts. *Democratic leadership* is a historical method in which the administrator tends to consider the employees as equals, considers the majority opinion, does not discriminate, and is people-centered. *Autocratic leadership* tends to be cooercive, authoritative, demanding, unyielding, and management-centered. In *paternalistic leadership*, the management assumes the "father" role in providing for its employees. Few progressive nursing homes will adhere to this idea, but it may be noted that fringe benefits, such as meals, discounts, etc., may owe their existence to it. *Laissez-faire* is synonymous with the "hands-off" attitude of government toward labor during the eighteenth and nineteenth centuries. Supervisors may be inclined to let the nursing home run itself when things are going well, merely coming forward when a problem develops.

Supervision Is Related to Authority

Authority is a means of exercising control. It has its foundation in the right of decision making. To the nursing home administrator, it is the rights he delegates to subordinates to accomplish the objectives of the nursing home. There are several types of authority, but they are not to be confused with leadership, which may use authority as one of the several tools to accomplish the tasks of the nursing home. *Authority is from top management flowing down the chain of command to the operating line. It is the right of the supervisor to give orders, expecting the obedience of the subordinates.* Authority presupposes that it has been delegated from higher management. Of course, the governing board has the final authority in the operation of the nursing home. It delegates authority to the administrator, who, in turn, delegates it to the supervisors, thereby multiplying his effective control over the nursing home.

Authority consists of the right to issue orders. expect obedience by the subordinates, and discipline those who breach those orders. When this authority is exercised within the limits of a particular function, it is said to be functional authority and consists of the assistance or advice of one not directly in the chain of command. Such a person may be given authority to issue orders, expect obedience, and may even mete out discipline when such orders are within the realm of his function. Line authority is that which exists within the chain of command.

Authority will usually exhibit itself, as we have discussed, in the procedures of leadership, e. g., democratic, autocratic, coercive, etc.

Supervision Is Related to Responsibility

If it is assumed that management has the right to order its employees to accomplish the nursing home objectives, then it must expect the employee to obey. If management has such a simple function as "making orders and getting obedience without question," the task is elementary. However, this is not how the delegation of authority works out. Modern nursing home operation has progressed to the point where other factors have become important.

The span of management will affect responsibility. There is a principle that says, there is a limit to the number of persons a supervisor can adequately supervise, owing to the increasing number of relationships that arise. Thus, a supervisor who may accept the responsibility for adequately supervising six nurse's aides may not be able to accept the responsibility for adequately supervising ten nurse's aides.

The division of work will affect responsibility. Employees will usually assume the responsibility for a fair share of the work load and will usually resist when they consider they are carrying an unfair part of the work load.

Responsibility is affected by the organizational balance. An organization is seldom better than its poorest unit. For example, the dietary staff cannot serve a good hot meal if the patient-care staff cannot get the patients dressed and at the breakfast table on time.

There should be an equal allotment of responsibility and authority. Workers will readily respond to needs when given the authority to act. Imagine the night aide who discovers a maintenance defect and, believing that she lacks authority, decides it is not within her responsibility to act. The result may be a very expensive repair cost because of the delay in getting attention.

The nursing home objectives must be the same for all employees before they will accept full responsibility to perform their assigned tasks. The administrator must relay the same goals to all employees, or he will discover cross-currents of opinion developing. The team spirit will win the loyalty of the employees, but the team must be striving for the same purpose. For example, if the supervisor of nurses allows certain employees to skirt certain nursing standards, it is not long before the whole nursing staff is skirting these same standards.

Finally, orders must issue from a properly designed source in order to elicit compliance. Too many "chiefs," we are told, cause confusion. Actually, what often occurs is that the employee does not know whom to obey and decides to do nothing. Workers seldom respond in this way when they know what they are expected to do. Responsible command evokes responsible action.

Chapter 3

Labor Relations
in the Nursing Home

Everyone labors. However, there are different levels of labor: professional, such as the administrator or the registered nurse; supervisory, such as a director of nurses; and the operator, which would be equivalent to the nurse's aide. Historically, we have identified labor as skilled and unskilled, or, more popularly, "white-collar" and "blue-collar"; however, this is not a true description. Many so-called blue-collar workers have developed a high degree of skill. We may use the services of an electrician, a plumber, or a carpenter and discover quickly that they are skilled workers.

Our labor heritage begins with antiquity. In the case of the nursing home worker, we find references to medical care even in ancient times. The ancient Egyptians, Assyrians, and Greeks were highly skilled in the healing arts. The position of physician was prominent in these and many other ancient countries. The midwife, who attended at the time of birth, is noted in every century, although she was usually nothing more than a gifted person. During the second century, the Greek, Galen, gave us the first book on the medical arts as he practiced them in Rome. His work was the standard until the sixteenth century. Nursing had some organization in the hospitals of the early centuries; however, it was in the religious orders that it developed.

The greatest obstacle in the development of nursing and medicine was the status of labor. Prior to the fifteenth century, labor as we recognize it today, did not exist. The pattern was feudalism, and the laborers were known as serfs. In short, labor was chattel, owned by the feudal lord. The laborer's position was so restricted that, though he might till the soil, he could not snare a rabbit, cut down a tree, or hook a fish, lest he be guilty of theft from his master. It is ironical that the breakup of the feudal pattern of labor was brought about as a result of the bubonic and pneumonic plagues which swept Europe in the fourteenth century. When this contagion wiped out nearly one-half the population, men began to sell their services to the highest bidder.

Almost simultaneously, there was a burst of scientific interest, and medicine began to develop. *Surprisingly enough, organized nursing did not develop until the eighteenth and nineteenth centuries, but was left to the social and religious orders, such as "missions of charity."* Most crafts and trades organized themselves into guilds, but the care of the infirm and aged did not share in the rising professionalism. Physicians usually attached themselves to the great universities, and few rose to meet the challenge of improving the healing arts. While hospitals trace their history to the second century, the modern hospital was born during the Crimean war, owing largely to the efforts of a single nurse, Florence Nightingale.

Labor has gone through several other phases in its rise toward recognition. Certainly, the condition of the serf of the Middle Ages was the height of domination by management. Even during this period, however, there was resistance to the system. In 1350 A.D. the English passed the Statutes of Laborers, which fixed wages and required the laborer to work, so great had been the resistance to the system. With the Black Plague—a second major plague was recorded in the seventeenth century—men began to sell their services and organize into mutual benefit associations called guilds. With the industrial revolution there was a breakdown in the numbers of one-craft laborers, and a rise of assembly-line methods. Piece work, child-labor abuse, long hours, and conflicts of labor and management contributed to the need for labor to unify its voice. By the late eighteenth century, a group of craftsmen united in the first labor union.

At first, workmen in the various crafts joined together to protect wages. These early organizations were largely craft-oriented, a practice that has carried over to the present day nursing home. The first known demand in the United States on the part of an organization to management was made in 1799, in Philadelphia, by the shoemakers. It is noteworthy that the first modern hospital was organized in Philadelphia in 1791. A second hospital there claims an even earlier date, beginning with a convalescent unit.

These early unions soon became political. About 1822, the workers' organizations, having found that they had a large voice at the polls, began to enter into politics. By 1832, the National Trades Union became a political influence in New York. Undoubtedly the attitude of government, which had been laissez-faire, "hands-off" toward labor, was an influential factor. At the same time, hospitals were developing a philosophy of humanitarianism that would preclude union activity for nearly a hundred years. The workers of the hospitals organized themselves into professional groups, but the idea of the hospital's serving "public interest" discouraged union organization.

The first unions, as we know them today, did not come into existence until after the Civil War. In 1869, the Noble Order of Knights of Labor was organized. It was soon disrupted by the advocates of the two schools of thought: political activity vs. bargaining with management. In 1886, Samuel Gompers organized the American Federation of Labor. It actually arose from the Federation of Organizing Trades and Labor Unions of 1881. As did all the early organizations of labor, it was based on crafts. A number of independent unions were organized according to particular industries, such as mine workers and auto workers. However, it was not until 1935 that a purely industrial union was organized, one that comprised large segments of the industrial labor force, without regard to specific crafts.

It is with the crossing or craft lines that organization of union activity within hospitals and nursing homes has resulted. While it appeared for many years that professionalism would preclude union organization within the health-care field, unions have now demonstrated that not only will the workers of nursing homes and hospitals organize, but also that they will participate in all known phases of the bargaining process, including the strike. It is with this fact in mind that the administrator should learn the correct procedures of dealing with the union. Unions are a way of life for the American laborer. His position has benefited greatly from his union membership, and he now expects to participate in it, to make his voice heard. The administrator has to deal with him on the basis of his labor heritage, that is, within the framework of the techniques common to an industrial union. Legal statutes that strengthen the worker's position and bargaining power are two of the union's tools. Unionism is a fact of life which the administrator may deal with one day. He may have to sit at the bargaining table with the representatives of his labor force and "bargain in good faith."

Collective Bargaining

Unions are bound by similar aims. These are higher wages, shorter hours, better working conditions, and job security. There is one other not generally thought of as an aim: union recognition. The union believes higher wages will improve the status of the individual wage earner and that wages are a rightful product of commerce. Shorter hours are usually identified with the shorter workweek, but they also deal with the proper definition with the working day, i.e., check-in, lunch, breaks, portal-to-portal, etc. Working conditions are the union's term covering any and all circumstances of labor imposed by management. It may be the place, supervision, safety, materials, equipment, and a host of other items, including a multitude of fringe benefits. Job security usually relates to hiring and firing practices, but also includes intimidation, promotion, discrimination, etc. Union recognition is, of course, the process of establishing the union as the bargaining agent.

When the union is organizing the work force of the nursing home, there are certain laws which apply such as the "right-to-work" law, "fair-labor" laws, "right-to-bargain" laws, etc. The administrator would be wisely advised to seek counsel on special labor relations law before he begins to deal with the union organizer.

If the management is opposed to organizing, it has the right to say so, and to criticize the union when the facts warrant it. On the other hand, the administrator and his supervisory staff cannot make threats, interrogate employees concerning union activities, and engage in surveillance of union activities. The administrator cannot prohibit or interfere with union solicitation during lunch breaks, rest periods, or off-time. He should in no way attempt to coerce any of his employees to organize and join a union. He may present his case, i.e., benefits, working conditions, etc., so long as the employees have free choice to join or not to join a union.

Determining who is the representative of labor to bargain with management is a process that must be accomplished before collective bargaining can begin. It may be an area of dispute within itself and sometimes will result in a jurisdictional strike, that is, one union strikes a business to force its recognition over another union. *The adminis-trator may have the use of the services of the National Labor Relations Board to provide a fair election of representatives.* Unless it has been clearly established that a union organizer is, in fact, the true rep-resentative of the nursing home employees, the administrator would do well to refer any contact with anyone claiming to be the represen-tative of his employees to his labor counsel. When such an identity has been legally established, the administrator is compelled to bargain in good faith.

The legal considerations for the administrator to remember are spelled out in about 25 different federal laws and, of course, additional state laws. Three federal laws are of significance: The National Labor Relations Act (Wagner Act) of 1935, the Labor-Management Relations Act (Taft-Hartley) of 1947, and the Labor-Management Reporting and Disclosure Act (Landrum-Griffin) of 1959.

The National Labor Relations Act forbids a refusal to bargain and any interference with bargaining. It further forbids the employer from discriminating against the union member.

The Labor-Management Relations Act regulates labor as well as management. Normally, it is thought of as the act prohibiting the closed shop and permitting states to pass "right-to-work" laws.

The Labor-Management Reporting and Disclosure Act requires unions to disclose their activities, policies, contracts, etc. It further requires an annual financial report by the union and reports by employers of any expenditures for the purpose of preventing organizing activities.

The collective bargaining procedure is not a complicated one, although it may be, when labor and management are at completely uncompromising odds. The administrator and governing board will select their representatives. The union will select theirs. When it has been ascertained that each is legally representing the respective sides, bargaining meetings will be set. Usually, the first meeting is to agree on rules for negotiation, the subjects to be discussed, and a schedule for the negotiation. After the preliminary meeting should come the presentation of proposals. Subsequent meetings will then consider the proposals, with the management presenting its arguments, and labor presenting its demands. There is no rule for conducting these meetings except, perhaps, to agree to use Robert's *Rules of Order*, a parliamentary procedure.

When the agreement is reached, it will be documented with a "Labor Agreement," which is legally binding. It should be signed by the legal representatives of each side, and can be recognized in any court when properly negotiated and written. The agreement may be between single nursing homes and a union, or groups of nursing homes and a union. It may be on an area-wide basis, covering the jurisdiction of the union, in which case negotiations may be by an association of nursing homes.

The actual labor agreement should specify the employees for whom the document was negotiated. It should state the conditions agreed upon. A time limit for the agreement should be set. Procedures for settling future conflicts should be included.

There are a number of terms that may be included. These may be wages, giving the base rate, the differential, overtime, sick pay, etc. Wages should be stated in specific terms, for instance, $3.50 per hour. Hours are usually stated per day or per week. Overtime is stated specifically. Working conditions that have been negotiated should be stated in clear, concise, yet comprehensive terms. Fringe benefits may be added; in fact, this is often the big package within the labor agreement. Hiring and firing procedures may be included. Grievances and their presentation and settlement procedures may be outined. It is well to place in the document a plan for renewing the agreement. A renewal plan may include the time each party is to be notified of the expiration date, the meetings established, and the time limits set.

Settlement of Disputes

When an agreement is not reached, the administrator will become involved in a labor dispute. The negotiation period should not be viewed as a period of dispute; it is merely a time of collective bargaining. While tempers may flare, as long as progress is being made it should not be considered a dispute. In fact, every possible measure should be taken to ensure that administration and labor not reach a deadlock, which is the beginning of a dispute. When deadlock is threatened, there are several things that may help. A cooling-off period of perhaps a weekend or a few days may give time for reconsideration. However, this should be mutually agreed upon lest either party should be considered as "refusing to bargain." Another possible step is to call in a third party. When such a party is called in, mediation, conciliation, or arbitration takes place.

Conciliation or mediation occurs when, nonagreement being evident, a third party is called in and uses advice, counsel, and moral persuasion to get both sides to make concessions to reach an agreement. There is nothing binding legally on either side. The third party is a respected, impartial, and skilled mediator, accepted by the two sides.

The federal government offers some assistance in mediation through the Federal Mediation and Conciliation Board. They may enter any case where the public interest is threatened. The Board also offers some services when requested by parties in nonagreement. Certain conditions must prevail, such as work stoppage, public interest, etc.

Should mediation fail, an arbitrator may be called in. Unlike the mediator or conciliator, *the arbitrator does have legal powers to judge and render a decision. Both sides agree in advance to accept the decision of the arbitrator.* Should arbitration be required by law, it is known as compulsory arbitration.

The National Labor Relations Board was established to correct certain unfair labor practices, secondary boycotts, and violations of collective bargaining. It provides for the election of legal representatives of labor, and may enter a dispute when the public interest is threatened. It may require arbitration. Usually, only a cooling-off period is recommended. It should be pointed out to the administrator that he may press for arbitration, should he reach a deadlock with the union. When agreeable, an arbitrator is selected; each side then submits its case for decision. The decision of the arbitrator becomes legally binding on both parties.

A word should be said about "public interest," since the nursing home qualifies under this concept, as would the hospital. To threaten the public interest means to place in jeopardy the health of citizens, health care services, and related health care facilities. "Health" is usually thought of as the right of the citizen to enjoy relative freedom from infirmity, disease, and contagion. To deny the citizen the use of facilities and services that assist him in exercising this right would threaten his interest. While "interest" may be broadly interpreted, the administrator can be assured that he would have little difficulty in convincing a court to grant an injunction in the public interest.

The Nursing Home Administrator Dealing with a Union

Nursing homes increasingly are being brought within the realm of organized labor, and it is well to recognize that points of conflict will arise. *These points of conflict could be summarized under four headings: costs vs. production, return on investment, worth of risk to the investor, and the aims of the union regarding wages, shorter hours, working conditions, and job security.* By cost vs. production, we mean the desire of management to make an operation economically feasible by keeping production high and costs down, in order to compete in the nursing home market. The management has two other objectives which the union may claim as debatable. By setting the due return on investment too high, a feeling of inequity develops between workers and owners. Such remarks as "rich nursing home owners" can only magnify this feeling. On the other hand, the investor may consider the risk great, and thus the profit again must be set high to ensure that financial difficulty does not overwhelm the business. The aims of labor are also understandable, yet in relation to costs, production, profit, etc., they become points for negotiation and agreement.

There are a number of things the two parties, and more especially the administrator can do to ease conflict. Appeal to reason. The conflict may be more imagination than fact. When the facts are openly discussed, the bitterness may dissolve. Appeal to the sense of service and humanity. Since you are dealing with the health care of the aged and infirm, great pains should be taken that such a dispute may not endanger or cause neglect of the patients. Present the facts. Each side should arm themselves with every fact they can assemble. Remember, you are attempting to enlighten the opposition as to your position, and facts speak loudly. Opinions are always debatable.

Chapter **4**

Medicare: Title XVIII

The student of health care services will be interested in the beginning of medical care legislation. The enactment of Medicare (Public Law 89–97) is a historic departure by the American government, which previously had left health care to private enterprise. Other governments have long had such practices. The German Empire under Otto von Bismarck (1815–1898) passed health care legislation. The United Kingdom passed health care legislation in 1911 entitled National Health Insurance. As early as 1893, John Graham Brooks, U.S. Commissioner of Labor, published a report, "Compulsory Insurance in Germany."

The American Association for Labor Legislation was founded in 1906 to lobby for compensation laws for both unemployment and medical expense. They developed a model bill in 1912 for states to adopt; however, none did. In 1927, a Committee on Costs on Medical Care was formed; subsequently it advised against compulsory medical legislation. President Roosevelt appointed a Committee on Economic Security, which failed to recommend health legislation, although it was considered. The Social Security Act of 1935, in section 702, was charged with making recommendations on "related subjects." The original act did not mention health care, however.

The original Social Security Act of 1935 covered the aged, dependent children, and the blind. The totally disabled were added in 1950. Health insurance was not added until 1965.

Of the early proposals, a number of questions were raised. Who would be covered: all workers? the aged? dependents of workers? Who would administer the program, the states? the federal government? Who would pay the cost: the workers? the public? the employers? How would the costs be paid: by contributions? by taxes?

Finally, what form would benefits take: compensation? medical payments?

As these questions were debated, some opposition developed owing to the stigma of "socialized medicine" and "compulsory health insurance." This opposition came not only from the medical profession and insurance groups, but even labor was for many years opposed to such a plan.

It is not easy to trace the history of the enactment of medical care legislation because of the multitude of such proposals; however, several efforts stand out, beginning with the Roosevelt administration. Franklin D. Roosevelt established the Interdepartment Committee to Coordinate Health and Welfare Activities. Then, 1938, he sponsored the National Health Conference. Several legislative proposals gained the floor of both the House and the Senate, but were not passed. These included the Wagner Bill, the Wagner-Murray-Dingell Bills, the Green-Elliot Bill, and the Taft Bill.

Other administrations subsequently made a variety of proposals, such as the Forand Bill, "Reinsurance" by the Eisenhower administration, the Javits plan, the Kennedy plan, etc. It was, however, the Kennedy administration that began a concerted effort to develop health care legislation. It sought definite legislation under Old Age, Survivors, and Disabled Insurance (OASDI) in which amendments to the Social Security Act of 1935 would be made to include health care benefits. Early leaders of this administration effort were Senators Clinton P. Anderson and Jacob Javits whose proposals were defeated in 1962. In 1963, the King-Anderson Bill was introduced, but also was not passed. In 1964, the Johnson adminstration continued the effort for health care legislation. Proposals included the Gore amendment, the Javits amendment, and the Ribicoff amendment, but none passed, and a deadlock developed.

In 1965, the legislative bodies considered several versions of the same basic proposal for health care legislation. Mainly, these versions were incorporated in proposals by the King-Anderson Bill, the Eldercare Bill, and the Byrnes Bill. When the actual legislative work got underway to write the final bill, the House Ways and Means Committee used these three versions to outline the legislation. This final version passed the House of Representatives and, with some slight modification, the United States Senate. The resultant act is known as the Social Security Act as amended, Public Law 89–97.

Almost immediately, it was recognized that the legislation, although good, was not adequate. Because of the aroused concern for health care, efforts were begun to develop a complete, balanced, and coordinated program, comprehensive in nature, for every person. Medicare was envisaged as an insurance program for the aged, Medicaid as an assistance program for the medically indigent, and comprehensive health care planning for every citizen as a basic right. Public Law 90–248 strengthened the Medicaid portion of the original legislation, and Public Law 89–749 set as a national goal comprehensive health care planning.

Comprehensive Health Care Planning

Comprehensive health care planning has as its aim that every individual, regardless of status, position, finances, or race has a right to good health care. Efforts are usually focused on an adequate distribution of facilities and emergency health care; the maintenance of reasonable cost; sufficient manpower; and the sharing of information and planning for the use of resources. An agency of comprehensive health care planning attempts to identify community health needs through research, coordination, goal setting, and the implementation of plans.

Most local and area agencies are an integral part of a larger state agency operating within the framework of section 314(b) of Public Law 89-749. While funding is available for each local, regional, or state effort, it should be noted that voluntary participation by individuals, governing agencies, or the health care industry will supplement the limited funds available.

The purpose and intent of the act is to bring together the combined efforts of many "voluntary" and/or formal government health planning bodies into a uniform and comprehensive effort. No attempt is made to usurp the responsible efforts of informal citizens' groups, voluntary health organizations, fund-raising groups, health and welfare groups, or any agency doing health care planning. The purpose of comprehensive health care planning is to focus on the unmet needs, a fair distribution of resources, and coordination of the many efforts.

An agency's effort may also focus on factors related to health, i.e., economic, social, educational and environmental factors, mental health, physical health services, and manpower. A typical area-wide planning effort might include:

Identification of health problems.
Identification of health needs.

Identification of goals, services, or policies.
Providing mechanisms for cooperative efforts.
Providing an information service.
Conducting periodic evaluations.
Collecting and sharing health care data.
Review of health care grant applications.

A prime consideration is the creation of a health advisory council representative of all groups within the planning area. The structure of the council is flexible, but should contain a majority of consumers and should reflect the geographic, economic, ethnic, and social constituency. It may be noted that teachers or those engaged in research are excluded from the class of consumers. Nursing home administrators are likewise not classed as consumers, but nevertheless are eligible to serve.

Medical Eligibility

Eligibility for Hospital Insurance (Part A) benefits under Medicare applies to "individuals age 65 or over who are entitled to monthly social security benefits; qualified railroad retirement beneficiaries age 65 or over; and uninsured persons age 65 or over who meet the requirements of a special transitional provision." Those declared permanently disabled were given eligibility in 1972 by Public Law 92-603 (H.R.-1).

"Entitled" means one who has established eligibility. The elderly person, 65 or over, must apply, and establish with the Social Security Agency, that he is entitled to benefits before any benefits are payable. In such cases, where the eligibility is not established by age 65 but is delayed to a later age, benefits may be made retroactive, but not to exceed one year. Protection begins at age 65, but has been interpreted to begin on the first calendar day of the month in which one becomes 65. Dependents may qualify for benefits as well as the survivors of deceased workers. Even aliens who have met certain resident requirements may qualify.

The individual is also eligible for supplementary Medical Insurance (Part B). Effective July 1973, a person deemed eligible for hospital insurance is enrolled automatically. For Hospital Insurance (Part A), no enrollment restrictions are made, other than the 12-month limitation of retroactive benefits. Withdrawal from the supplementary Medical Insurance program (Part B) may be made at the end of any calendar quarter. Termination is possible for nonpayment of premiums; however, a ninety-day grace period is allowed. Once a person withdraws from the program, he has the opportunity of re-enrolling in general enrollment periods which are set during the first quarter of each year. Late enrollment is penalized by a 10% increase in premiums for each year.

Premiums for Part B are reviewed and revised annually. The federal government pays one-half of this premium. An annual deductible for Part B is set by law; in 1973 it was set at $60.00. A deductible payable to a hospital for each "spell of illness" is revised annually, as are deductible amounts for the daily rates after a certain number of benefit days are used. See the discussion on benefits. Employer-employee contributions are also set by law.

The student should learn to distinguish between Part A and Part B, to know something about eligibility and benefits. Reference is made to two publications available from the Superintendent of Documents, U.S. Printing Office, Washington, D.C. The first is the *Social Security Handbook* and the second is the *Medicare Handbook*. Because of the changing of the original law, the annual review, and the transitional provision for enrollment, an accurate interpretation should always be made in light of the current rules and regulations.

Medicare Benefits

According to the *Social Security Handbook*, "hospital insurance protection" means that the individual protected may have benefits paid on his behalf or, in certain cases, paid to him for the covered hospital and related health care services. The Medical Insurance plan builds upon the protection provided by the basic hospital insurance plan by covering a substantial part of the cost of physicians' services (including surgery) and a number of other health items and services.

The benefit period includes 90 days of hospital care plus an additional "lifetime reserve" of 60 days. A "benefit period" begins when a person enters a hospital and terminates when a person has no longer been a patient for 60 consecutive days in the hospital or skilled nursing facility. The original act used the phrase, "spell of illness," and included skilled nursing care even if it was not in a skilled nursing facility. However, benefits are normally paid only to participating hospitals and skilled nursing facilities. Hospital insurance will cover the cost of general hospital care, room and board, operations, drugs, medical supplies, diagnostic tests, laboratory fees, and physical therapy. Some services are excluded, i.e., telephone, television, private room (except as a medical necessity), and personal items. The cost to the patient includes the initial hospital deductible (as reviewed and set annually), a supplemental payment from the 61st to 90th day (this payment is 25% of the initial deductible fee), and payment for or replacement of the first 3 pints of blood used. The lifetime reserve of 60 days will be supplemented at a rate set at 50% of the initial deductible fee for each day used. A new benefit period (spell of illness) will renew all benefits except the lifetime reserve.

Benefits in the Skilled Nursing Facility (SNF) include room and board, nursing care, therapy, drugs, a semi-private room, social services, and medical supplies. SNF benefits are available after three consecutive days of hospitalization, but must begin within 14 days of discharge from the hospital. A twenty-eight day period is allowed for those persons who are not permitted because of the nonavailability of SNF beds. The illness for which extended care benefits are paid must be the same illness for which admission was made to the hospital, or an illness developed in the skilled nursing facility during the time benefits were being paid. In other words, benefits are paid when the stay in the skilled nursing facility is a normal continuation of the illness requiring hospitalization. The skilled nursing facility must meet the "conditions of participation." The cost for the patient is nothing during the first 20 days in the SNF, with a supplemental payment for the 21st through the 100th day. This supplement is set at 12½% of the amount set for the initial hospital deductible fee.

Benefits are paid under Medical Insurance once a person has established that he has personally paid for medical services in the amount set by law as an annual deductible. This amount is now $60.00. The individual should claim all expenditures so that the first $60.00 deductible can be established with Medicare. In addition, the beneficiary is paid only 80% of a reasonable charge. He must pay directly to the provider the additional 20% plus any charges not considered reasonable and customary.

Medical Insurance benefits include the payment of the physician for his services whether in the hospital or elsewhere, surgical procedures by dental surgeons and podiatrists, the rental of medical devices and equipment, ambulance services when found to be an emergency medical necessity, blood after the first three pints, outpatient services at hospitals, and certain special medical needs. With the passage of the 1972 revision of the Social Security Act, H.R.1, Medicare benefits were extended to disability beneficiaries, those needing kidney transplants, and those with kidney disease requiring renal dialysis.

The patient should consult his Medicare Handbook or his local office of Social Security to determine the exact services for which benefits are payable.

Persons connected in any way with the operation of a nursing home should certainly be familiar with the standards for certification of such a facility as set forth in 1974 by the Department of Health, Education, and Welfare. Toward that end, the major portion of these standards has been reproduced in the following pages.

Skilled Nursing Facilities*

Standards for Certification and Participation in Medicare and Medicaid Programs

Title 20—Employees' Benefits

CHAPTER III—SOCIAL SECURITY ADMIN-ISTRATION, DEPARTMENT OF HEALTH, EDUCATION, AND WELFARE

[Regs. 5, further amended]

PART 405—FEDERAL HEALTH INSURANCE FOR THE AGED AND DISABLED

Skilled Nursing Facilities

On July 12, 1973, there was published in the FEDERAL REGISTER (38 FR 18620) a notice of proposed rulemaking which set forth proposed amendments to regulations relating to the conditions of participation for skilled nursing facilities, the certification procedures for providers and suppliers of services, the provider and supplier appeals processes, and implementation of provisions of the Social Security Amendments of 1972 (Pub. L. 92–603) affecting the foregoing.

Interested parties were given the opportunity to submit within 30 days data, views, or arguments on the proposed amendments. The comment period was extended by the Secretary for an additional 30 days to September 13, 1973, and notice of this extension appeared in the FEDERAL REGISTER of August 14, 1973.

Comments were received from many sources (including representatives of national, State and local organizations) concerned with skilled nursing services and with the qualifications and duties of health care personnel rendering services under Medicare. All of the comments received on the proposed regulations have been carefully considered.

The most substantive comments received recommended the inclusion of requirements for: (1) A medical director or organized medical staff for skilled nursing facilities; (2) 7-day registered nurse services; (3) a discharge planning program; and (4) a "bill of rights" for patients in such facilities. Since these items were not included in the proposed regulations as published, and are of considerable impact, they are not included in these final regulations. However, they will be published with notice of proposed rulemaking at a later date to afford ample opportunity for comments. Furthermore, under another notice of proposed rulemaking, to be published at a later date, additional changes in the utilization review standards will be issued.

A number of the comments recommended that: (1) Patient care policies

* A reproduction of the *Federal Register* Vol. 39, No. 12, Part III (Thursday, January 17, 1974), pp. 2238–2249. The sponsor of these standards is the Department of Health, Education and Welfare: Social and Rehabilitation Service and Social Security Administration.

be available to the public; (2) the frequency of physician visits be clearly defined; (3) all nursing service staff receive training in rehabilitative nursing; (4) the definition of qualifications of certain health specialists be clarified; (5) there should be a requirement for daily rounds by the charge nurse; and (6) the director of nursing services participates at least annually in continuing education. These comments were accepted and the regulations clarified accordingly.

The following changes have been made to reflect other comments that were received:

(1) The director of nursing services may not serve as a charge nurse in a facility with an average daily total occupancy of 60 or more. This requirement had been an average daily occupancy of 50 or more. This brings the requirement in line with most other Federal and State standards.

(2) In the case of patients needing laboratory and radiological services in a facility not providing such services, the requirement was added that the facility assist the patient in arranging for transportation to the provider of such services. This addition reflects a similar requirement for dental services; as with the dental services provision, transportation of patients for laboratory and radiological services is not covered under Medicare.

(3) The paragraph concerning approved drugs and biologicals which lack substantial evidence of effectiveness for all indications has been deleted. Department-wide regulations on this subject, applicable to all providers and suppliers participating in Federal programs, will be published in the near future. In the meantime, current regulations and policies relating to drugs and biologicals remain in effect.

(4) Those provisions concerning the term of a provider agreement were revised to extend the term of agreement to 60 days after the date specified for the correction of deficiencies to enable the State agency to survey and process their recommendation to the Secretary before the agreement expires.

(5) The definition of a social worker has been revised to include a graduate of a school of social work approved or accredited by the Council on Social Work Education. This will permit a social worker with either a master's or baccalaureate degree in social work to serve as a qualified consultant.

(6) The definitions of qualified professionals in § 405.1101 frequently make reference to the standards of various national professional organizations. The Department has examined the current standards of those organizations and is adopting them. The Secretary will examine future changes in the standards of these organizations and determine whether such changes should be reflected in regulations.

(7) Several provisions of existing regulations which were not included in the proposed regulations as published on July 12, 1973, have now been reinstated after reviewing comments that their deletion could have an adverse effect on patient care. These were: Time requirements for physical examination of the patient at admission; the attending physician must arrange for the medical care of the patient in his absence; duties assigned food service employees outside the dietetic service cannot interfere with their dietetic work assignments; and space, supplies, and equipment must be provided for a patient activities program.

(8) A provision was added to require the retention of the medical records of minors until 3 years after the patient becomes of age under State law. The regulations had been silent on this point. State laws typically provide opportunity for an individual to personally enforce rights accruing during their minority once majority is reached. While this change may require retention of records for a considerable length of time, protection for both the minor patient and the facility is provided, should litigation occur:

The following summarizes those substantive comments that were not accepted.

(1) The suggestion that the time for consultation for the dietitian or pharmacist consultant be specified either in hours or number of visits weekly was not accepted because a rigidly accepted number of hours or visits is no assurance of quality of the service provided. The regulations are, to the extent possible, performance standards, and rely upon the

professional judgment of the surveyor in determining whether quality service inherent in the standard has been achieved.

(2) Concern was expressed about the requirement that a facility assume financial responsibility when arranging with an outside resource to provide therapy and certain other services. It was suggested that the patient be billed directly by the person(s) furnishing the services. The provision was retained because these services are part of extended care services under Part A and billing for other services under Part A is done by the facility. Furthermore, the Part A payment mechanism provides safeguards against overutilization and exorbitant fees, and focusing responsibility on the facility enables the surveyor to readily review the circumstances under which the services are offered.

(3) Request was made that during the appeals process, benefits should continue to be paid to a facility that had been terminated from participation in the program. This request was rejected because facilities are terminated from program participation when the health and safety of patients can no longer be assured and only after the facility has been given notice of the nature of its deficiencies and been given ample time to make the necessary improvements. When this decision has been made, it is not possible to justify continuing payment to a facility beyond the 30-days benefits provided in the statute for those beneficiaries admitted to the facility prior to the effective date of termination.

(4) Request was also made that Medicaid provide hearings for all facilities that had been terminated or where agreements had not been renewed. This appeals process will be determined by State practices consonant with Medicaid being a State-administered program.

(5) Numerous comments were received from social workers, consumer groups and organizations, protesting the optional provision of social services by skilled nursing facilities. This change is the result of amendments found in section 265 of Pub. L. 92–603, the Social Security Amendments of 1972; hence, no action could be taken to reinstate this as a mandatory requirement without further legislative action.

(6) The suggestion that there be a specific ratio of nursing staff to patients was not accepted because the variation from facility to facility in the composition of its nursing staff, physical layout, patient needs and the services necessary to meet those needs precludes setting such a figure. A minimum ratio could result in all facilities striving only to reach that minimum and could result in other facilities hiring unneeded staff to satisfy an arbitrary ratio figure. However, as a means of closely monitoring the adequacy of staffing in skilled nursing facilities, Medicare has adopted a provision that now appears in title XIX regulations thereby further achieving uniformity between the two programs. This provision calls for the facility to submit quarterly staffing reports to the State agency, and this is reflected in these amendments in Subpart K, § 405.1121 (b).

(7) Several suggestions were made that there was insufficient provision for protection of the patient's rights. The regulations do specifically provide that the facility must have rules on the protection of the personal and property rights of patients; and that patient care policies include provisions to protect these rights. Additionally, discriminatory treatment in skilled nursing facilities would be barred by the continued requirement that the facilities must be in compliance with title VI of the Civil Rights Act of 1964. However, as previously indicated, a "bill of rights" for patients will be published under the notice of proposed rulemaking procedures.

Some criticism of the revised format of the conditions of participation was expressed. The skilled nursing facility regulations are designed as performance standards; greater specificity would diminish their applicability to all facilities. Additionally, State agency surveyors have recently undergone extensive training to enhance their understanding of the program and the survey process. These performance-oriented requirements will provide these surveyors criteria on which to base their assessment of an individual facility's performance. Further, certification requirements for all providers and suppliers of services (hospitals, skilled nursing facilities, home health agencies, providers of outpatient physical therapy services, independent laboratories, and portable X-ray services) are now centralized in the new Subpart T.

In the definition found in § 405.1101

(a)(2), administrator of skilled nursing facility, the length of supervisory management experience required was revised from one year to three years to assure adequate experience to direct administrative activities in such health facilities. This technical change reflects current title XIX requirements for administrators and thereby further achieves conformance between the two programs.

The amendments as announced under the notice of proposed rulemaking (38 FR 18620) are adopted, with the noted changes. In addition, some parts of the regulations were redrafted for clarification purposes, in line with the comments received.

(Secs. 1102, 1814, 1832, 1833, 1861, 1863, 1865, 1866, 1871, 49 Stat. 647, as amended, 79 Stat. 294, as amended, 79 Stat. 313–327, as amended, 79 Stat. 331 (42 U.S.C. 1302, 1395f, 1395k, 1395l, 1395x, 1395z, 1395bb, 1395cc, 1395hh))

Effective date. These amendments shall be effective February 19, 1974.

(Catalog of Federal Domestic Assistance Program No. 13.800, Health Insurance for the Aged and Disabled-Hospital Insurance)

Dated: December 19, 1973.

J. B. CARDWELL,
Commissioner of Social Security.

Approved: December 27, 1973.

CASPAR W. WEINBERGER,
Secretary of Health, Education, and Welfare.

Regulation No. 5 of the Social Security Administration, as amended (20 CFR Part 405), are further amended as set forth below:

Subpart F—Agreements, Elections, Contracts, Nominations, and Notices

1. The heading for Subpart F is revised to read as set forth above.

§ 405.601, 405.602   [Amended]

2. In §§ 405.601 and 405.602, the words "extended care facility" are revised to read "skilled nursing facility."

3. A new § 405.604 is added to read as follows:

§ 405.604   Term agreements with skilled nursing facilities.

Effective with respect to provider agreements accepted for filing on or after October 30, 1972, an agreement with a skilled nursing facility shall be for a specified term and such term shall be determined by the Secretary in the following manner:

(a)(1) The term of an agreement may be for a period of 12 full calendar months where the facility is in full compliance with the standards contained in Subpart K of this part.

(2) Where the facility is not in full compliance with standards contained in Subpart K of this part the term of an agreement may:

(i) Be restricted to a term that ends no later than the 60th day following the end of the time period specified for the correction of deficiencies in a written plan which the Secretary has approved: *Provided,* That such term shall not exceed 12 full calendar months; or

(ii) Provide a conditional term of 12 full months, subject to an automatic cancellation clause that the agreement will terminate at the close of a predetermined date which shall be no later than the 60th day following the end of the time period specified for the correction of deficiencies: *Provided,* That such date will occur within such 12-month term, unless the Secretary determines that all required corrections have been satisfactorily completed or that the facility has made substantial effort and progress in correcting such deficiencies and has resubmitted in writing a plan of correction acceptable to the Secretary.

(b)(1) Where the Secretary determines that the health and safety of program beneficiaries will not be jeopardized thereby, the term of an agreement may be extended for a period of 2 full calendar months, if the Secretary finds that such extension is necessary to:

(i) Prevent irreparable harm to such facility; or

(ii) Prevent hardship to the program beneficiaries being furnished items and services by such facility; or

(2) If the Secretary finds it impracticable within such term to determine whether such facility is complying with the provisions of the Act and regulations issued thereunder.

(c)(1) Except as provided in paragraph (b) of this section, the term of an agreement may not be extended and such agreement shall terminate at the close of the last day of its specified term and will not be automatically renewable from term to term.

(2) The nonrenewal of an agreement

under the conditions described in this section is not a termination of the agreement by the Secretary pursuant to the provisions discussed in § 405.614. A determination by the Secretary not to accept such facility for participation following the end of such term shall be an initial determination relating to the facility's qualifications as a provider of services for the period immediately following such term and the facility shall be entitled to a hearing with respect to such determination. (See Subpart O of this part.)

(3) Where the Secretary determines that he will not accept an agreement with a skilled nursing facility for the period immediately following the end of the term of such facility's existing agreement, the Secretary shall give notice of such determination to the facility at least 30 days and to the public at least 15 days before the end of such term. Each notice by the Secretary shall state the reasons for such determination, the effective date for the termination of the existing agreement, and the applicability of such termination as it relates to the services of the facility.

(d) Notwithstanding the preceding provisions of this section, an agreement filed by an extended care facility (now defined as a skilled nursing facility) which was accepted by the Secretary prior to October 30, 1972, and which was in effect on such date, shall be for a specified term ending at the close of December 31, 1973.

4. Section 405.605 is revised to read as follows:

§ 405.605   Provider of services; scope of term.

As used in section 1866 of the Act and this Part 405, the term "provider of services" (or "provider") refers only to a hospital, a skilled nursing facility, or a home health agency (see Subparts J, K, and L of this part) and, for the limited purposes of furnishing outpatient physical therapy or speech pathology services a clinic, rehabilitation agency, or public health agency (see Subpart Q of this part).

5. Section 405.606 is amended by revising paragraph (b), and adding a new paragraph (c) to read as follows:

§ 405.606   Acceptance of provider as a participant.

*   *   *   *   *

(b) If the provider wishes to participate in the program, both copies of the agreement shall be signed by an authorized official of the organization and filed with the Secretary and, upon acceptance for filing by the Secretary, a copy of such agreement shall be returned to the provider with the Secretary's written notice of acceptance. Such notice shall indicate the date on which the agreement was signed by the authorized official of the provider and the date on which the agreement was accepted by the Secretary; specify the effective date of the agreement; and, in the case of an agreement filed by a skilled nursing facility, the term of such agreement as determined in accordance with the provisions of § 405.604.

(c) The participation of a hospital, skilled nursing facility, or home health agency which voluntarily files an agreement to participate in the health insurance program contemplates that such hospital, facility, or agency will accept program beneficiaries for care and treatment. If a participating hospital, facility, or agency has any restrictions on the types of services it will make available and/or the type of health conditions that it will accept, or has any other criteria relating to the acceptance of persons for care and treatment, it is expected that such restrictions or criteria, if made applicable to program beneficiaries, will be applied in the same manner in which they are applied to all other persons seeking care and treatment by such hospital, facility, or agency. A provider's admission policies and practices that are inconsistent with the provider agreement objectives set forth in this paragraph (c) may be the basis for termination of participation by the Secretary pursuant to § 405.614(a)(1).

6. Paragraph (a) of § 405.613 is revised to read as follows:

§ 405.613   Termination by provider of services.

(a) A provider may terminate a section 1866 agreement (and in the case of a skilled nursing facility, prior to the end of the specified term of such agreement—see § 405.604) by filing with the Secretary a written notice of its intention to terminate such agreement. The notice of intent to terminate shall state the date for the termination of the agreement (the date must be the first day of a month). The Secretary may accept the termination date stated in the notice or he may set a different date. If the notice of termination does not specify the date for the termination of the agreement, the date shall be set by the Secretary. However, if the termination date is set by the Secretary, such date shall not be more than 6 months from the date the notice is filed. In addition to giving notice to the Secretary, the provider also gives at least 15 days notice to the public by publishing in one or more local newspapers a statement of the date of termination of the provider agreement with the Secretary. The notice also shall inform the public of the applicability of termination (see § 405.615) as it relates to services of the provider.

*   *   *   *

7. Paragraph (a) of § 405.614 is revised to read as follows:

§ 405.614   Termination by the Secretary.

(a) *Cause for termination.* The Secretary may terminate an agreement (and in the case of a skilled nursing facility, prior to the end of the specified term of such agreement—see § 405.604) if the Secretary determines that the provider of services:

(1) Is not complying substantially with the provisions of title XVIII and this Part 405, or with the provisions of the agreement entered into pursuant to § 405.606; or

(2) No longer meets the appropriate conditions of participation necessary to qualify as a hospital (see Subpart J of this part), skilled nursing facility (see Subpart K of this part), home health agency (see Subpart L of this part), or a rehabilitation agency, clinic, or public health agency as a provider of outpatient physical therapy or speech pathology services (see Subpart Q of this part), as the case may be; or

(3) Fails to furnish information as the Secretary finds to be necessary for a determination as to whether payments are due or were due under this Part 405 and the amounts thereof; or

(4) Refuses to permit examination of its fiscal or other records by, or on behalf of, the Secretary as may be necessary for verification of information furnished as a basis for payment under the health insurance benefits program.

*   *   *   *   *

8. Paragraph (a) of § 405.615 is revised to read as follows:

§ 405.615   Applicability of termination.

A termination of an agreement under the conditions described in §§ 405.604, 405.613, or 405.614 shall be applicable:

(a) In the case of inpatient hospital services (including inpatient tuberculosis hospital services and inpatient psychiatric hospital services), or posthospital extended care services furnished to any individual after the effective date of such termination, except that payment may be made for up to 30 days with respect to such services furnished to any beneficiary who was admitted to the hospital or skilled nursing facility prior to the effective date of the termination.

*   *   *   *

9. Section 405.616 is amended to read as follows:

§ 405.616   Reinstatement of provider as participant after termination.

(a) Subject to the provisions of paragraph (b) of this section, where an agreement between a provider of services and the Secretary is terminated by the Secretary under the conditions described in §§ 405.604 and 405.614, such institution or agency shall not file another agreement to participate in the health insurance benefits program unless the Secretary finds that the reason for the termination of the prior agreement has been removed and that there is reasonable assurance that it will not recur.

(b) Where an agreement between a provider of services and the Secretary is terminated under conditions described in § 405.604, § 405.613, or § 405.614, such institution or agency shall not file another agreement to participate in the health insurance benefits program unless the Secretary finds that such institution or agency has fulfilled (or has made arrangements satisfactory to the Secretary to fulfill) all of the statutory and regulatory responsibilities of its prior agreement with the Secretary.

*   *   *   *

10. Section 405.685 is amended by adding a paragraph (d) to read as follows:

§ **405.685** Agreements with States pursuant to section 1864; general.

The Secretary shall enter into an agreement with any State which is able and willing to do so, under which the services of the State health agency or other appropriate State agency (or the appropriate local agencies) will be utilized by the Secretary:

* * * *

(d) To review statements obtained from each skilled nursing facility setting forth (from payroll records) the average numbers and types of personnel (in full-time equivalents) on each tour of duty during at least 1 week of each quarter, such week to be selected by the survey agency and to occur irregularly in each quarter of a year.

Subpart K—Conditions of Participation; Skilled Nursing Facilities

11. Subpart K is amended by deleting §§ 405.1101 through 405.1110. These sections are superseded by new Subpart T. Subpart K is further amended by revising the heading as set forth above, adding a new § 405.1101 and §§ 405.1120 through 405.1137 to read as follows:

Sec.
405.1101 Definitions.

* * * * *

405.1120 Compliance with Federal, State, and local laws.
405.1121 Governing body and management.
405.1122 Patient care policies.
405.1123 Physician services.
405.1124 Nursing services.
405.1125 Dietetic services.
405.1126 Specialized rehabilitative services.
405.1127 Pharmaceutical services.
405.1128 Laboratory and radiologic services.
405.1129 Dental services.
405.1130 Social services.
405.1131 Patient activities.
405.1132 Medical records.
405.1133 Transfer agreement.
405.1134 Physical environment.
405.1135 Infection control.
405.1136 Disaster preparedness.
405.1137 Utilization review.

§ 405.1101 Definitions.

As used in this subpart, the following definitions apply:

(a) *Administrator of skilled nursing facility.* A person who:

(1) Is licensed as required by State law; or

(2) If the State does not have a Medicaid program, and has no licensure requirement, is a high school graduate (or equivalent), has completed courses in administration or management approved by the appropriate State agency, and has 3 years of supervisory management experience in a skilled nursing facility or related health program; or

(3) If the administrator of a hospital in which there is a hospital-based distinct-part skilled nursing facility, in a State that does not license skilled nursing facility administrators, meets the requirements of § 405.1021(f).

(b) *Approved drugs and biologicals.* Only such drugs and biologicals as are:

(1) In the case of Medicare:

(i) Included (or approved for inclusion) in the United States Pharmacopoeia, National Formulary, or United States Homeopathic Pharmacopoeia; or

(ii) Included (or approved for inclusion) in AMA Drug Evaluations or Accepted Dental Therapeutics, except for any drugs and biologicals unfavorably evaluated therein; or

(iii) Not included (nor approved for inclusion) in the compendia listed in paragraphs (b)(1)(i) and (b)(1)(ii) of this section, may be considered approved if such drugs:

(A) Were furnished to the patient during his prior hospitalization, and

(B) Were approved for use during a prior hospitalization by the hospital's pharmacy and drug therapeutics committee (or equivalent), and

(C) Are required for the continuing treatment of the patient in the facility.

(2) In the case of Medicaid, those drugs approved by the State Title XIX agency.

(c) *Charge nurse.* A person who is:

(1) Licensed by the State in which practicing as a:

(i) Registered nurse; or

(ii) Practical (vocational) nurse who:

(A) Is a graduate of a State-approved school of practical (vocational) nursing; or

(B) Has 2 years of appropriate experience following licensure by waiver as a practical (vocational) nurse, and has achieved a satisfactory grade on a proficiency examination approved by the Secretary, or on a State licensure examination which the Secretary finds at least equivalent to the proficiency examination, except that such determinations of proficiency shall not apply with respect to persons initially licensed by a State or seeking initial qualifications as a practical (vocational) nurse after December 31, 1977; and

(2) Is experienced in nursing service administration and supervision and, in areas such as rehabilitative or geriatric nursing, or acquires such preparation through formal staff development programs.

In the case of skilled nursing facility services in an institution for the mentally retarded or in an institution for those with mental diseases, or a distinct part thereof, a person licensed in another category of health care discipline who has special training in the care of such patients may serve as charge nurse provided that such person is licensed in such category by the State following completion of a course of training which included at least the number of classroom and practice hours in all the nursing subjects included in the program of a State-approved school of practical (vocational) nursing, as evidenced by a report on comparison of the courses in the respective curricula to the State agency by the agency(ies) of the State responsible for the licensure of such personnel. (An institution primarily engaged in the care of the mentally retarded or in the treatment of mental diseases cannot qualify as a participating skilled nursing facility under Medicare.)

(d) *Controlled drugs.* Drugs listed as being subject to the Comprehensive Drug Abuse Prevention and Control Act of 1970 (Pub. L. 91–513) as set forth in 21 CFR Part 308.

(e) *Dietetic service supervisor.* A person who:

(1) Is a qualified dietitian; or

(2) Is a graduate of a dietetic technician or dietetic assistant training program, corresponding or classroom, approved by the American Dietetic Association; or

(3) Is a graduate of a State-approved course that provided 90 or more hours of classroom instruction in food service supervision and has experience as a supervisor in a health care institution with consultation from a dietitian; or

(4) **Has training and experience in** food service supervision and management in a military service equivalent in content to the program in paragraph (e) (2) or (e) (3) of this section.

(f) *Dietitian (qualified consultant).* A person who:

(1) Is eligible for registration by the American Dietetic Association under its requirements in effect on the publication of this provision.

(2) Has a baccalaureate degree with major studies in food and nutrition, dietetics, or food service management, has 1 year of supervisory experience in the dietetic service of a health care institution, and participates annually in continuing dietetic education.

(g) *Director of nursing services.* A registered nurse who is licensed by the State in which practicing, and has 1 year of additional education or experience in nursing service administration, as well as additional education or experience in such areas as rehabilitative or geriatric nursing, and participates annually in continuing nursing education.

(h) *Drug administration.* An act in which a single dose of a prescribed drug or biological is given to a patient by an authorized person in accordance with all laws and regulations governing such acts. The complete act of administration entails removing an individual dose from a previously dispensed, properly labeled container (including a unit dose container), verifying it with the physician's orders, giving the individual dose to the proper patient, and promptly recording the time and dose given.

(i) *Drug dispensing.* An act entailing the interpretation of an order for a drug or biological and, pursuant to that order, the proper selection, measuring, labeling, packaging, and issuance of the drug or biological for a patient or for a service unit of the facility.

(j) *Existing buildings.* For purposes of ANSI Standard No. A117.1 and minimum patient room size (see § 405.1134 (c) and (e)) in skilled nursing facilities or parts thereof whose construction plans are approved and stamped by the appropriate State agency responsible therefore before the date these regulations become effective.

(k) *Licensed nursing personnel.* Registered nurses or practical (vocational) nurses licensed by the State in which practicing.

(l) *Medical record practitioner (qualified consultant)*. A person who:
(1) Is eligible for certification as a registered record administrator (RRA), or an accredited record technician (ART), by the American Medical Record Association under its requirements in effect on the publication of this provision; or
(2) Is a graduate of a school of medical record science that is accredited jointly by the Council on Medical Education of the American Medical Association and the American Medical Record Association.

(m) *Occupational therapist (qualified consultant)*. A person who:
(1) Is a graduate of an occupational therapy curriculum accredited jointly by the Council on Medical Education of the American Medical Association and the American Occupational Therapy Association; or
(2) Is eligible for certification by the American Occupational Therapy Association under its requirements in effect on the publication of this provision; or
(3) Has 2 years of appropriate experience as an occupational therapist, and has achieved a satisfactory grade on a proficiency examination approved by the Secretary, except that such determinations of proficiency shall not apply with respect to persons initially licensed by a State or seeking initial qualifications as an occupational therapist after December 31, 1977.

(n) *Occupational therapy assistant.* A person who:
(1) Is eligible for certification as a certified occupational therapy assistant (COTA) by the American Occupational Therapy Association under its requirements in effect on the publication of this provision; or
(2) Has 2 years of appropriate experience as an occupational therapy assistant, and has achieved a satisfactory grade on a proficiency examination approved by the Secretary, except that such determination of proficiency shall not apply with respect to persons initially licensed by a State or seeking initial qualification as an occupational therapy assistant after December 31, 1977.

(o) *Patient activities coordinator (qualified consultant)*. A person who:
(1) Is a qualified therapeutic recreation specialist; or
(2) Has 2 years of experience in a social or recreational program within the last 5 years, 1 year of which was full-time in a patient activities program in a health care setting; or
(3) Is a qualified occupational therapist or occupational therapy assistant.

(p) *Pharmacist.* A person who:
(1) Is licensed as a pharmacist by the State in which practicing, and
(2) Has training or experience in the specialized functions of institutional pharmacy, such as residencies in hospital pharmacy, seminars on institutional pharmacy, and related training programs.

(q) *Physical therapist (qualified consultant)*: A person who is licensed as a physical therapist by the State in which practicing, and
(1) Has graduated from a physical therapy curriculum approved by the American Physical Therapy Association, or by the Council on Medical Education and Hospitals of the American Medical Association, or jointly by the Council on Medical Education of the American Medical Association and the American Physical Therapy Association; or
(2) Prior to January 1, 1966, was admitted to membership by the American Physical Therapy Association, or was admitted to registration by the American Registry of Physical Therapists, or has graduated from a physical therapy curriculum in a 4-year college or university approved by a State department of education; or
(3) Has 2 years of appropriate experience as a physical therapist, and has achieved a satisfactory grade on a proficiency examination approved by the Secretary, except that such determinations of proficiency shall not apply with respect to persons initially licensed by a State or seeking qualification as a physical therapist after December 31, 1977; or
(4) Was licensed or registered prior to January 1, 1966, and prior to January 1, 1970, had 15 years of full-time experience in the treatment of illness or injury through the practice of physical therapy in which services were rendered under the order and direction of attending and referring physicians; or

(5) If trained outside the United States, was graduated since 1928 from a physical therapy curriculum approved in the country in which the curriculum was located and in which there is a member organization of the World Confederation for Physical Therapy, meets the requirements for membership in a member organization of the World Confederation for Physical Therapy, has 1 year of experience under the supervision of an active member of the American Physical Therapy Association, and has successfully completed a qualifying examination as prescribed by the American Physical Therapy Association.

(r) *Physical therapist assistant.* A person who is licensed as a physical therapist assistant, if applicable, by the State in which practicing, and

(1) Has graduated from a 2-year college-level program approved by the American Physical Therapy Association; or

(2) Has 2 years of appropriate experience as a physical therapist assistant, and has achieved a satisfactory grade on a proficiency examination approved by the Secretary, except that such determinations of proficiency shall not apply with respect to persons initially licensed by a State or seeking initial qualification as a physical therapist assistant after December 31, 1977.

(s) *Social worker (qualified consultant).* A person who is licensed, if applicable, by the State in which practicing, is a graduate of a school of social work accredited or approved by the Council on Social Work Education, and has 1 year of social work experience in a health care setting.

(t) *Speech pathologist or audiologist (qualified consultant).* A person who is licensed, if applicable, by the State in which practicing, and

(1) Is eligible for a certificate of clinical competence in the appropriate area (speech pathology or audiology) granted by the American Speech and Hearing Association under its requirements in effect on the publication of this provision; or

(2) Meets the educational requirements for certification, and is in the process of accumulating the supervised experience required for certification.

(u) *Supervision.* Authoritative procedural guidance by a qualified person for the accomplishment of a function or ac-

tivity within his sphere of competence, with initial direction and periodic inspection of the actual act of accomplishing the function or activity. Unless otherwise stated in regulations, the supervisor must be on the premises if the person does not meet assistant-level qualifications specified in these definitions.

(v) *Therapeutic recreation specialist (qualified consultant).* A person who is licensed or registered, if applicable, by the State in which practicing, and is eligible for registration as a therapeutic recreation specialist by the National Therapeutic Recreation Society (Branch of National Recreation and Park Association) under its requirements in effect on publication of this provision.

§ 405.1120 Condition of participation— compliance with Federal, State, and local laws.

The skilled nursing facility is in compliance with applicable Federal, State, and local laws and regulations.

(a) *Standard: Licensure.* The facility, in any State in which State or applicable local law provides for licensing of facilities of this nature:

(1) Is licensed pursuant to such law; or

(2) If not subject to licensure, is approved by the agency of the State or locality responsible for licensing skilled nursing facilities as meeting fully the standards established for such licensing, and

(3) Except that a facility which formerly met fully such licensure requirements, but is currently determined not to meet fully all such requirements, may be recognized for a period specified by the State standard-setting authority.

(b) *Standard: Licensure or registration of personnel.* Staff of the facility are licensed or registered in accordance with applicable laws.

(c) *Standard: Conformity with other Federal, State, and local laws.* The facility is in conformity with all Federal, State, and local laws relating to fire and safety, sanitation, communicable and reportable diseases, postmortem procedures, and other relevant health and safety requirements.

§ 405.1121 Condition of participation— governing body and management.

The skilled nursing facility has an effective governing body, or designated persons so functioning, with full legal authority and responsibility for the operation of the facility. The governing body adopts and enforces rules and regulations relative to health care and safety of patients, to the protection of their personal and property rights, and to the general operation of the facility. The governing body develops a written institutional plan that reflects the operating budget and capital expenditures plan.

(a) *Standard: Disclosure of ownership.* The facility supplies full and complete information to the survey agency as to the identity (1) of each person who has any direct or indirect ownership interest of 10 per centum or more in such skilled nursing facility or who is the owner (in whole or in part) of any mortgage, deed of trust, note, or other obligation secured (in whole or in part) by such skilled nursing facility or any of the property or assets of such skilled nursing facility, (2) in case a skilled nursing facility is organized as a corporation, of each officer and director of the corporation, and (3) in case a skilled nursing facility is organized as a partnership, of each partner; and promptly reports any changes which would affect the current accuracy of the information so required to be supplied.

(b) *Standard: Staffing patterns.* The facility furnishes to the State survey agency information from payroll records setting forth the average numbers and types of personnel (in full-time equivalents) on each tour of duty during at least 1 week of each quarter. Such week will be selected by the survey agency.

(c) *Standard: Bylaws.* The governing body adopts effective patient care policies and administrative policies and bylaws governing the operation of the facility, in accordance with legal requirements. Such policies and bylaws are in writing, dated, and made available to all members of the governing body which ensures that they are operational, and reviews and revises them as necessary.

(d) *Standard: Independent medical evaluation (medical review).* The governing body adopts policies to ensure that the facility cooperates in an effective program which provides for a regular program of independent medical evaluation and audit of the patients in the facility to the extent required by the programs in which the facility participates (including, at least annually, medical evaluation of each patient's need for skilled nursing facility care).

(e) *Standard: Administrator.* The governing body appoints a qualified administrator who is responsible for the overall management of the facility, enforces the rules and regulations relative to the level of health care and safety of patients, and to the protection of their personal and property rights, and plans, organizes, and directs those responsibilities delegated to him by the governing body. Through meetings and periodic reports, the administrator maintains ongoing liaison among the governing body, medical and nursing staffs, and other professional and supervisory staff of the facility, and studies and acts upon recommendations made by the utilization review and other committees. In the absence of the administrator, an employee is authorized, in writing, to act on his behalf.

(f) *Standard: Institutional planning.* The institutional plan:

(1) Provides for an annual operating budget which includes all anticipated income and expenses related to items which would, under generally accepted accounting principles, be considered income and expense items (except that nothing in this paragraph shall require that there be prepared, in connection with any budget, an item-by-item identification of the components of each type of anticipated expenditure or income),

(2) Provides for a capital expenditures plan for at least a 3-year period (including the year to which the operating budget described in paragraph (1) of this section is applicable) which includes and identifies in detail the anticipated sources of financing for, and the objectives of, each anticipated expenditure in excess of $100,000 related to the acquisition of land, the improvement of land, buildings, and equipment, and the replacement, modernization, and expansion of the buildings and equipment which would, under generally accepted accounting principles, be considered capital items,

(3) Provides for review and updating at least annually, and

(4) Is prepared, under the direction of the governing body of the institution, by a committee consisting of representatives of the governing body, the ad-

ministrative staff, and the organized medical staff (if any) of the institution.

(g) *Standard: Personnel policies and procedures.* The governing body, through the administrator, is responsible for implementing and maintaining written personnel policies and procedures that support sound patient care and personnel practices. Personnel records are current and available for each employee and contain sufficient information to support placement in the position to which assigned. Written policies for control of communicable disease are in effect to ensure that employees with symptoms or signs of communicable disease or infected skin lesions are not permitted to work, and that a safe and sanitary environment for patients and personnel exists and incidents and accidents to patients and personnel are reviewed to identify health and safety hazards. Employees are provided, or referred for, periodic health examinations, to ensure freedom from communicable disease.

(h) *Standard: Staff development.* An ongoing educational program is planned and conducted for the development and improvement of skills of all the facility's personnel, including training related to problems and needs of the aged, ill, and disabled. Each employee receives appropriate orientation to the facility and its policies, and to his position and duties. Inservice training includes at least prevention and control of infections, fire prevention and safety, accident prevention, confidentiality of patient information, and preservation of patient dignity, including protection of his privacy and personal and property rights. Records are maintained which indicate the content of, and attendance at, such staff development programs.

(i) *Standard: Use of outside resources.* If the facility does not employ a qualified professional person to render a specific service to be provided by the facility, there are arrangements for such a service through a written agreement with an outside resource—a person or agency that will render direct service to patients or act as a consultant. The responsibilities, functions, and objectives, and the terms of agreement, including financial arrangements and charges, of each such outside resource are delineated in writing and signed by an author-

ized representative of the facility and the person or the agency providing the service. The agreement specifies that the facility retains professional and administrative responsibility for the services rendered. The financial arrangements provide that the outside resource bill the facility for covered services (either Part A or B for Medicare beneficiaries) rendered directly to the patient, and that receipt of payment from the program(s) to the facility for the services discharges the liability of the beneficiary or any other person to pay for the services. The outside resource, when acting as a consultant, apprises the administrator of recommendations, plans for implementation, and continuing assessment through dated, signed reports, which are retained by the administrator for follow-up action and evaluation of performance. (See requirement under each service—§§ 405.1125 through 405.1132.)

(j) *Standard: Notification of changes in patient status.* The facility has appropriate written policies and procedures relating to notification of the patient's attending physician and other responsible persons in the event of an accident involving the patient, or other significant change in the patient's physical, mental, or emotional status, or patient charges, billings, and related administrative matters. Except in a medical emergency, a patient is not transferred or discharged, nor is treatment altered radically, without consultation with the patient or, if he is incompetent, without prior notification of next of kin or sponsor.

§ 405.1122   Condition of participation— patient care policies.

The skilled nursing facility has written policies to govern the continuing skilled nursing care and related medical or other services provided.

(a) *Standard: Development and review of patient care policies.* The facility has policies, which are developed with the advice of (and with provision for review of such policies from time to time, but at least annually, by) a group of professional personnel including one or more physicians and one or more registered nurses, to govern the skilled nursing care and related medical or other services it provides. The policies, which are available to admitting physicians, sponsoring agencies, patients, and the public, reflect awareness of, and provision for, meeting the total medical and psychosocial needs of patients, including admission, transfer, and discharge planning; and the range of services available to patients, including frequency of physician visits by each category of patients admitted. These policies also include provisions to protect patients' personal and property rights. Medical records and minutes of staff and committee meetings reflect that patient care is being rendered in accordance with the written patient care policies, and that utilization review committee recommendations regarding the policies are reviewed and necessary steps taken to ensure compliance.

(b) *Standard: Execution of patient care policies.* The facility has a physician, a registered nurse, or a medical staff, designated in writing, to be responsible for the execution of such policies. If the responsibility for day-to-day execution of patient care policies has been delegated to a registered nurse, the facility makes available an advisory physician from whom she receives medical guidance.

§ 405.1123 Condition of participation—physician services.

Patients in need of skilled nursing or rehabilitative care are admitted to the facility only upon the recommendation of, and remain under the care of, a physician. To the extent feasible, each patient or his sponsor designates a personal physician.

(a) *Standard: Medical findings and physicians' orders at time of admission.* There is made available to the facility, prior to or at the time of admission, patient information which includes current medical findings, diagnoses, and orders from a physician for immediate care of the patient. Information about the rehabilitation potential of the patient and a summary of prior treatment are made available to the facility at the time of admission or within 48 hours thereafter.

(b) *Standard: Patient supervision by physician.* The facility has a policy that the health care of every patient must be under the supervision of a physician who, based on a medical evaluation of the

patient's immediate and long-term needs, prescribes a planned regimen of total patient care. Each attending physician is required to make arrangements for the medical care of his patients in his absence. The medical evlauation of the patient is based on a physical examination done within 48 hours of admission unless such examination was performed within 5 days prior to admission. The patient is seen by his attending physician at least once every 30 days for the first 90 days following admission. The patient's total program of care (including medications and treatments) is reviewed during a visit by the attending physician at least once every 30 days for the first 90 days, and revised as necessary. A progress note is written and signed by the physician at the time of each visit, and he signs all his orders. Subsequent to the 90th day following admission, an alternate schedule for physician visits may be adopted where the attending physician determines and so justifies in the patient's medical record that the patient's condition does not necessitate visits at 30-day intervals. This alternate schedule does not apply for patients who require specialized rehabilitative services, in which case the review must be in accordance with § 405.1126(b). At no time may the alternate schedule exceed 60 days between visits. If the physician decides upon an alternate schedule of visits of more than 30 days for a patient, (1) in the case of a Medicaid benefits recipient, the facility notifies the State Medicaid agency of the change in schedule, including justification, and (2) the utilization review committee or the medical review team (see § 405.1121(d)) promptly reevaluates the patient's need for monthly physician visits as well as his continued need for skilled nursing facility services (see § 405.1137(d)). If the utilization review committee or the medical review team does not concur in the schedule of visits at intervals of more than 30 days, the alternate schedule is not acceptable.

(c) *Standard: Availability of physicians for emergency patient care.* The facility has written procedures, available at each nurses station, that provide for having a physician available to furnish necessary medical care in case of emergency.

§ 405.1124   Condition of participation— nursing services.

The skilled nursing facility provides 24-hour service by licensed nurses, including the services of a registered nurse at least during the day tour of duty 5 days a week. There is an organized nursing service with a sufficient number of qualified nursing personnel to meet the total nursing needs of all patients.

(a) *Standard: Director of nursing services.* The director of nursing services is a qualified registered nurse employed full-time who has, in writing, administrative authority, responsibility, and accountability for the functions, activities, and training of the nursing services staff, and serves only one facility in this capacity. If the director of nursing services has other institutional responsibilities, a qualified registered nurse serves as her assistant so that there is the equivalent of a full-time director of nursing services on duty. The director of nursing services is responsible for the development and maintenance of nursing service objectives, standards of nursing practice, nursing policy and procedure manuals, written job descriptions for each level of nursing personnel, scheduling of daily rounds to see all patients, methods for coordination of nursing services with other patient services, for recommending the number and levels of nursing personnel to be employed, and nursing staff development (see § 405.1121(h)).

(b) *Standard: Charge nurse.* A registered nurse, or a qualified licensed practical (vocational) nurse, is designated as charge nurse by the director of nursing services for each tour of duty, and is responsible for supervision of the total nursing activities in the facility during each tour of duty. The director of nursing services does not serve as charge nurse in a facility with an average daily total occupancy of 60 or more patients. The charge nurse delegates responsibility to nursing personnel for the direct nursing care of specific patients during each tour of duty, on the basis of staff qualifications, size and physical layout of the facility, characteristics of the patient load, and the emotional, social, and nursing care needs of patients.

(c) *Standard: Twenty-four-hour nursing service.* The facility provides 24-hour nursing service which is sufficient to meet nursing needs in accordance with the policies developed as provided in § 405.1122(a) on patient care policies. The policies ensure that each patient receives treatments, medications, and diet as prescribed, and rehabilitative nursing care as needed; receives proper care to prevent decubitus ulcers and deformities, and is kept comfortable, clean, well-groomed, and protected from accident, injury, and infection; and encouraged, assisted, and trained in self-care and group activities. Nursing personnel, including at least one registered nurse on the day tour of duty 5 days a week, licensed practical (vocational) nurses, nurse aides, orderlies, and ward clerks, are assigned duties consistent with their education and experience, and based on the characteristics of the patient load and the kinds of nursing skills needed to provide care to the patients. Weekly time schedules are maintained and indicate the number and classification of nursing personnel, including relief personnel, who worked on each unit for each tour of duty.

(d) *Standard: Patient care plan.* In coordination with the other patient care services to be provided, a written patient care plan for each patient is developed and maintained by the nursing service consonant with the attending physician's plan of medical care, and is implemented upon admission. The plan indicates care to be given and goals to be accomplished and which professional service is responsible for each element of care. The patient care plan is reviewed, evaluated, and updated as necessary by all professional personnel involved in the care of the patient.

(e) *Standard: Rehabilitative nursing care.* Nursing personnel are trained in rehabilitative nursing, and the facility has an active program of rehabilitative nursing care which is an integral part of nursing service and is directed toward assisting each patient to achieve and maintain an optimal level of self-care and independence. Rehabilitative nursing care services are performed daily for those patients who require such service, and are recorded routinely.

(f) *Standard: Supervision of patient nutrition.* Nursing personnel are aware of the nutritional needs and food and fluid intake of patients and assist promptly where necessary in the feeding of patients. A procedure is established to inform the dietetic service of physicians' diet orders and of patients' dietetic problems. Food and fluid intake of patients is observed, and deviations from normal are recorded and reported to the charge nurse and the physician.

(g) *Standard:* *Administration of drugs.* Drugs are administered in compliance with State and local laws. Procedures are established by the pharmaceutical services committee (see § 405.1127 (d)) to ensure that drugs are checked against physicians' orders, that the patient is identified prior to administration of a drug, and that each patient has an individual medication record and that the dose of drug administered to that patient is properly recorded therein by the person who administers the drug. Drugs and biologicals are administered as soon as possible after doses are prepared, and are administered by the same person who prepared the doses for administration, except under single unit dose package distribution systems. (See § 405.1101(h).)

(h) *Standard: Conformance with physicians' drug orders.* Drugs are administered in accordance with written orders of the attending physician. Drugs not specifically limited as to time or number of doses when ordered are controlled by automatic stop orders or other methods in accordance with written policies. Physicians' verbal orders for drugs are given only to a licensed nurse, pharmacist, or physician and are immediately recorded and signed by the person receiving the order. (Verbal orders for Schedule II drugs are permitted only in the case of a bona fide emergency situation.) Such orders are countersigned by the attending physician within 48 hours. The attending physician is notified of an automatic stop order prior to the last dose so that he may decide if the administration of the drug or biological is to be continued or altered.

(i) *Standard: Storage of drugs and biologicals.* Procedures for storing and disposing of drugs and biologicals are established by the pharmaceutical services committee. In accordance with State and Federal laws, all drugs and biologicals, are stored in locked compartments under proper temperature controls and only authorized personnel have access to the keys. Separately locked, perma-

nently affixed compartments are provided for storage of controlled drugs listed in Schedule II of the Comprehensive Drug Abuse Prevention & Control Act of 1970 and other drugs subject to abuse, except under single unit package drug distribution systems in which the quantity stored is minimal and a missing dose can be readily detected. An emergency medication kit approved by the pharmaceutical services committee is kept readily available.

§ 405.1125 **Condition of participation— dietetic services.**

The skilled nursing facility provides a hygienic dietetic service that meets the daily nutritional needs of patients, ensures that special dietary needs are met, and provides palatable and attractive meals. A facility that has a contract with an outside food management company may be found to be in compliance with this condition provided the facility and/ or company meets the standards listed herein.

(a) *Standard: Staffing.* Overall supervisory responsibility for the dietetic service is assigned to a full-time qualified dietetic service supervisor. If the dietetic service supervisor is not a qualified dietitian he functions with frequent, regularly scheduled consultation from a person so qualified. (See § 405.1121(i).) In addition, the facility employs sufficient supportive personnel competent to carry out the functions of the dietetic service. Food service personnel are on duty daily over a period of 12 or more hours. If consultant dietetic services are used, the consultant's visits are at appropriate times, and of sufficient duration and frequency to provide continuing liaison with medical and nursing staffs, advice to the administrator, patient counseling, guidance to the supervisor and staff of the dietetic service, approval of all menus, and participation in development or revision of dietetic policies and procedures and in planning and conducting inservice education programs (see § 405.1121(h)).

(b) *Standard: Menus and nutritional adequacy.* Menus are planned and followed to meet nutritional needs of patients in accordance with physicians' orders and, to the extent medically possible, in accordance with the recommended dietary allowances of the Food and Nutrition Board of the National

Research Council National Academy of Sciences.

(c) *Standard: Therapeutic diets.* Therapeutic diets are prescribed by the attending physician. Therapeutic menus are planned in writing, and prepared and served as ordered, with supervision **or consultation from the dietitian and advice from the physician whenever necessary. A current therapeutic diet manual approved by the dietitian is readily available to attending physicians and nursing and dietetic service personnel.**

(d) *Standard: Frequency of meals.* At least three meals or their equivalent are served daily, at regular hours, with not more than a 14-hour span between substantial evening meal and breakfast. To the extent medically possible, bedtime nourishments are offered routinely to all patients.

(e) *Standard: Preparation and service of food.* Foods are prepared by methods that conserve nutritive value, flavor, and appearance, and are attractively served at the proper temperatures and in a form to meet individual needs. If a patient refuses food served, appropriate substitutes of similar nutritive value are offered.

(f) *Standard: Hygiene of staff.* Dietetic service personnel are free of communicable diseases and practice hygienic food-handling techniques. In the event food service employees are assigned duties outside the dietetic service, these duties do not interfere with the sanitation, safety, or time required for dietetic work assignments. (See § 405.1121(g).)

(g) *Standard: Sanitary conditions.* Food is procured from sources approved or considered satisfactory by Federal, State, or local authorities, and stored, prepared, distributed, and served under sanitary conditions. Waste is disposed of properly. Written reports of inspections by State and local health authorities are on file at the facility, with notation made of action taken by the facility to comply with any recommendations.

§ 405.1126 **Condition of participation— specialized rehabilitative services.**

In addition to rehabilitative nursing (§ 405.1124(e)), the skilled nursing facility provides, or arranges for, under written agreement, specialized rehabilitative services by qualified personnel (i.e., physical therapy, speech pathology and audiology, and occupational therapy) as needed by patients to improve and maintain functioning. These services are provided upon the written order of the patient's attending physician. Safe and adequate space and equipment are available, commensurate with the services offered. If the facility does not offer such services directly, it does not admit nor retain patients in need of this care unless provision is made for such services under arrangement with qualified outside resources under which the facility assumes professional and financial responsibilities for the services rendered. (See § 405.1121(1).)

(a) *Standard: Organization and staffing.* Specialized rehabilitative services are provided, in accordance with accepted professional practices, by qualified therapists or by qualified assistants or other supportive personnel under the supervision of qualified therapists. Written administrative and patient care policies and procedures are developed for rehabilitative services by appropriate therapists and representatives of the medical, administrative, and nursing staffs.

(b) *Standard: Plan of care.* Rehabilitative services are provided under a written plan of care, initiated by the attending physician and developed in consultation with appropriate therapist(s) and the nursing service. Therapy is provided only upon written orders of the attending physician. A report of the patient's progress is communicated to the attending physician within 2 weeks of the initiation of specialized rehabilitative services. The patient's progress is thereafter reviewed regularly, and the plan of rehabilitative care is reevaluated as necessary, but at least every 30 days, by the physician and the therapist(s).

(c) *Standard: Documentation of services.* The physician's orders, the plan of rehabilitative care, services rendered, evaluations of progress, and other pertinent information are recorded in the patient's medical record, and are dated and signed by the physician ordering the service and the person who provided the service.

(d) *Standard: Qualifying to provide outpatient physical therapy services.* If the facility provides outpatient physical therapy services, it meets the applicable health and safety regulations pertaining to such services as are included in Subpart Q of this part. (See §§ 405.1719;

405.1720; 405.1722 (a) and (b) (1), (2), (3) (i), (4), (5), (6), (7), and (8); and 405.1725.)

§ 405.1127 Condition of participation—pharmaceutical services.

The skilled nursing facility provides appropriate methods and procedures for the dispensing and administering of drugs and biologicals. Whether drugs and biologicals are obtained from community or institutional pharmacists or stocked by the facility, the facility is responsible for providing such drugs and biologicals for its patients, insofar as they are covered under the programs, and for ensuring that pharmaceutical services are provided in accordance with accepted professional principles and appropriate Federal, State, and local laws. (See § 405.1124 (g), (h), and (i).)

(a) *Standard: Supervision of services.* The pharmaceutical services are under the general supervision of a qualified pharmacist who is responsible to the administrative staff for developing, coordinating, and supervising all pharmaceutical services. The pharmacist (if not a full-time employee) devotes a sufficient number of hours, based upon the needs of the facility, during regularly scheduled visits to carry out these responsibilities. The pharmacist reviews the drug regimen of each patient at least monthly, and reports any irregularities to the medical director and administrator. The pharmacists submits a written report at least quarterly to the pharmaceutical services committee on the status of the facility's pharmaceutical service and staff performance.

(b) *Standard: Control and accountability.* The pharmaceutical service has procedures for control and accountability of all drugs and biologicals throughout the facility. Only approved drugs and biologicals are used in the facility, and are dispensed in compliance with Federal and State laws. Records of receipt and disposition of all controlled drugs are maintained in sufficient detail to enable an accurate reconciliation. The pharmacist determines that drug records are in order and that an account of all controlled drugs is maintained and reconciled.

(c) *Standard: Labeling of drugs and biologicals.* The labeling of drugs and biologicals is based on currently accepted professional principles, and includes the appropriate accessory and cautionary instructions, as well as the expiration date when applicable.

(d) *Standard: Pharmaceutical services committee.* A pharmaceutical services committee (or its equivalent) develops written policies and procedures for safe and effective drug therapy, distribution, control, and use. The committee is comprised of at least the pharmacist, the director of nursing services, the administrator, and one physician. The committee oversees pharmaceutical service in the facility, makes recommendations for improvement, and monitors the service to ensure its accuracy and adequacy. The committee meets at least quarterly and documents its activities, findings, and recommendations.

§ 405.1128 Condition of participation—laboratory and radiologic services.

The skilled nursing facility has provision for promptly obtaining required laboratory, X-ray, and other diagnostic services.

(a) *Standard: Provision for services.* If the facility provides its own laboratory and X-ray services, these meet the applicable conditions established for certification of hospitals that are contained in §§ 405.1028 and 405.1029, respectively. If the facility itself does not provide such services, arrangements are made for obtaining these services from a physician's office, a participating hospital or skilled nursing facility, or a portable X-ray supplier or independent laboratory which is approved to provide these services under the program. All such services are provided only on the orders of the attending physician, who is notified promptly of the findings. The facility assists the patient, if necessary, in arranging for transportation to and from the source of service. Signed and dated reports of a clinical laboratory, X-ray, and other diagnostic services are filed with the patient's medical record.

(b) *Standard: Blood and blood products.* Blood handling and storage facilities are safe, adequate, and properly supervised. If the facility provides for maintaining and transfusing blood and blood products, it meets the conditions established for certification of hospitals that are contained in § 405.1028(j).

If the facility does not provide its own facilities but does provide transfusion services alone, it meets at least the requirements of § 405.1028(j) (1), (3), (4), (6), and (9).

§ 405.1129 Condition of participation—dental services.

The skilled nursing facility has satisfactory arrangements to assist patients to obtain routine and emergency dental care (See § 405.1121(i).) (The basic Hospital Insurance Program does not cover the services of a dentist in a skilled nursing facility in connection with the care, treatment, filling, removal, or replacement of teeth or structures supporting the teeth; and only certain oral surgery is included in the Supplemental Medical Insurance Program.)

(a) *Standard: Advisory dentist.* An advisory dentist participates in the staff development program for nursing and other appropriate personnel (see § 405.-1121(h)), and recommends oral hygiene policies and practices for the care of patients.

(b) *Standard: Arrangements for outside services.* The facility has a cooperative agreement with a dental service, and maintains a list of dentists in the community for patients who do not have a private dentist. The facility assists the patient, if necessary, in arranging for transportation to and from the dentist's office.

§ 405.1130 Condition of participation—social services.

The skilled nursing facility has satisfactory arrangements for identifying the medically related social and emotional needs of the patient. It is not mandatory that the skilled nursing facility itself provide social services in order to participate in the program. If the facility does not provide social services, it has written procedures for referring patients in need of social services to appropriate social agencies. If social services are offered by the facility, they are provided under a clearly defined plan, by qualified persons, to assist each patient to adjust to the social and emotional aspects of his illness, treatment, and stay in the facility.

(a) *Standard: Social service functions.* The medically related social and emotional needs of the patient are identified and services provided to meet them, either by qualified staff of the facility, or by referral, based on established procedures, to appropriate social agencies. If financial assistance is indicated, arrangements are made promptly for referral to an appropriate agency. The patient and his family or responsible person are fully informed of the patient's personal and property rights.

(b) *Standard: Staffing.* If the facility offers social services, a member of the staff of the facility is designated as responsible for social services. If the designated person is not a qualified social worker, the facility has a written agreement with a qualified social worker or recognized social agency for consultation and assistance on a regularly scheduled basis. (See § 405.1121(i).) The social service also has sufficient supportive personnel to meet patient needs. Facilities are adequate for social service personnel, easily accessible to patients and medical and other staff, and ensure privacy for interviews.

(c) *Standard: Records and confidentiality of social data.* Records of pertinent social data about personal and family problems medically related to the patient's illness and care, and of action taken to meet his needs, are maintained in the patient's medical record. If social services are provided by an outside resource, a record is maintained of each referral to such resource. Policies and procedures are established for ensuring the confidentiality of all patients' social information.

§ 405.1131 Condition of participation—patient activities.

The skilled nursing facility provides for an activities program, appropriate to the needs and interests of each patient, to encourage self care, resumption of normal activities, and maintenance of an optimal level of psychosocial functioning.

(a) *Standard: Responsibility for patient activities.* A member of the facility's staff is designated as responsible for the patient activities program. If he is not a qualified patient activities coordinator, he functions with frequent, regularly scheduled consultation from a person so qualified. (See § 405.1121(i).)

(b) *Standard: Patient activities program.* Provision is made for an ongoing program of meaningful activities appropriate to the needs and interests of patients, designed to promote opportunities for engaging in normal pursuits, including religious activities of their choice, if any. Each patient's activities program is approved by the patient's attending physician as not in conflict with the treatment plan. The activities are designed to promote the physical, social, and mental well-being of the patients. The facility makes available adequate space and a variety of supplies and equipment to satisfy the individual interests of patients (see § 405.1134(g)).

§ **405.1132 Condition of participation— medical records.**

The facility maintains clinical (medical) records on all patients in accordance with accepted professional standards and practices. The medical record service has sufficient staff, facilities, and equipment to provide medical records that are completely and accurately documented, readily accessible, and systematically organized to facilitate retrieving and compiling information.

(a) *Standard: Staffing.* Overall supervisory responsibility for the medical record service is assigned to a full-time employee of the facility. The facility also employs sufficient supportive personnel competent to carry out the functions of the medical record service. If the medical record supervisor is not a qualified medical record practitioner, this person functions with consultation from a person so qualified. (See § 405.1121(i).)

(b) *Standard: Protection of medical record information.* The facility safeguards medical record information against loss, destruction, or unauthorized use.

(c) *Standard: Content.* The medical record contains sufficient information to identify the patient clearly, to justify the diagnosis and treatment, and to document the results accurately. All medical records contain the following general categories of data: Documented evidence of assessment of the needs of the patient, of establishment of an appropriate plan of treatment, and of the care and services provided; authentication of hospital diagnoses (discharge summary, report from patient's attending physician, or transfer form), identification data and consent forms, medical and nursing history of patient, report of physical examination(s), diagnostic and therapeutic orders, observations and progress notes, reports of treatments and clinical findings, and discharge summary including final diagnosis and prognosis.

(d) *Standard: Physician documentation.* Only physicians enter or authenticate in medical records opinions that require medical judgment (in accordance with medical staff bylaws, rules, and regulations, if applicable). Each physician signs his entries into the medical record.

(e) *Standard: Completion of records and centralization of reports.* Current medical records and those of discharged patients are completed promptly. All clinical information pertaining to a patient's stay is centralized in the patient's medical record.

(f) *Standard: Retention and preservation.* Medical records are retained for a period of time not less than that determined by the respective State statute, the statute of limitations in the State, or 5 years from the date of discharge in the absence of a State statute, or, in the case of a minor, 3 years after the patient becomes of age under State law.

(g) *Standard: Indexes.* Patients' medical records are indexed according to name of patient and final diagnoses to facilitate acquisition of statistical medical information and retrieval of records for research or administrative action.

(h) *Standard: Location and facilities.* The facility maintains adequate facilities and equipment, conveniently located, to provide efficient processing of medical records (reviewing, indexing, filing, and prompt retrieval).

§ **405.1133 Condition of participation— transfer agreement.**

The skilled nursing facility has in effect a transfer agreement with one or more hospitals approved for participation under the programs, which provides the basis for effective working arrangements under which inpatient hospital care or other hospital services are available promptly to the facility's patients when needed. (A facility that has been unable to establish a transfer agreement with the hospital(s) in the community or service area after documented attempts to do so is considered to have such an agreement in effect.)

(a) *Standard: Patient transfer.* A hospital and a skilled nursing facility shall be considered to have a transfer agreement in effect if, by reason of a written agreement between them or (in case the two institutions are under common control) by reason of a written undertaking by the person or body which controls them, there is reasonable assurance that:

(1) Transfer of patients will be effected between the hospital and the skilled nursing facility, ensuring timely admission, whenever such transfer is medically appropriate as determined by the attending physician, and

(2) There will be interchange of medical and other information necessary or useful in the care and treatment of individuals transferred between the institutions, or in determining whether such individuals can be adequately cared for otherwise than in either of such institutions, and

(3) Security and accountability for patients' personal effects are provided on transfer.

Any skilled nursing facility which does not have such agreement in effect, but which is found by a State agency (of the State in which such facility is situated) with which an agreement under section 1864 is in effect (or, in the case of a State in which no such agency has an agreement under 1864, by the Secretary) to have attempted in good faith to enter into such an agreement with a hospital sufficiently close to the facility to make feasible the transfer between them of patients and the information referred to in paragraph (a)(2) of this section, shall be considered to have such an agreement in effect if and for so long as such agency (or the Secretary, as the case may be) finds that to do so is in the public interest and essential to ensuring skilled nursing facility services for persons in the community who are eligible for payments with respect to such services under the programs.

§ 405.1134 Condition of participation— Physical environment.

The skilled nursing facility is constructed, equipped, and maintained to protect the health and safety of patients, personnel, and the public.

(a) *Standard: Life safety from fire.* The skilled nursing facility meets such provisions of the Life Safety Code of the National Fire Protection Association (21st Edition, 1967) as are applicable to nursing homes; except that, in consideration of a recommendation by the State survey agency, the Secretary may waive, for such periods as deemed appropriate, specific provisions of such Code which, if rigidly applied, would result in unreasonable hardship upon a skilled nursing facility, but only if such waiver will not adversely affect the health and safety of the patients; and except that the provisions of such Code shall not apply in any State if the Secretary finds, in accordance with applicable provisions of section 1861(j)(13) of the Social Security Act, that in such State there is in effect a fire and safety code, imposed by State law, which adequately protects patients in skilled nursing facilities. Where waiver permits the participation of an existing facility of two or more stories which is not of at least 2-hour fire resistive construction, blind, nonambulatory, or physically handicapped patients are not housed above the street level floor unless the facility is of 1-hour protected noncombustible construction (as defined in National Fire Protection Association Standard No. 220), fully sprinklered 1-hour protected ordinary construction, or fully sprinklered 1-hour protected wood-frame construction. Nonflammable medical gas systems, such as oxygen and nitrous oxide, installed in the facility comply with applicable provisions of National Fire Protection Association Standard No. 56B (Standard for the Use of Inhalation Therapy) 1968 and National Fire Protection Association Standard No. 56F (Nonflammable Medical Gas Systems) 1970.

(b) *Standard: Emergency power.* The facility provides an emergency source of electrical power necessary to protect the health and safety of patients in the event the normal electrical supply is interrupted. The emergency electrical power system must supply power adequate at least for lighting in all means of egress; equipment to maintain fire detection, alarm, and extinguishing systems; and life support systems. Where life support systems are used, emergency electrical service is provided by an emergency generator located on the premises.

(c) *Standard: Facilities for physically handicapped.* The facility is accessible to, and functional for, patients, personnel, and the public. All necessary accommodations are made to meet the needs of persons with semiambulatory disabilities, sight and hearing disabilities, disabilities of coordination, as well as other disabilities, in accordance with the American National Standards Institute (ANSI) Standard No. A117.1, American Standard Specifications for Making Buildings and Facilities Accessible to, and Usable by, the Physically Handicapped. The Secretary (or in the case of a facility participating as a skilled nursing facility under title XIX only, the survey agency—see § 249.33(a)(1)(i) of this title) may waive in existing buildings, for such periods as deemed appropriate, specific provisions of ANSI Standard No. A117.1 which, if rigidly enforced, would result in unreasonable hardship upon the facility, but only if such waiver will not adversely affect the health and safety of patients.

(d) *Standard: Nursing unit.* Each nursing unit has at least the following basic service areas: Nurses station, storage and preparation area(s) for drugs and biologicals, and utility and storage rooms that are adequate in size, conveniently located, and well lighted to facilitate staff functioning. The nurses station is equipped to register patients' calls through a communication system from patient areas, including patient rooms and toilet and bathing facilities.

(e) *Standard: Patient rooms and toilet facilities.* Patient rooms are designed and equipped for adequate nursing care and the comfort and privacy of patients, and have no more than four beds, except in facilities primarily for the care of the mentally ill and/or retarded where there shall be no more than 12 beds per room. (An institution primarily engaged in the care of the mentally retarded or in the treatment of mental diseases cannot qualify as a participating skilled nursing facility under Medicare.) Single patient rooms measure at least 100 square feet, and multipatient rooms provide a minimum of 80 square feet per bed. The Secretary (or in the case of a facility participating as a skilled nursing facility under title XIX only, the survey agency—see § 249.33(a)(1)(i) of this title) may permit variations in individual cases where the facility demonstrates in writing that such variations

are in accordance with the particular needs of the patients and will not adversely affect their health and safety. Each room is equipped with, or is conveniently located near, adequate toilet and bathing facilities. Each room has direct access to a corridor and outside exposure, with the floor at or above grade level.

(f) *Standard: Facilities for special care.* Provision is made for isolating patients as necessary in single rooms ventilated to the outside, with private toilet and handwashing facilities. Procedures in aseptic and isolation techniques are established in writing and followed by all personnel. Such areas are identified by appropriate precautionary signs.

(g) *Standard: Dining and patient activities rooms.* The facility provides one or more clean, orderly, and appropriately furnished rooms of adequate size designated for patient dining and for patient activities. These areas are well-lighted and well-ventilated. If a multipurpose room is used for dining and patient activities, there is sufficient space to accommodate all activities and prevent their intereference with each other.

(h) *Standard: Kitchen and dietetic service areas.* The facility has kitchen and dietetic service areas adequate to meet food service needs. These areas are properly ventilated, and arranged and equipped for sanitary refrigeration, storage, preparation, and serving of food as well as for dish and utensil cleaning and refuse storage and removal.

(i) *Standard: Maintenance of equipment, building, and grounds.* The facility establishes a written preventive maintenance program to ensure that equipment is operative and that the interior and exterior of the building are clean and orderly. All essential mechanical, electrical, and patient care equipment is maintained in safe operating condition.

(j) *Standard: Other environmental considerations.* The facility provides a functional, sanitary, and comfortable environment for patients, personnel, and the public. Provision is made for adequate and comfortable lighting levels in all areas, limitation of sounds at comfort levels, maintaining a comfortable room temperature, procedures to ensure water to all essential areas in the event of loss of normal water supply, and adequate ventilation through windows or mechanical means or a combination of both.

§ 405.1135 Condition of participation—infection control.

The skilled nursing facility establishes an infection control committee of representative professional staff with responsibility for overall infection control in the facility. All necessary housekeeping and maintenance services are provided to maintain a sanitary and comfortable environment and to help prevent the development and transmission of infection.

(a) *Standard: Infection control committee.* The infection control committee is composed of memers of the medical and nursing staffs, administration, and the dietetic, pharmacy, housekeeping, maintenance, and other services. The committee establishes policies and procedures for investigating, controlling, and preventing infections in the facility, and monitors staff performance to ensure that the policies and procedures are executed.

(b) *Standard: Aseptic and isolation techniques.* Written effective procedures in aseptic and isolation techniques are followed by all personnel. Procedures are reviewed and revised annually for effectiveness and improvement.

(c) *Standard: Housekeeping.* The facility employs sufficient housekeeping personnel and provides all necessary equipment to maintain a safe, clean, and orderly interior. A full-time employee is designated responsible for the services and for supervision and training of personnel. Nursing personnel are not assigned housekeeping duties. A facility that has a contract with an outside resource for housekeeping services may be found to be in compliance with this standard provided the facility and/or outside resource meets the requirements of the standard.

(d) *Standard: Linen.* The facility has available at all times a quantity of linen essential for proper care and comfort of patients. Linens are handled, stored, processed, and transported in such a manner as to prevent the spread of infection.

(e) *Standard: Pest control.* The facility is maintained free from insects and rodents through operation of a pest control program.

§ 405.1136 Condition of participation—disaster preparedness.

The skilled nursing facility has a written plan, periodically rehearsed, with procedures to be followed in the event of an internal or external disaster and for the care of casualties (patients and personnel) arising from such disasters.

(a) *Standard: Disaster plan.* The facility has an acceptable written plan in operation, with procedures to be followed in the event of fire, explosion, or other disaster. The plan is developed and maintained with the assistance of qualified fire, safety, and other appropriate experts, and includes procedures for prompt transfer of casualties and records, instructions regarding the location and use of alarm systems and signals and of fire-fighting equipment, information regarding methods of containing fire, procedures for notification of appropriate persons, and specifications of evacuation routes and procedures. (See § 405.1134(a).)

(b) *Standard: Staff training and drills.* All employees are trained, as part of their employment orientation, in all aspects of preparedness for any disaster. The disaster program includes orientation and ongoing training and drills for all personnel in all procedures so that each employee promptly and correctly carries out his specific role in case of a disaster. (See § 405.1121(h).)

§ 405.1137 Condition of participation—utilization review.

The skilled nursing facility carries out utilization review of the services provided in the facility at least to inpatients who are entitled to benefits under the program(s). Utilization review has as its overall objectives both the maintenance of high quality patient care and assurance of appropriate and efficient utilization of facility services. There are two elements to utilization review: medical care evaluation studies that identify and examine patterns of care provided in the facility, and review of extended duration cases which is concerned with efficiency, appropriateness, and cost effectiveness of care. If the Secretary determines that the utilization review procedures established pursuant to title XIX are superior in their effectiveness to the procedures required under this section, he may, to the extent that he deems it appropriate, require for purposes of this title that the procedures established pursuant to title XIX be utilized instead of the procedures required by this section.

(a) *Standard: Written plan of utilization review activity.* The facility has a written, currently applicable utilization review plan, approved by the governing body and the medical director or organized medical staff (if applicable), which includes at least the following: (1) procedures for medical care evaluation studies, and for dissemination and followup of study findings and committee recommendations; (2) definition of the period(s) of extended duration and procedures for review of individual cases of extended duration; (3) a method for identifying patients other than by name (e.g., medical record number); and (4) provision for maintaining written records of committee activities.

(b) *Standard: Composition and organization of utilization review committee.* The committee or group responsible for utilization review is composed of two or more physicians and, optionally, other professional personnel. All medical determinations are made by the physician members of the committee. No physician reviews any case in which he was professionally involved.

(c) *Standard: Medical care evaluation studies.* Medical care evaluation studies are performed to promote the most effective and appropriate use of available health facilities and services consistent with patient needs and professionally recognized standards of health care. Studies, which could include assessment of findings resulting from periodic medical review, emphasize identification and analysis of patterns of patient care and changes indicated to maintain consistent high quality of services. Each medical care evaluation study (whether medical or administrative in emphasis) identifies and analyzes factors related to the patient care rendered in the facility, and serves as the basis for recommendations for change beneficial to patients, staff, the facility, and the community. Studies, on a sample or other basis, include but need not be limited to, admissions, durations of stay, and professional services (including drugs and biologicals) furnished. At least one study is in progress at any given time.

(d) *Standard: Review of cases of extended duration.* Periodic review is made of each current inpatient skilled nursing facility beneficiary case of continuous extended duration, the length of which is defined in the utilization review plan, to determine whether further inpatient stay is necessary. Reviews may also be applied to patients not covered by the program, and/or to cases where duration of stay has not yet reached the definition(s) of extended duration. The plan may specify a different number of days for different diagnostic classes of cases, or may use the same number of days for all cases. In any event, the period(s) specified bears a reasonable relationship to current average length-of-stay statistics, and does not exceed 21 days from admission. An exception to this 21-day limit may be made where the specific diagnostic classes of cases have average lengths of stay exceeding 21 days, in which instances the plan specifices the extended duration period for each specific diagnostic class. In cases for which advance approval of payment has been made, the period(s) of extended duration may be defined as that period for which payment has been approved. After the initial review, reviews for medical necessity for further inpatient stay are made at least every 30 days for the first 90 days and at least every 90 days thereafter. A review is made and a final determination regarding the patient's further care is reached no later than 7 days following the time period specified as the period of extended duration in the utilization review plan.

(e) *Standard: Admission or further stay not medically necessary.* Final determination regarding the necessity for admission or for further stay, including stay beyond the period of extended duration, is limited to physician members of the committee, and may be made by the full physician complement, a subcommittee, or a single committee physician. When a single committee physician has decided that admission is not medically necessary or is inappropriate, or that further stay is no longer medically necessary, further concurrence is obtained as specified in the plan (to include at least a second committee physician) within the 7-day period. If committee members determine, from an extended duration review or a medical care evaluation study, that further stay is not medically necessary, the attending physician is consulted or given the opportunity for consultation, and notification is made in writing within 48 hours by the committee to the administration, the attending physician, and the patient or his representative.

(f) *Standard: Administrative responsibilities.* The administrative staff of the facility is kept directly and fully informed of committee activities to facilitate support and assistance. The administrator studies and acts upon recommendations made by the committee, coordinating such functions with appropriate staff members.

(g) *Standard: Utilization review records.* Written records of committee activities are maintained. Appropriate reports, signed by the committee chairman, are made regularly to the medical staff, administrative staff, governing body, and sponsors (if any). Minutes of each committee meeting are maintained and include at least:

(1) Name of committee,

(2) Date and duration of meeting,

(3) Names of committee members present and absent,

(4) Description of activities presently in progress to satisfy the requirements for medical care evaluation studies, including the subject and reason for study, dates of commencement and expected completion, summary of studies completed since the last meeting, conclusions, and followup on implementation of recommendations made from previous studies, and

(5) Summary of extended duration cases reviewed, including the number of cases, case identification numbers, admission and review dates, and decisions reached, including the basis for each determination and action taken for each case not approved for extended care.

Home Health Services

Home health services are available under insurance and include such benefits as a visiting nurse, therapy, and restorative services. One hundred home health visits (each single service counts as a visit) are allowed within a year of discharge from the hospital. Starting a new benefit period will terminate home care. Medicare will pay for home health care under either Hospital Insurance (Part A) or Medical Insurance (Part B). Benefits are paid at 100% of the reasonable cost.

When the patient's medical condition warrants further treatment of a condition for which he was treated in a hospital or skilled nursing facility, he may receive benefits. However, Medical Insurance will also pay for services to treat a medical condition for which hospitalization is not deemed necessary. Such treatment and services must be provided by an authorized home health agency. The patient must be confined to his home (a nursing home will disqualify him if it provides mainly skilled nursing care because the services of skilled nursing facilities should include restorative services). The home health agency must document three basic conditions to be eligible for reimbursement: (1) the patient's medical need, (2) services to meet this need, and (3) qualified health personnel. Essentially, such services must be under a physician's plan of care for the patient, must include the need of skilled nursing services on an intermittent basis, or physical or speech therapy, and must be administered by qualified personnel. The physician's plan of care for the patient must relate the prescribed services to the patient's condition by diagnosis.

Health Maintenance Organization

A new concept of total health care in the health maintenance organization was authorized by Congress as part of the Medicare legislation. While it is still in the experimental stages, this is a promising new way to control costs yet provide quality care. Patterned after the Kaiser Plan in California, the Health Maintenance Organization (HMO) may emerge as the predominating method of providing total care for a fixed fee.

The Secretary of Health, Education, and Welfare defines a health maintenance organization as: "a legal entity which provides or arranges for the provision of basic and supplemental health services to its members in the manner prescribed by, is organized and operated in the manner prescribed by, and otherwise meets the requirements of,

section 1301 of the Act (Sec. 215, 58 Stat. 690, 42 U.S.C. 216; sec. 1301)."
Basic health services mean:
> Physicians services.
> Outpatient services.
> Inpatient hospital services.
> Crisis intervention mental health services.
> Medical treatment of alcohol or drug abuse.
> Diagnostic laboratory.
> Therapeutic radiology.
> Home health services.
> Preventive health services.

Certain supplemental services are included:
> Intermediate and long-term care facilities.
> Vision care.
> Dental services.
> Physical medicine and rehabilitative services.
> Prescription drugs (prescribed in basic health services).
> Family planning.

Each HMO would define its service geographically and provide services directly to its members. It may use its own resources or make arrangements with other providers in the area.

To become a member of the HMO, a person would enter into a contractual arrangement. In certain cases, i.e., welfare recipients, a contract may be made on behalf of the member. The term "subscriber" is applied to a member who has entered into a contractual relationship with the HMO.

Undergirding the philosophy of the HMO is the practice of health professionals, i.e., physicians, dentists, nurses, podiatrists, optometrists, physicians' assistants, clinical psychologists, social workers, pharmacists, nutritionists, occupational therapists, physical therapists, to compose a medical group. The group generally coordinate their practices by pooling income, arranging salaries or prearranged drawing accounts, sharing health records, equipment, and administrative staff. The Secretary requires such professionals to devote over 50% of their professional activity to the HMO.

In addition to the primary organization, individual practice associations may enter into a written services agreement with the HMO. Such an agreement will include a fixed fee for services. The fee will be set by a system of fixing rates of payment for health services within that community.

Individual subscribers of services will pay a fixed fee for basic services, such fee to be paid periodically without regard to the services used. This fee will also be fixed by a community rating system. Payment plans include options of copayment plans for rendered services or a no copayment plan. Medicare and Medicaid may agree to use HMO services through a contractual agreement on behalf of beneficiaries.

Utilization Review

Federal regulations have been established for skilled nursing homes participating in federal programs to establish a program of utilization review of the services provided in the facility. "Utilization review has as its overall objectives both the maintenance of high quality patient care and the assurance of appropriate and efficient utilization of facility services."

There are two elements of utilization review: medical care evaluation studies that identify and examine patterns of care provided in the facility, and the review of extended duration cases, one which is concerned with efficiency, appropriateness, and cost effectiveness of care.

Each facility is required to have a written plan of utilization review. The plan shall include:

Organization of the committee.
Frequency of meetings.
The type of records.
Definition of extended duration cases.
Methods of selection of cases.
Third party relationships.
Dissemination of reports.
Responsibilities of the administrative staff

Normally, the committee shall have at least two or more physicians, other professional personnel, and such other necessary personnel, but the review is not to be made by persons employed by the facility or anyone in the facility having a financial interest, including a professional involvement in care.

The purpose of medical care evaluation studies is to promote the most effective and efficient use of available health facilities and services consistent with a patient's needs and professionally recognized standards of health care. Such studies may include:

Identification of patterns of patient care.
Changes in health care procedures.
Factors related to patient care in the facility.
Sample studies of admissions.
Durations of stay.
Ancillary services.
Professional services.

The Secretary requires one study to be in progress at any time and at least one study being completed per year. Data for the study may be compiled from records, statistics, profile data, and cooperative endeavors with Professional Standard Review Organizations, fiscal intermediaries, providers of services, or other agencies. Accurate documentation shall be maintained.

All cases of extended duration will be periodically reviewed. The first review is made after a specific interval of time selected for each diagnosis or a period of time the same for all diagnoses of cases. It is suggested that extended duration cases be reviewed each 30 days for 90 days and each 90 days thereafter. However, the facility is charged with developing supporting data to justify review periods for each diagnosis.

When the review committee finds that the further stay of a patient is not medically necessary, they are required to give proper notification to the attending physician, the facility, and the next of kin. Such notice is to be given in writing within two days. In extended duration cases, three working days after the end of the extended duration period are allowed.

The Professional Standards Review Organization is yet another requirement to be imposed by the Secretary of Health, Education, and Welfare to bring about a fair and equitable use of health care services and manpower with geographical areas. Certain regulations will describe the function, composition, and relationship for any designated PSRO so designated with each geographical area. All functioning agencies concerned with health care services will become a part of the professional review. Objectives are: the educational, effective manpower use; the quality of care criteria; and other data gathering functions. With the utilization review within each facility functioning independently, little continuity can be expected; however, the PSRO will coordinate efforts within areas to meet high quality standards of health care.

Discharge Planning

It is generally accepted by regulatory and contracting agencies that a utilization review of patient care should include discharge planning. Such discharge planning should be in the form of an organized discharge planning program that will make available the results to the utilization review committee. Discharge planning will include all patients, but emphasis will be on the long-term cases. It should include information concerning the alternatives to nursing care that may be available in the community.

The Secretary of Health, Education, and Welfare requires the administrator of the facilities contracting for federal programs, i.e., Medicare or Medicaid, to delegate in writing the responsibility for discharge planning to one or more persons of the facility's staff. An alternate plan may call for the administrator to arrange for such planning with a local health, social, or welfare agency.

Procedures for discharge planning should be written to include how the discharge coordinator will function, and his authority and relationships with the facility's staff. The Secretary also requires such a plan to be in operation for each patient within 7 days after the day of admission. A maximum time period will be set for a re-evaluation for each patient's plan. He recommends the use of local resources to the facility, the patient's preferences, the attending physician's recommendations, and a periodic review of the total program.

The facility should provide at the time of discharge post-discharge information in the form of a summary about the discharged patient. The objective is the continuity of care from the facility to post-discharge status. Such a summary includes: the patients rehabilitation potential, information about diagnoses, prior treatments, the physician's orders, and pertinent social information. The summary may be given directly to the patient and/or his guardian.

Fiscal Intermediaries

The Social Security Administration is charged with the responsibility of selecting fiscal intermediaries to whom the participating hospitals, skilled nursing facilities, and other providers may submit requests for payment. However, participants may elect to deal directly with the Social Security Administration. A fiscal intermediary reimburses the providers under an interim reimbursal procedure, with an annual audit to verify cost factors. A fiscal intermediary usually provides utilization controls and supplies the Social Security Administration with experience data. Intermediaries are selected for their ability to provide controls and reimbursal procedures, and are responsible to the Social Security Administration.

Blue Cross Association (Blue Cross-Blue Shield, Hospital-Medical Insurance) and Mutual of Omaha Insurance Company are two typical fiscal intermediaries.

The intermediary is charged with determining the reasonable cost. This is done by compiling the normal cost for services within a given locality. Physician's fees were frozen at the 1968 level but are now being revised from time to time. There is some difficulty in correlating the costs of the nonprofit institution with those of the proprietary institution.

Valuable data are being gathered that may be projected into the future to reveal where Medicare is going. Data on the utilization of services, enrollment, types of providers, and cost factors are noteworthy indicators of future trends.

Chapter *5*

Insurance Liability
and Business Law

The student of nursing home administration will discover that every business is a risk. While risk is pure chance, in thinking of the insurability of a business, it is merely the uncertainty of loss. Loss takes many forms such as loss of life, loss of property, accident, etc. Also, with risk or the uncertainty of loss, there are considerations which are psychological in nature. There are anxiety, uncertainty, and emotional tension attached to the probability of loss. There are resultants, or side effects, to loss. For example, the loss of a nursing home to fire means probable loss of life, loss of employment, possessions, etc.

Because of the probability of loss, the administrator will discover ways of overcoming the results of accidental loss. He may assume the loss himself by paying the expense of such loss. He may defer or insure the probable loss. To defer it means to transfer the responsibility, for a premium, to another, i.e., an insurance company. The administrator may further reduce the probability of loss by establishing safety practices and by practicing good management.

Insurance companies are quite willing to accept the responsibility of paying for loss within the nursing home, if certain conditions are met. The loss must be purely accidental in nature. It must be measurable in order that it may be limited and compared to similar losses. The theory of modern insurance is, because of the risk of loss, the uncertainty of operation of business, the investment needed for continued operation, we insure against the probability of similar, measurable, but limited accidental loss.

The insurance contract will normally specify who or what is to be insured, the exact terms, the limits of the policy, and the amount of the premium and forfeiture for nonpayment. It will specify the time period covered and any exceptions to the contract.

When the administrator needs to make a claim under the terms of an insurance policy, he should be aware that most policies require a written notification of loss within a specified time. Proof of loss will be necessary. In most cases, an adjustor will be employed; however, in the case of death, a certificate of death will be necessary. In the case of illness, a physician's statement is required. A claim is voided by evidence of fraud, failure to offer proof, or submitting a claim not covered by the contract. A reasonable time of making the claim is usually specified, but it is well to remember that every day that transpires between the time of actual loss and making the claim may give rise to doubt. Cancellation of the contract will be different from voiding a claim. In this case, the entire contract is cancelled. This is an option written into the contract.

For the administrator, it is not important to know the mechanics of insurance, since a competent agent will normally look after the interests of his clients and will advise of changes, coverages, etc.; but it is very important for the administrator to know what coverage he has. Since there are many types of insurance, we will discuss briefly those related to the operation of the nursing home.

Fire insurance protection is one major concern and is usually written to include additional coverage for losses from windstorm, lightning, water, and hail. Normally, but not always, the fire protection policy has a coinsurance requirement of 80% of the actual value to be insured. When loss is incurred, the amount of insurance carried is divided by the insurance required (usually 80%), and then multiplied by the loss sustained to get the amount recovered. It is possible to acquire insurance that pays 100% of the loss. In computing the loss, the actual value is the original cost, plus inflation, less depreciation. Depreciation on permanent structures is usually, but not always, figured at 2% per year. The administrator should insure for the actual value of the facility, neither under nor over the fair market value.

The administrator will use an auto in his business and should know the types of insurance available for his protection. Naturally, he will carry *collision insurance,* a type policy that usually has a deductible clause ($50.00 to $100.00) for each accident), and *comprehensive in-*

surance which includes protection against fire, theft, glass breakage, hail, windstorm, flood, vandalism, etc. Additional coverage such as *bodily liability and property damage* may be added. This coverage is usually identified with such figures as $5,000/$20,000/$10,000 which means $5,000 to each person injured, $20,000 total bodily injury payments, and $10,000 property damage liability payment. In addition, for a small fee, *medical payments* or an amendment to cover transport of patients may be added. Without this latter amendment to the auto insurance policy,the transport of patients will be at the nursing home administrator's risk.

Theft insurance may be purchased to protect the nursing home against loss by larceny, theft, burglary, robbery, or felonious acts. Legally, any theft is larceny, burglary is against property, and robbery is against a person. Insurance is costly for coverage against all types of theft, but it may be the difference in staying in business after a serious loss.

Every employer should carry some form of *workman's compensation*. While this is usually not required, employee injury is probably the greatest risk sustained by the employer. A normal policy pays for medical expense—the amount is unlimited—and weekly compensation. Usually, rates and compensation are set by state law. The greatest value of the employer's carrying compensation insurance is that it limits the liability of the nursing home by deferring the risk to the insurance company. Coverage and benefits are carried on employees for accidental injury while on the job. "Injury" may include disease, respiratory difficulties, chemical burns, etc., whose cause can be traced to the place of employment.

Public liability insurance covers the legal liability incurred by the nursing home for nonoccupation accidents on the premises of the nursing home. Claims arising from negligence of nursing home employees resulting in injury to a third party while he is a visitor—this may be a tradesman, relative, governmental inspector, etc.—will be covered. In actual practice, a person is not negligent until a court of law declares him negligent and therefore liability must be established.

Malpractice insurance covers the legal liability incurred by the nursing home administrator and/or his employees for negligence in the practice of their profession and work. The injured third party is the patient. Many times the public liability and malpractice insurance are written as a package. When this is the case, the primary one protected is the nursing home owner. An employee may be held accountable for his own acts. Therefore, the employed administrator should provide his own malpractice insurance. One recommended means of obtaining coverage is for the nursing home administrator to join the American College of Nursing Home Administrators and thereby become eligible for group coverage at a nominal rate.

The nursing home may elect to institute coverage of its employees under a *group health insurance plan*. These plans, available from most health insurance companies, may specify a minimum number of employees in the group and offer coverage to meet the health needs of the employees. Premiums may be paid as a lump sum by the employer, who collects from the employee. As a fringe benefit, the employer may elect to share in the cost of the premium. The policy may include more than health protection for illness and disability and be amended to include death benefits, protection of family members, or loss of time.

There are occasions that would require the posting of a *performance or surety bond*. The treasurer, the administrator, or an employee may be required to place a performance bond. In the event of building a new addition, the builder or contractor should be required to purchase *builder's risk insurance*. When making a mortgage, *credit insurance* is usually required, and the deed is assured as valid by purchasing *title insurance*. Another type of insurance is the purchase of an *annuity* in connection with an employee's *pension plan*. A more recent innovation to insurance is called *business interruption insurance* for disaster, work stoppage, or accident.

Business Law

Law exists as statutes enacted by legislative bodies, either local, state, or national; or a body of rules, legal codes, and regulations by a legal agency. The nursing home will relate to many of these. For example, Senate Bill 388 of 1969 for the state of Texas forbids a nursing home to operate without the supervision of a full-time licensed administrator. A Skilled Nursing Facility offering extended care benefits will function under regulations of the Department of Health, Education, and Welfare, which gets its authority from Public Law 89-97 to govern such facilities. The handling of narcotics is heavily regulated, with stiff penalties for improper use and handling, the restrictions being imposed upon the nursing staff of the nursing home. The employees receive minimum wages as guaranteed under the Fair Labor Standards Act as amended in 1966 which the Secretary of Labor is empowered to enforce. When a nursing home rule such as requiring nurses to wear a uniform at their own expense threatened to reduce employee pay to below the minimum wage, the Secretary of Labor contested and found such practice in violation of the original legislation. Nurses and other uniformed employees are reimbursed the actual cost of wearing uniforms.

Civil law consists of the statutes enacted by duly constituted governmental bodies. These are the local ordinances, state laws, and federal statutes. Civil law regulates the relationships among people including business transactions.

Common law is a result of court decisions. Such decisions are the precedents established by court decrees. Frequently, precedent is established when a court rules on the true intent of a statute, rule or regulation. For example, the precedent of requiring employers to pay uniform allowance was the result of a cafe waitress who filed suit against her employer charging the requirement reduced her wages below the minimum rate per hour.

Public law deals with the government and its regulation of the individual. *Private laws* define the rights and liabilities between individuals or organizations. An example of public law is Medicare and Medicaid. An example of private law is the establishment of a legal guardianship.

Criminal law, of course, concerns misdemeanors or felonies. Assault and Battery injures the person of another while libel injures one's character.

Procedural law governs the conduct and procedures of lawsuits.

Constitutional law deals with the constitutionality of the law itself.

A code may be established for a series of laws concerning a singular subject. The Uniform Sales Act and the Uniform Commercial Code govern sales.

The Courts System

The courts system has been devised as the method citizens may use to resolve injustice and wrong. The administrator may sue for justice, becoming the plaintiff, or be sued, becoming the defendent. If the suit is for justice, that is damages, restoring property, etc., he may request a trial by jury. If the suit is for equity, i.e., enforcement of a rule, statute, regulation, etc., the judge will decide and either issue or deny an injunction. There are the equivalent of three court systems, all of which are interrelated. We have the federal system, i.e., the claims court, the custom court, the tax court, and the appeals court system consisting of the District Court, the Court of Appeals, and the United

States Supreme Court. The states also have a system of courts beginning with justice of the peace, the municipal courts, i.e., domestic,
juvenile, etc., the criminal court, and an appeals system including a
state Supreme Court. It is well to note that counties also have a court
system which is a part of the state system, such as County Court,
District Court, Superior Court, Appellate Court.

The nursing home administrator frequently enters into contract
with other parties. It may be to make a financial agreement for care of a
patient, admitting a patient for nursing care (see the sample form
that follows), make a transfer agreement with a hospital, purchase
or order supplies, contract for services with a welfare agency, rent,
lease, etc. In each, he exercises a legal contract, oral or written, that
is binding in a court of law. *A legal contract is a binding agreement between two competent persons for lawful purpose and supported by
consideration.*

ADMISSION AGREEMENT

The CEDAR CREST NURSING HOME and _____do hereby
agree to the following terms and conditions for the admission of
_____as a patient requiring medical and nursing care.

REQUIREMENTS FOR ADMISSION:
    The patient will be admitted by a licensed physician.
    The patient agrees to be seen regularly by said physician.
    The patient will have an examination within 14 days of admission.
    The physician will furnish diagnosis, current orders, and a report of
        examination, medical history, and other needs.
    An admission form will be completed at the time of admission.

FOR DISCHARGE OF PATIENT:
    The patient shall be dismissed by authority of the physician, the relative/
        guardian, the written consent of the patient, or by the nursing home.
    A significant change will be reported to the physician, relative/guardian,
        and Medicaid case-worker for assistance patients.
    The physician may transfer a patient to a hospital.
    Medicaid patients may be transferred to a facility matching the typing
        given to the patient by the medical assistance unit.

SERVICES SHALL INCLUDE:

General nursing care	Room and board	Laundry (washable type)
Hand and/or tube feeding	Linens and maid service	Clini-tests
	Skin care lotions	Emergency safety
Disposal pads	Sterile dressings	equipment
Hospital bed	Bed rails when ordered	

NOT INCLUDED IN OUR SERVICES (to be provided by the patient):

Physician's services	Oxygen	Drugs as prescribed
Clothing	Beautician's services	Transportation
Personal effects	Telephone service	

PLACEMENT IN ROOMS:

As space is available and with compatible roommates.

We abide by the Civil Rights Act of 1964.

PAYMENT OF ACCOUNTS:

Billing is at the end of the service period, monthly, and payable in full at that time.

Refund for unrendered services (when advance payment is made), for each unused day, 1/30 monthly rate.

FINANCIAL AGREEMENT:

To be paid by agency, insurance, other: $_____

To be paid by patient (or in behalf of):   _____

Total monthly payment   _____

_____

Nursing Home Representative

_____

Patient/guardian/relative

Date_____

A number of agreements are oral, while others are written. Normally, if an agreement is for the transfer of real estate, marriage, a third party, longer than one year, or for an executor, it is in writing. "Consideration" is anything of value and has nothing to do with "fair value." Certain types of agreements may be made without consideration, especially those considered pledges to religious and educational organizations. Restraint of trade, such as price fixing between nursing homes is illegal, as is gambling in most states.

When there is a breach of contract, the administrator may sue or be sued for compensatory damages to cover the loss. One may sue for performance of a contract, as in the case of the administrator who has a management contract; he may be held liable for failure to fulfill it. *One consideration in a breach of contract is the statutes of limitation imposed by all states. Limitation means the time lapse allowed before a legal claim of suit is instituted.* For example, the nursing home would forfeit its claim to collect an account if the claim were not made within the statutes of limitation. Since these vary from state to state, we give as an example the statutes of limitation for the state of Texas. For a nursing home account, the limitation is four years, for notes it is four years, for contracts it is four years, and for domestic judgments it is ten years. The administrator should consult legal counsel to determine his rights to enforcement of a contract.

Ownership of Property

Normally, a person may own property as sole owner, jointly with a partner, or as community property. Property is of two broad general classes, real and personal. When classed as real, it is called real estate and consists of land, buildings, mineral deposits, water, air, or anything attached to the soil. Personal property is said to be movable or temporary in nature. The building and the land on which the nursing home is situated are called real estate, while the equipment, machinery, fixtures, furniture, supplies, etc., are considered personal property. *Title to property is usually by deed, by quitclaim, by warranty, or by abstract of title.* Of course, one may inherit property. The author, inventor, and artist have special protection to ownership under rights of intellectual achievement or discovery. Property may be owned for specified times under terms of rental or lease.

Because the nursing home administrator is involved in ordering and purchasing, he should be aware of the Uniform Commercial Code, which attempts to establish uniform means of transferring title to goods ordered, shipped, and received. Since each sale may differ in contract and intent, a sale is said to have transpired when the title and possession of the goods is transferred to the buyer for consideration. The code attempts to define such terms as "on approval," "FOB," "installment sales," "cash sales," etc.

In addition, the nursing home administrator has some liability for safeguarding the patients' possessions. He must keep an accurate up-to-date inventory and surrender possessions of the deceased person to the legal representatives of the estate.

Business Ethics

Because the nursing home administrator will be contracting for services, making sales, purchasing real estate, renting and leasing, and dealing every day with people, he will be aware not only of the legal responsibility but the ethical responsibility. Some questions he might ask are: "Is it fair?", "Is this equitable?", "Is this honest?." He will need to determine whether there is a conflict of interest. Since ethics in business is essentially what is right and what is wrong, the administrator who deals fairly and justly will be an asset to his profession.

The concept of ethics comes to us from the moral fiber and tradition of the business community. However, there is another reason for a high ethical tone within the nursing home. Since service is the primary commodity, and because the individuals being served are sometimes not responsible persons by reason of disease or infirmities, far greater responsibility rests on the shoulders of the nursing home administrator and his staff. When an agreement is made to serve this type patient, the nursing home becomes the total provider of service, an awesome responsibility.

The nursing home administrator will find at times that his operation is open to criticism and that he is not always in a position to defend himself. He, therefore, has only one ultimate defense: good service. His honesty, integrity, and the fairness with which he deals with people will be used to judge his profession, his nursing home, and his work. Therefore, every contract or transaction he makes should reflect the highest professional ethics.

Ethics has become a prominent factor in the business world. We find business voluntarily regulating itself in many ways. The principles upheld by the Better Business Bureau, the Chamber of Commerce, civic clubs, and fraternal organizations, and the professional codes speak loudly for business ethics.

The individual administrator should develop a plan for the improvement of personal ethics. This may include his active participation in his church and in civic activities, his reading for personal improvement, and a diligent attempt to maintain a rigidly ethical position. He should educate himself to be professional, which is simply another way of saying he should discover the best way of conducting his business. If his goals of nursing home service are set beyond himself to include a belief in God, to encompass the needs of the aged, and to serve humanity, he can reach a level of business ethics worthy of praise. Should he choose to serve his own self-interest, to operate merely within the limits of the law, or to set his goal on material gain, he will never be a credit to the nursing home profession.

Legal Responsibility of the Administrator

This entire text, in a sense, discusses the responsibilities of the administrator, and many references are made to his various legal obligations. While it is not within the frame of reference of this book to give specific legal advice, it is nevertheless its intent to direct the administrator to abide strictly by the law. It is when the nursing home administrator takes his rightful place within the professional community that his true legal standing will be defined.

Legally, the administrator is bound by the same laws as are all citizens. However, since he is in a unique position to assist and serve others under less than normal conditions, and since he serves persons who by reason of physical, medical, and social decline in capacity are dependent, his legal responsibility is increased. It can be said that he may have greater accountability under the law. It is, however, to be noted that the nursing home profession is just beginning to achieve professional status, and conceivably its "greater accountability" may be less than that in other professions. Since licensing of administrators is relatively new, and because the profession is new in society, no great volume of court decisions concerning an administrator of a nursing home are on record. Nevertheless, it is reasonable to assume that the large bulk of decisions testing in court-related professions has been recorded.

Perhaps the highest legal responsibility of the administrator will evolve from his participation in his trade organization, the nursing home association, which has attempted to establish ethical responsibility. As the administrator subscribes to the code of ethics of his peers, he is establishing the legal climate in which he will function, under which he may be judged.

A code of ethics may define the curriculum which the administrator must master. Actually, such a code may be evolving now through the structure of the National Association of Boards of Examiners for Nursing Home Administrators, which subscribes to the core of knowledge recommended by the National Advisory Council to the Board of Licensure. This instrument was published in the Federal Register after it was compiled. To this date, however, except for the efforts of this text and a few select authors, little definition has been given to the core of knowledge. The implication is that what an administrator is supposed to know in order to carry out the functions of his profession has yet to be totally defined. This fact does not support the administrator who would take the position of ignorance. It merely points out that some confusion may result when a court attempts to decide how professional the administrator is supposed to be.

A profession may have its standards set for it in a number of ways. In the case of the nursing home, the regulations of a government agency are binding. Regulations imposed by contracts to provide services under the Medicare, Medicaid, and Veterans Administration nursing care programs will add to the amount of specialized knowledge required. Any rule, regulation, policy, or penalty imposed by a nursing home association on its membership will increase the degree of legal accountability on the part of administrators. Finally, the requirement to upgrade in-service training or to set a high entry standard of education for administrators will influence future legal decisions. In conclusion, it appears that the legal responsibility of the administrator will increase along with the demand for his professional upgrading.

Legal Responsibility of the Nurse

The legal responsibility of the employed nurse or nurse's aide rests with both the employee and the administration of the nursing home. The principle of law, respondent superior, or "Let the master answer" applies. It would be well, therefore, for the administrator to develop good hiring practices by his determination of ability, character, and work habits and to maintain them through his supervision of job assignments, job descriptions, and training.

Texas law specifically prohibits any infringement by the nurse's aide on the responsibilities of the licensed vocational nurse, the registered nurse, and the physician. However, the law calls one to account only for his own specific acts of negligence. Specific acts may be limited by training, supervision, or by law. There are some areas where the legal responsibility is critical, as in the administration of medications, therapy, treatment, etc. There are also areas of ethical responsibility, such as counseling, advising the patient, giving relatives reports, or "taking charge."

Legal Papers in Nursing Home Administration

In one sense, all clinical and administrative papers compiled with respect to specific patients are confidential and legal in nature. Therefore, we list those considered confidential, which must be safeguarded so that only those for whom they are intended shall have legal access to them.

> Admission agreement.
> Consent for care.
> Power of attorney.
> Clothing and valuables list.

Financial receipts.
Physician's order, signed.
Narcotics record.
Release from responsibility for leave of absence.
Release from responsibility for discharge.
Release of information.
Permission to use a patient's picture.
Death certificate.
Autopsy report.
Legal contracts.
Legal judgments.
Daily clinical records and reports.
Transfer of ownership and transfer of records.
Subpoena of records by judicial body.

Release of Information

Several principles apply to the release of information that will guide the establishment of a policy. Since the law varies from state to state, the advice of legal counsel is recommended. *Generally, information is considered privileged and confidential, is owned by the facility, and may be released by the consent of the one whom it concerns, and without consent, by an order of a court for a legitimate purpose.*

Records are transferred to a new owner of the facility upon a written authorization of the licensing agency.

While doctors, state agencies, welfare agencies, and hospitals will have frequent use of information concerning the patient, it will be well to meet all legal requirements. To provide information for insurance companies or another agency, it is necessary to get written consent. Even if the patient wishes to see his own records, one should obtain written consent or let him get a court order.

The existence of psychiatric records usually implies incompetency; unless a legal guardian can sign the consent, information should be withheld.

Always get written consent before releasing information to the press, radio, or television. Get the patient's written consent to use his picture for advertising or publicity.

Chapter *6*

On-the-Job Training

and Motivation

In this section we discuss the training of new employees and their motivation. Later we discuss in-service training as an up-grading process for all employees of the nursing home.

The administrator's interest in training should undergird his entire plan of supervision. Training in the nursing home is nothing more than teaching the employee to do his job better. A better job means better service. Better service means greater success in caring for the aged. Service will be in direct ratio to the training and motivation of the nursing home staff. While there are several types of training available to the administrator, the best will be one in which the administrator assumes the role of leader of the training program. He may not be the instructor, but he will correlate the program to his staff meetings, and the supervision and motivation of employee service.

Apprenticeship

The method of apprenticeship is one of our oldest forms of training. It is a combination of formal training and on-the-job training for the development of a skill. In the plan, a master craftsman usually supervises the training while the learner is actually working at the job for which he is preparing. At the same time, he is studying a specific curriculum, usually in a formal classroom, off the job. Notoriously, apprenticeship has been by crafts; however, the technique is not entirely foreign to the professions. The registered nurse has "floor duty," the doctor completes an "internship," and the nursing home administrator may be required to gain a year or more of experience under the direction of a "preceptor-teacher" before he is licensed.

Apprenticeship is founded upon the ability of the master craftsman to guide the student in learning a skill. It may be akin to the nursing home administrator taking a young assistant, and, over a period of time, training him in the skills of administration. It is customary in apprenticeship to set a time limit, usually from two to five years, for the period of instruction. Health skills now being taught this way include those of the pharmacist, laboratory technician, registered nurse, physician, x-ray technician, inhalation therapist, physical therapist, nursing home administrator, and others.

None of these apprentice programs is registered with the Bureau of Apprenticeship or the U.S. Department of Labor, but all are similar to its program, although different terms are sometime used, e.g., internship, floor duty, laboratory, etc. This is a modification of the principle of apprenticeship.

Formal Training

Formal training is also involved in the method of internship. A definite curriculum of study is established and is scheduled in the classroom. This classroom study may be at the place of employment, where several trainees can learn together. In some cases, individual study such as a correspondence course may be accomplished. Perhaps the apprentice's simplest means of acquiring the formal training to supplement on-the-job training is to go to the local high school, trade school, or junior college. The two-year junior college provides an excellent institutional setting for formal training. Such schools are assuming the responsibility of technical and vocational training both in accredited plans and nonaccredited plans. Whether the school is called a junior college, a community college, or an institute is of little consequence, since the purpose is usually the same for all two-year institutions: equiping the student with a marketable skill.

Degree plans may lead to a transferrable degree that will become the basis for acquiring a four-year bachelor of arts or bachelor of science degree. However, the goal may be a terminal degree that certifies the student with skills of a specific nature.

The National Association of Boards of Examiners for Nursing Home Administrators recommends a degree plan for candidates for licensure. From the beginning of the licensure movement in 1969, most state licensure boards have set a minimum number of class-hours, varying from 50 to 400, as a requirement for licensure. This minimum requirement changes to a two-year associate degree in 1975 in many states. Their degree recommendations include an internship in an approved nursing home work-station for which college credit will be granted. Their "Suggested Curriculum for Associate in Applied Science Degree in Long Term Health Care" is:

First semester, freshman year	Semester Hours
English Composition & Rhetoric	3
Introduction to Sociology	3
Business Speech & Communication	3
Introduction to Nursing Home Administration	3
Approved Elective	3
	15

Second semester, freshman year	Semester Hours
State & Federal Government	3
Mental Hygiene & Personality Adjustment	3
Psychology of Patient Care	3
Technology of Patient Care	3
Rehabilitation & Recreation	3
	15

First semester, sophomore year	Semester Hours
Nursing Home Internship (with seminar)	6
Principles of Accounting	4
Human Relations & Personnel Management	3
Approved Elective	3
	16

Second semester, sophomore year	Semester Hours
Nursing Home Internship II (with seminar)	6
Nursing Home Administration Law	3
Financial Management of the Nursing Home	3
Nutrition & Quantity Foods (with laboratory)	4
	16

Approved Electives:
Introduction to Psychology
Business Math
Report Writing
General Administrative Problems
Supervision
Safety and First Aid

The position of the National Association of Boards of Examiners is the same as that recommended by the National Advisory Council for Nursing Home Administration in its report to the Secretary of Health, Education, and Welfare. It was recommended that all states proceed with an associate degree program for qualifying a nursing home administrator for a license by July 1, 1975. In this recommendation a future requirement would increase the educational level to that of a bachelor of arts or science degree.

Care should be taken to abide with the law concerning hours, pay, and apprenticeship training. Programs may be registered with the Department of Labor, Bureau of Apprenticeship. Personnel trained by these programs to serve the nursing home are cooks, bakers, dietary aides, nurse's aides, maintenance and laundry workers, and others.

This discussion concerns the worker training on the job while studying formally in classroom instruction. It is possible to train by on-the-job training alone.

On-the-Job Training

On-the-job training is probably the most useful of all methods for the training of nursing home personnel. This method teaches a skill as the student actually performs the work for which he is employed. Inasmuch as the nursing home is required by the licensing agency and by both Medicaid and Medicare contracts to provide a continuous training program, this is the most logical method. It also permits the employment of unskilled workers with the possibility of upgrading them.

Orientation is essentially a method of on-the-job training. The nursing home administrator will make this method an integral part of his training program. *Orientation is a method of acquainting the new employee with his responsibilities.* It may also be used for instituting a new program or service within the functions of the nursing home. However, orientation is also short-term training for a specific purpose. If the instruction is detailed, logical, and orderly, the employee should have no difficulty in becoming well acquainted with his new job in a short period of time.

On-the-job training involves prolonged training of the individual worker. The assignment of the new worker to an experienced worker is the first step in on-the-job training. Care should be taken, however, not to overwhelm the new employee. While he should be guided closely, it should be the elementary steps of his job that are covered until the supervisor is reasonably sure that the job is mastered. There are several plans for making this assignment, but first some method of enlisting and training the worker chosen as teacher should be instituted.

If the orientation involves several new employees, a full week should be scheduled; and if they are to work as nurse's aides and are also without previous nursing home experience, the orientation should be expanded to two or more weeks. If, on the other hand, one is orienting experienced nurse's aides, the trainer is concerned with acquainting the new employee with the policies and procedures of the nursing home. When only one new employee is placed on the job, her orientation could best be accomplished by placing her as an extra person on the assigned shift (or in some cases another shift), where an experienced worker would acquaint her with the methods and procedures of the nursing home. After three to five days of working as an extra and when the supervisor's evaluation determines her to be indoctrinated successfully, she could then be placed on the job as a regular staff member.

The administrator is concerned with two interrelated aspects of training: to see that the new employee is well trained for his job, and to acquaint the new employee with those policies and procedures of the nursing home that relate to his job. On-the-job training will accomplish the first, and orientation will accomplish the second. In fact, orientation may serve to acquaint all workers with new precedures, methods, or equipment. Orientation of the new employee should be accomplished with on-the-job training. After the employee is familiarized with the policies and procedures of the nursing home, her orientation should be considered closed. On-the-job training in new skills should continue. The administrator should see that the trainee has a genuine on-the-job training in skills and not just an orientation program. The on-the-job program is quite exhaustive in content. The administrator is interested in knowing that the employee can do the job, that he continues to improve at his job, and that he is acquainted with new policies, procedures, and methods relating to his job. Whichever of these is the goal will determine the curriculum of on-the-job training. Below we have outlined both a plan for orientation and a plan for on-the-job training so that the administrator can compare them as to content and purpose.

PLAN OF ORIENTATION FOR NEW EMPLOYEES

Introduction to the supervisory staff.
Location of employee facilities, as locker, washroom.
Employees' services, i.e., meals, breaks, assistance.

Review of hours, time clock, meal schedule.
Review of *Employee's Manual.*
Review of Job Description.
Tour of the nursing home.
Introduction to fellow employees.
Review of safety requirements and disaster plan.
Miscellaneous.

PLAN FOR SHORT ON-THE-JOB TRAINING PROGRAM

Short description of training program, schedule, etc.
Statement of the philosophy of the training program.
Statement of objectives of the program.
Outline of subject matter.
Texts, procedure manual, written material.
Instructional and training methods.
Training aids.
Evaluation of training.
Reference books.

PLAN OF EXTENDED NURSE'S AIDE TRAINING PROGRAM:

A. The nurse's aide training program consists of both practical training and curriculum study, requiring a student's workbook. It deals with the admission and discharge of patients, A.M. and P.M. nursing care, assistance to the patient, assisting the professional nurse, and alertness to changes in a patient's condition.
B. The nurse's aide trainee performs an increasing number of duties, such as bedmaking, feeding, bathing, taking temperature elevation, and assisting the patient. She studies related curriculum by her workbook to provide additional insight into the care of the aged and infirm. She develops a working relationship with her fellow workers, one that promotes mutual respect and a sharing of the work load. She develops love and compassion for serving the elderly as a nurse's aide.
C. Specifically, the objectives of the training program are:
    a. Develop the techniques and procedures of nursing devices and equipment.
    b. Develop an understanding of geriatrics.
    c. Develop a sense of service to the aged.

      d. Develop an ability to communicate with people related to nursing care, including the patient, relatives/guardians, visitors, and the nursing staff.

      e. Develop an awareness of problem solving and some of the techniques for sharing.

   D. Outline of curriculum:

      a. Introduction to nursing.

      b. Anatomy and physiology.

      c. Admission and discharge of patients.

      d. Bedmaking, including positioning and turning patient.

      e. Personal hygiene, bathing, grooming.

      f. Nurse's notes and observations of vital signs.

      g. Assisting the professional nurse.

      h. Assisting in therapy, exercise, and ambulation.

      i. Assisting the critical or dying patient.

      j. Assistance in feeding.

      k. Assistance in dressing.

      l. Dietary and fluid intake, elimination, and output.

      m. Environmental sanitation, safety, coping with disaster.

      n. Maintenance of linens, equipment, etc.

      o. Social problems in geriatrics.

      p. Psychological and emotional problems.

      q. Treatment and respect of patient's rights.

      r. Review of licensing agencies' standards.

      s. Public relations.

      t. Legal consideration.

  E. Training held in the nursing classroom uses the bed and other nursing equipment for demonstration. The teacher first leads a discussion of the lesson material and then illustrates the application of principles. Emphasis falls on the terminology of nursing so as to improve communication and understanding, the mastery of techniques, and the practical application of nursing principles.

  F. Training aids are: the demonstration nursing unit, audio materials, filmstrips, slides, the chalkboard, crafts, leaflets, and daily lesson sheets. The class size should be limited to 20.

  G. Performance in demonstration and on-the-job serves as the evaluation method.

  H. Reference books selected by the instructor.

In comparing the above outlines, certain aspects stand out. In the orientation plan, the outline concerns the circumstances in which the employee will be working. In the second plan very little is said about the actual training techniques, since this is left to the experienced worker who directs the on-the-job training. In the last plan for extended training, the material is arranged for classroom instruction. This plan may be like an in-service training program, which we will discuss in the next chapter. However, it should be noted that all three plans emphasize the upgrading of the employee, while the last two emphasize improvement of the employee's skill.

Methods of Training On-the-Job

We have shown the use of classroom instruction and demonstration. Something further should be said about the actual methods of training on-the-job. As previously mentioned, the more practical method allows the new employee to work over and above the regular staffing pattern for a number of days, perhaps a week, under the supervision of an experienced worker.

A plan should be developed to detail properly the tasks to be performed. By using the methods developed by job analysis, the various functions of a task are broken into component segments. Each segment of a task is then demonstrated by the leader and practiced by the new employee. Time should be allowed for mastering each step before proceeding to the next. Also, the leader should progress from the simpler steps to the more difficult.

The amount of detail needed to define a task is related to the type of student, the amount of material to be covered, and the objective of the learning situation. Naturally, the leader will assume that the experienced employee already has working skills and needs merely a demonstration of methods used by the particular nursing home and an evaluation of his level of skill. On the other hand, the inexperienced employee will need a detailed explanation of each task and adequate practice. There are a number of basic functions performed in the nursing home that belong in a patient-care manual which could serve as the basis for on-the-job training. Some tasks are bedmaking, positioning, ambulation, medical asepsis, serving and feeding, personal care, skin care, admission and discharge, charting, vital signs, collecting specimens, etc. Take, for example, turning the bed patient:

Objective: To prevent bed sores, to stimulate circulation, and to restore the ability of the patient to assist himself. Patients who are immobile are turned at least every two hours.
Safety rules: Use assistance where necessary, avoid undue strain, protect the patient during the move.

Prepare the bed for the turning procedure:
   a. raise it to a comfortable working height,
   b. lower bed rail and head of bed,
   c. check for catheter tubing, or other devices,
   d. remove nurse-call cord, drape bedding to side of bed.
Position of aide:
   a. stand with feet slightly apart, close to bed,
   b. keep back straight, don't twist or bend it,
   c. bend knees and hips,
   d. use smooth coordinated motions.
Move the patient toward you:
   a. place one hand gently under shoulders,
   b. place other hand under the small of back,
   c. move patient's upper body toward you,
   d. lift, don't drag, to avoid friction burn,
   e. repeat for hips and feet.
Turning the patient:
   a. bend the patient's knees,
   b. move arm and patient up,
   c. see that bed rail opposite is up,
   d. with your arm under hips and shoulder roll the patient gently
      over.
Explain to the patient each step
Reposition bed:
   a. put up bed rails,
   b. reconnect devices,
   c. place pillows for patient's comfort.

An evaluation follow-up should be developed. These checkups should be periodic, perhaps at the end of the first day, the end of the first week, and the end of each month. However, checkups may occur at the completion of each unit or segment of the job. For example, the administrator developing on-the-job training for nurse's aides may choose to evaluate progress at the completion of each phase of the new employee's work assignment.

Motivation Research in the Nursing Home

A simple definition of motivation is "why people act the way they do." In the nursing home, it is important, because the primary work of the nursing home is concerned with people. The administrator supervises workers who are offering service to the patients.

There are several methods of discovering what motivates people. When one considers the hundreds of factors which may impel a person to action, he may become bewildered. However, psychologists have done research on "human drives" and have discovered that they can be grouped in several general areas. Sigmund Freud identified two drives as the need to belong and the need of self-preservation. Others, such as Dr. Edward Thorndike and Dr. Abraham H. Maslow, have advanced other theories of needs. The administrator, however, does not have to be a psychologist to know that his employees are motivated for various reasons, whether social, biological, or self-preservative. His primary problem is to know why his employees act as they do, and then to formulate working conditions that utilize such motives as may improve the operation of the home.

The in-depth interview is one method of determining motives. For example, a licensure board for nursing home administrators may conduct an oral examination of candidates for license. The interviewer selects a number of questions to be asked the candidate. The manner of response, the answers given, and the cooperation the candidate gives the interviewer may reveal, for example, whether he is motivated to become a nursing home administrator because of compassion and concern for the elderly. The interviewer not only must be able to ask questions skillfully, but also to recognize the information he is seeking.

The group interview is similar to an in depth interview with an individual, except that two or more participate. The group is led into conversation concerning a specific subject which has been assigned by the interview leader. The interviewer will be looking for: responses and participation by the group members; likes, dislikes, prejudices; interests and knowledge responses; and clues to problem personalities.

A word of caution should be sounded for the administrator. While the interview is revealing as to problems and motivation, it also has some pitfalls. One is a possible inability of the leader skillfully to guide and interpret the results. Another is the tendency to jump to conclusions or to magnify out of proportion what may seem at the time pertinent to the problems. As an example, take the student enrolled in a class of nursing home administration but apparently with a negative attitude, so that for weeks the teacher accepted this as the true attitude; however, discussions of various subjects relating to nursing home administration began to draw out the personality of the student. In the end, it was discovered that he had a deep compassion for the ill and elderly, was well grounded in human relations, and had perhaps the keenest interest in his profession of any student in the class. In one sense, any conversation with an individual, or any group meeting, has elements of the interview. A student of human nature would constantly be looking for motivating factors.

There are certain other projective techniques that may be used when the administrator possesses the necessary skill to interpret their results. These would include tests for preference, for role playing, and other expressive techniques. Normally, these would be employed by a trained psychologist, for they are effective only in the hands of the skilled interviewer. The administrator should beware of the amateurish use of such tools. He should, however, apply himself to developing some of the tried and proved techniques of motivation, i.e., improving working skills and giving recognition to workers.

Motivation and Working Conditions

Employees are motivated by their likes and dislikes, their beliefs, goals, ideals, and needs. The place of employment or the conditions under which they work will encourage them or discourage them. Working conditions are important. If the home is clean, odorless, and sanitary, it will affect the employees' mental attitude. If they have a lounge, a scheduled break, or personal privileges, they respond more willingly. Employees are motivated by those with whom they work. If they are respected and find a harmonious team led by a supervisor they respect, it is reflected in their work. The type of supervision is important to them. Nursing home employees favor a fair, direct, and efficient supervisor. Seldom do they do their best work for someone who is harsh in his manner.

Work security is very important to the employee. He wants steady employment with an opportunity for promotion. A nurse prefers a regular vacation, will be concerned about sick leave or other fringe benefits. The nursing home employee will not differ much from the average employee in American business. When he is satisfied that he has the best available job, he will have a greater incentive to develop stable work habits.

The nursing home employee may respond favorably to the working conditions; however, the best work is done when there is a challenge. Workers like to take pride in their work and will respond when good quality work is respected in the nursing home. Employees who are free to excel and improve will find their motivation to work. In a nursing home where new ideas are respected and used, the employees usually come to work more eagerly. Finally, workers do best the things they like to do. The aide who has a keen interest in older people will be more willing to deal with the problems that arise in patient care. Because they care, they are proud of their work. *In summary, we can say the things that motivate the worker are: a good nursing home, good supervision, the respect of fellow workers, a job he likes, a job that promises work security, and a challenging assignment.*

Motivation and Recognition

Recognition is one of the basic drives that motivates the nursing home worker. While it may not be the most important one, it is high among incentives. The nursing home administrator should establish certain practices of recognition. These need not be "showy," "flowery," or "flattering." In every instance, the administrator will proceed with sincerity. He should determine the motivation that stimulates each worker to perform his duties. The administrator then would do well to take recognition of this aspect, either directly or indirectly. Discovering this basic drive in each employee will pay dividends. The administrator should find out what each employee wishes to do in the nursing home and, insofar as is possible, place him in that position. He should then be encouraged to perfect his work and be praised when he does.

A form of recognition is criticism, but it should always be used constructively. The employee will resent embarrassment. The fact that the supervisor will take the time to make observations about an employee's work is in itself recognition. Constructive criticism is always objective, never personal.

Personal criticism: "Jim, I think you have your nerve taking Fred's parking place."

Constructive criticism: "Jim, our company policy is to assign parking places. Would you check at the office to where you have been assigned?"

A simple but subtle type of recognition is consideration. A worker appreciates understanding and a second chance. Every employee will sooner or later make a mistake and, of course, some make more than others. By developing a constructive attitude, recognizing the potential of the individual, and supervising only as closely as is necessary, a supervisor may develop an employee. However, the employee will respond only so long as he feels the supervisor is being considerate of him, and is not singling him out for harder work and inconsiderate supervision.

Every worker wants due credit for his performance. Administrators soon learn that an employee will respond to praise. It may not be more than the use of the pronoun "we" or a kind remark to a relative concerning the employee's good performance. It might be public citation for proficiency. Care should be taken to see that it is always sincere and is genuinely deserved. Normally, there are several ways to praise a worker. It may be by spoken word directly to the individual or to another in the presence of the worker. It may be by stating the fact, either directly to the individual, or publicly, as in the nursing home newspaper, or a news release. Some supervisors prefer the team approach to praise of a worker. No one worker is singled out, but the unit is. A department, a shift, or a work group is recognized for its achievement. In any event, praise should not be used too frequently, and never in such a way as to draw attention to the praiser.

More than anything else perhaps, the worker wants the friendship of the administrator and supervisor. Friendliness need not mean involvement in the personal affairs of the employee, but only assurance that the supervisor has the employee's best interest at heart. An occasional question about the employee's family, first names used at least privately, or a short conversation with him will court his friendship. Occasionally an employee may be taken into limited confidence when the supervisor or administrator needs his help in planning.

There are several other means of recognizing the worth and usefulness of an employee. Perhaps the best is the pay check. Workers work for money, primarily because our society demands it for survival, and not because it is of first magnitude as a motivator. In fact, *employees are more likely to appreciate their pay check as a form of recognition of their labor than for the money itself.* However, money and work are inseparable in our economic system, and the administrator should view it for what it is: a motivator to get the job done.

Chapter 7

In-Service Training

An ongoing training program is required for each nursing home. It must be well planned to be effective in maintaining the proficiency of the employees. In contrast with the on-the-job training program, which is primarily for new employees, in-service training is for all employees. To be effective, all employees should be in continual training. Of course, the supervisor may have priority in training; however, all employees need it.

Setting Training Goals

The first goal should be a survey of training needs. Ask, "Is performance good? Is the occupancy up? Is the public relations image good? Are we having supervisory problems?" Jot down any factor that may relate to training: problems, performance, communication, equipment utilization, skills, supervision, personnel organization, operation, procedure, attitudes, etc. Need for improvement in these areas becomes the basis of a training plan. Write out the training plan. Keep it simple, but be specific. Divide it into units and lessons which become progressively more difficult and thorough. These divisions relate to more specific goals of training. Note the progressive breakdown of general goals into specific objectives in the following plan:

> General aim: Training nurse's aides.
> Unit aim: Aides assisting in admission.
> Lesson title: Showing the new patient his room.

Similar plans of the overall training program are developed for each job catagory, each having several units. For example, the nurse's aide training program covers such subjects as patient orientation, bed-making, nurse's observations, assistance in feeding, etc. Each of these may be subdivided into one or more lessons.

It is necessary, once a training plan has been devised, to decide upon a supervisor of training, on methods and training aids, and on site, before making a schedule.

Scheduling of training is difficult, but once it has achieved a definite place in the activities of the home, it becomes no problem. One never will satisfy every person and fit every personal schedule. The administrator has to weigh every factor, every activity, every duty schedule, and then make his decision as to when he can best hold the training classes. Once scheduled, the employees will make the time to train.

Finally, give the training program a big send-off. Start with a lot of fanfare. Make it sound important. Use every method of publicity to make it sound great and then plan and work to keep it great. Do not disappoint the employees with a dull, dreary course. Make it live up to its billing.

Supervision of the Training Program

There is no doubt that the supervisor of the training program will be one of the secrets of its success. A dynamic, challenging attitude can make the program. The administrator will want to give him every bit of assistance at his disposal and back him one hundred percent. Management has a vital role in training, since it is responsible for setting the training goals, approving the program, and selecting the leadership. The administrator will need to accept his full responsibility as the head of management. Otherwise, the training program will never get started.

The administrator selects the training leader and assigns his position on the management team. The training leader, while that of a staff position, is introduced to all personnel as a staff member acting for the administrator. His title may be assistant administrator in charge of training.

The training leader must be personally qualified. His character and personality should command respect; his education must include some study of training techniques; his experience in the field in which he is teaching should strengthen his position; finally, he should be loyal to the nursing home administrator. Perhaps no one else in the entire nursing home organization develops a program based on goals set by the administrator. He advises on the teaching methods and techniques. He may also advise on the division of units and lessons. The administrator will do well to set the goals, and then let the training leader develop the program.

If the leader is qualified, he may teach. If he is not, he obtains competent teachers for specific units or lessons. For a seminar type of teaching, experts are usually called in from time to time to lecture on their specialty. Classroom teachers may be trained by sending them to seminars and conferences, or even by sending them to a local junior college for specific courses.

An Adequate Place for Training

The administrator and the nursing home owners should provide an adequate place for training. It need not be elaborate, and is usually available from the facilities within the nursing home, but it is important to the training program.

There are some advantages in using on-the-job facilities, since the average employee learns best in a natural setting. An unoccupied patient room will make an excellent demonstration unit. It would, however, dictate the size of the class; if the room available constantly changes, confusion results. The advantage of having the equipment readily available and set up for demonstrations dealing with patient-care techniques does have some value, especially when the program has another meeting area. A training room is perhaps the best solution. While it does entail a capital outlay, it is both necessary and sometimes is required by the contracting agencies. It may be a room for multiple use, such as the day room. In this event, a certain section is designated for training equipment. Cabinets for storage, a chalk board, and training aids need to be provided. Such a room could also be used for improvement classes for the patients in the facility. It is possible, however, to have a training program without a designated training room. It would then be necessary to schedule several sections of the training classes to meet the space problem where no special training room was designated.

In addition to the obvious advantage which is afforded the program with a classroom of its own—that of being able to maintain permanent displays and to post necessary information—this special facility tends to enhance the importance of the training program. Also, it makes possible the use of various types of special equipment, such as audio, visual aids, and a library. Suggestions for books for the classroom library are found among those listed at the end of many chapters of this text, under the heading, "For Further Study." To these may be added books dealing with specific equipment, techniques, and training.

Selecting the Methods of Training

The nursing home training leader must be acquainted with and skilled in the methods of training. While the full understanding of educational processes is a full-time vocation requiring at least the Bachelor of Arts degree, knowledge of specific techniques may be acquired though study and observation. Not every home will be able to afford a specialist; it may have to utilize other management personnel. Those persons with educational backgrounds in other fields could acquire the necessary training in teaching and learning techniques to perform acceptably.

Some methods of teaching are more adaptable than others to in-service training. *Correspondence courses* are good for self-study, but they are the most difficult to correlate specifically to the training goals of the nursing home. *Personal instruction* and *training classes* are better. When supported with seminars, guest speakers, demonstrations, and discussions, these form the basis for good in-service training. A *teaching booth or carrell*, with personal assignments, is excellent. Finally, testing, either oral, written, or by observation of performance, is necessary for evaluation.

Some methods lend themselves to the classroom. The *lecture* is the most common, and is good when done effectively. In fact, a good lecturer can arouse interest, gain understanding, and even acquire a response. The method is, however, much abused. Telling is not teaching. The *discussion,* when skillfully led by the teacher, is perhaps the best. It has all the elements of the philosophy of teaching, i.e., imparting knowledge, seeking change, and gaining a response. The *question and answer* method seeks the correct response, while *panel discussion* emphasizes imparting knowledge as well as eliciting response. The use of several *forum* methods is based on the presentation of assigned materials by one or more persons, followed by a discussion. One may use *workshop* methods to great effect when the classes are small. Usually, small groups will be assigned projects or subjects to be researched and discussed.

Other instructional methods are better suited to the large group. The lecture and forum methods are better when the size of the group limits individual response. The use of projected aids, such as slides, filmstrips, and movies, is excellent. A panel of experts also is popular with larger group instruction. It is noteworthy that some types of curriculum can better be taught in a small class. Usually, the more detailed or the more practical the curriculum is, the more necessary it is to have a small class or workshop.

Generally speaking, learning may take place when the following are true:

> The learner is interested in the learning situation.
> The learner has the right attitude.
> The learner is exposed to knowledge.
> The learner gains some understanding.
> The learner can apply his new knowledge.

Each of these principles is oversimplified, and learning may not take place in the order given; however, any learning situation has each principle present. The student will note that of the five steps only one deals primarily with the teacher's part in the learning situation; the other four are pupil-centered. True, the teacher has a key role in gaining the interest of the pupil; however, the student has to allow himself to become interested in the learning situation, his attitude being the key. He needs the correct attitude toward himself and his need, the learning situation, the class or teaching situation, and the teacher. The teacher's part is primarily to expose the student to information and to inspire the pupil to gain some understanding. Again, it should be noted that it is the pupil who ultimately gains understanding; this he may do through exposure to the teaching situation, the repetition or application of it. Finally, he can be assured of mastery of the subject when he can give a correct response or can apply what he learns.

Any method the training leader uses is an application of the above principles. A review of those methods available to the training leader includes:

> *Personal study and research* by assignment.
> *Programmed instruction* on teaching machines.
> *Lecture* by an expert.
> *Panel of experts* who engage in conversation with a moderator interpreting the *question and answer* or free exchange of questions.

Discussion in which the audience participates.
Symposium in which several persons give speeches.
Forum in which speeches are followed by discussion.
Seminar or directed study in a group situation.
Buzz session of small groups simultaneously.
Workshop or small work groups.
Demonstration or simulation of an actual situation.
Visual aids, such as film, filmstrip, slides.
Audio aids, listening combined with discussion.
Field trip, visiting an actual situation.

General Training Aids

A training aid is just what its name implies, an aid to instruction and teaching. Generally, there are three types: nonprojected, projected, and audio. The nonprojected aids are static displays, which are either flat in construction or are simulated three-dimensional mock-ups. Projected aids include movies, filmstrips, slides, and television. Audio aids include cassette, tape deck, and records.

Any time a visual aid is used, it improves understanding; in fact, the simple addition of visual aids to a teaching situation is said to double the effectiveness and retention of the information imparted. It is also said, that if you add activity to hearing and seeing, you will again double the effectiveness of the learning situation.

There are several types of general training aids that should be made available to the learning situation. By far the best and most versatile aid is the *chalk board.* Its usefulness is limited only by the skill of the leader, i.e., his writing legibly, accurately, and interestingly. Close to the chalk-board in usefulness is the *tackboard.* Any type of flat charts, maps, posters, banners, etc., may become semipermanent for purposes of instruction.

Charts and graphs are examples of static displays. Progress may be noted easily by a graph. Charts are merely the listing, cataloging, or correlating of information. They may be either pictorial or worded.

Posters are excellent. They usually give a short pithy message that may tell the same message over and over until replaced. With the availability of movable lettering and the use of pictures from any good magazine, anyone can make a simple poster. Posters may show simple strip sentences, e.g. "THINK." A good sign kit on the market makes any instructor an "expert." *Pictures,* with or without wording or captions, teach a visual concept. Since pictures are usually found just about any place, they can become an effective aid to training. One variation is the *cartoon.* A cartoon gives a message with a smile.

While *books* are not static displays, nevertheless they are permanent, in that their message is always available as a part of the instructional process. The administrator needs to develop a reference library of books related to the nursing home, its operation and functions. Such books may fill only a single shelf or a whole cabinet. They should, of course, be available to the training class and the students. The training leader would encourage the use of the books by making assignments, suggestions, and inspiration. *Notebooks* are an integral part of training. Any instructor can encourage learning by assigning notebook projects to the students. Coupled with research, notebooks are one of the best aids.

Finally, audio aids have become very useful with the recent adaptability of magnetic tape. Magnetic tape in reels is gradually being replaced by a cassette type of players because of the ease in selection. However, the reel recorder and player will be preferred in high fidelity recording, such as music, while the cassette seems adequate for voice reproduction. Records have some advantage ·over tapes, in that selection is even more quickly made when a section of a record is desired.

Projected Training Aids

There are four types of projected training aids, with a possible fifth being developed. They are: *films, filmstrips, slides, and transparencies.* The fifth is *microfilm or microfiche,* used primarily in research. It is noteworthy that another innovation possibly useful is *television cassettes.* Already out of the experimental stage, these are accepted in the home entertainment field.

The use of films will continue to be popular; however, they are stereotyped, in that the message a film contains is difficult to key specifically to a curriculum. With some research on the part of the training leader, however, he can find many useful films to meet his training needs. Normally, there are two types available: 16 mm sound, and 8 mm, which is silent, unless synchronized with other devices such as cassettes or "Film-O-Sound." Some instruction is necessary for the proper operation of the projectors. Usually, a minimal few minutes will acquaint a person for their operation. Practically every projector has a threading and operation guide attached to the case, but respect for the film is needed, since it is fragile and must be handled with care. Every film should be previewed by the training leader or class instructor before being shown. The first reason is to test the equipment, and the second is to evaluate the film for purposes of learning. A poor film or one poorly related to learning objectives will, at best, only waste time. In evaluation of the film, note what discussion subjects may be stimulated by viewing it. Any film can have its learning value increased by a proper introduction, noting points for the class to watch for and to discuss at the conclusion. Finally, do respect the return date of a borrowed or rented film. Because of the cost of films, they are usually rented or obtained on free loan.

A checklist for film use might be:

Order the film, giving first and second preferences as to showing date.

Assemble equipment, such as screen, projector, extension cord, etc.

Preview the film and note discussion subjects.

Introduce the film by telling students what to look for.

Show the film. First turn on the projector, then turn out the lights.

Hold a discussion at the close of the film.

Store the equipment.

Return the film the next day.

Another very useful aid is the use of the filmstrip. These are short edited scenes, usually 36 frames, projected on the screen. The viewer also hears a script, either read by the training leader or taken from a record. The cost of a good filmstrip is far less than that of a sound movie and has some advantages. It can be stopped at any place for additional comment, may be edited on the spot, and is relatively inexpensive to purchase or rent, or to secure equipment. However, the selection of the filmstrip must be done with great care so as to relate it to training needs. Slides, 35 mm in size, are becoming very popular because of their small cost, their versatility, and their adaptability to production by amateurs. A teacher may make slides, since any good slide camera will do. When the student poses for a slide, and then sees himself, it is a learning activity he will remember. Because of the projected image dominating the darkened room, a projected message will command the greatest attention. Combining visual aids with audio, and then relating both to teaching form a major asset to effective teaching.

In recent years, both the opaque and transparency overhead projectors have come into wide usage. The opaque is normally quite bulky, owing to increased lighting requirements, but it does have the advantage that anything flat may be projected on the screen. Any illustration, even in color, may be used. Any available written material goes well, if the type size is 14 points or more. The second type, called a transparency, uses clear film, usually one to two mils in thickness, on which the leader may print, write, or draw his own message. A number of educational publishers are now preparing transparencies on a variety of subjects. However, the leader, with a minimum of ability, may make his own. Several office copy machines are now equipped to produce transparencies much as they reproduce other materials.

Problems in Training

With in-service training, there are related problems in establishing and maintaining the training program. The largest single problem is scheduling the training opportunities. Training does involve time, which most nursing homes find very precious, because of the 7-day, 24-hour work week. Unless a fair share of time is allotted, a definite schedule cannot be kept. It is no wonder administrators find it difficult to keep training in a prominent position with the many activities required of a well-run nursing home.

Guarding the place for training will be difficult. If other activities such as recreation and entertainment utilize the room assigned for training, displays may get taken down and misplaced, then training aids will be scattered.

Priorities need to be determined. Obviously, the administrator will be unable to involve 100% of his staff all the time. He may wish to grant preference to training supervisors, who, in turn, will assist in training department workers.

Scheduling may be a problem, but getting a maximum attendance from busy workers will equal it. Work schedules may interfere, and supervisors may not be cooperative in getting their workers to attend. To keep interest in training is another problem needing constant attention. If the administrator does not promote training, or if the supervisor will not support it, the workers will not expect it.

Motivating employees to train is the responsibility of the administrator and the supervisors. Education is hard to sell, since it requires discipline. Far too many employees feel they are "too old to learn" and let this attitude defeat their opportunities to train. Equally as difficult is the defeat of the "too busy to learn" attitude. These attitudes can be overcome, however.

The greatest problem is leadership. Far too many administrators hire their employees with no thought of promoting training. Consequently, when a program is being considered, it is discovered that no one has the necessary qualifications to develop it. The administrator will be on the lookout for a good assistant who has some training ability. He will cultivate him and encourage him. He may even send him back to school to learn training techniques. By all means, he will send him to every appropriate seminar available. Finally, the administrator will keep his training assistant busy teaching or developing training programs. This may be by assignment or encouragement; but whatever the means, these will be constant until his nursing home develops a good training program.

The location of workers with teaching ability may be easier than the administrator would believe. Churches have used members as their teaching staff. Civic clubs, social organizations, and fraternities develop a surprising number of persons who can lead discussion groups. Finally, a supervisor in the nursing home may serve, but only if she possesses the necessary skills.

Evaluating Training By Testing

The administrator or his training assistant needs to develop methods of evaluation in order to ascertain the effectiveness of the program. One important means is testing.

There are many types of tests, all of which may be combined. One may be superior to another; but the circumstances in which it is used and the purpose for which it is given will define its value. Such tests may include:

> True or false questions.
> Completion or recall statements.
> Multiple choice.
> Essays.
> Visual observations.
> Audio testing (oral).
> Psychological testing.
> Interview.
> Rating of statements.

Each type of test has its own significant purpose. Tests are valuable in organizing our thinking. The statement which says, "describe," "discuss," or "define" compels one to organize his thoughts before answering. Tests are useful in encouraging the recall of facts and information such as one might use in learning new methods. Multiple choice, matching, and completion tests give a more objective evaluation. True or false tests are also helpful, but do not demand full recall. One may use testing to discover the interests a person has. The interview, observation, or certain other tests reveal much about a person. Some tests, when skillfully used, will reveal attitudes, personal attributes, and personality defects. The administrator should use these sparingly, since they are psychological in nature and take a trained psychologist to interpret results.

Testing is a tool of learning and teaching. By probing for a student's understanding after a period of instruction, the teacher can determine future goals. They are not, however, an end within themselves.

Evaluating Training By Analysis

The administrator or training supervisor has at his command an excellent method of evaluating training progress. This is by analysis. It is not only helpful in evaluating training, but also in evaluating the progress of the business.

Analysis is based upon scientific methods, of which there are several variations. For our purposes, it is enough to illustrate only two of their simpler forms.

First, *scientific analysis* presupposes the collection of data from various sources concerning the area of evaluation. Data may be in several forms, including the statistical and the graphic. To some extent, statements and observations may become a part of the data. Some of the data may be evolved into other forms, such as norms, averages, percentages, ratios, etc. After sufficient data have been collected, they are arranged into units, patterns, groups, or structures for analysis. Finally, the data are evaluated for conclusions.

A variation of scientific analysis is *inductive analysis*. In this, one first assumes a norm or standard and then collects the data. The data are, as in scientific analysis, grouped and evaluated. However, the purpose is to assess the variants to the assumed norm. In other words, one assumes a factor and then collects data to prove the hypothesis.

The evaluation of data is no exact science; but for practical purposes in the nursing home it may be refined. Several questions might be asked, but two give the administrator some insight:

"What are the results of the analysis?"
"How do they compare with the beginning condition?"

From the data collected, it is possible to develop an achievement guide. Such a standard could be based on class hours, test results, research activities, personal observation, or interview results. Evaluation of the standard might compare individual results, grades of various groups, production, attitudes, etc. In one sense, the administrator is constantly evaluating. He should develop a flow of data and train himself in their analysis.

Inaugurating the Training Program

In order for the training program to gain prominence in the eyes of the nursing home employees, it is necessary to magnify it. The administrator's attitude toward training is the first step. There are also concrete measures to be taken.

Training plans should be published. Starting with a guidebook of the total training program, one should list all training policies. This list should be published, at least in a condensed form, if a more elaborate one is not feasible. The larger nursing home chain can develop more refined guidelines. However, even the smallest home, in which the administrator takes an active part in training, a set of policies should be established and published. It may be a simple memo, a section of the employees' manual, a printed brochure, or one typed and mimeographed in the nursing home office.

Plans for specific training opportunities must be publicized. A number of specific ways are available to the administrator and the training supervisor. When plans are ready, make a formal announcement. Use the bulletin board, give the information at a staff meeting, use the public address system, or send a memo to each supervisor and/or worker. A news release will help to stress its importance. If a nursing home paper is published, write an article. Publish a special training paper or send an article to the local newspaper. The administrator, certainly, will want to repeat the announcement by several methods. Posters attract attention when strategically placed, e.g., near the time clock. Of course, a second and third memo to the workers will remind them of the training opportunity.

Assign the supervisory staff the responsibility of enlisting the trainees personally. Then intensify their help through recognition.

Finally, make the first training night a meaningful experience. Recognize the teacher and the students by various means, such as making an announcement or taking pictures. It may be well to plan some social event. If an expert speaker can be enlisted, it will add prestige. Above all, training must be made meaningful to succeed. Back up publicity with good, sound, inspiring teaching.

Chapter *8*

Human Relations
and Problem Solving

Management-Worker Relationships

The development of a close relationship between the management of the nursing home and its employees is a fundamental prerequisite for solving problems. When harmony exists, problem solving becomes routine. When it does not exist, one problem seems to spawn another.

The administrator should make problem solving an overall goal. It is an obligation he assumes when he hires personnel. It may be said that he has hired the employees to solve the problems of the patients. Since service is the primary function of the nursing home, the administrator will devise methods and techniques to accomplish this.

The employee accepts the role of problem solver when he accepts employment in the organization of the nursing home. He is implying by his acceptance of employment that he can solve problems. His work might be assembling heterogeneous factors into organized and efficient patterns of service. For example, the patient who is helpless and in bed has a problem of hygiene, which the employee solves by assembling the necessary materials, learning the correct procedures, and making the necessary application.

The employee is the first-line problem solver. He is nearest the conflict; he is in the place where most problems exist. He cannot, however, serve effectively in his assigned capacity without the cooperation of the administrator, who assists in organizing, planning, delegating, etc.

The tools of problem solving then are several. Cooperation between the administrator and the employee is the first. It may involve the one knowing and then doing an efficient job to support the efforts of the other. Communication is another tool. The relaying of facts is a must. The proper delegation of authority is equally important. Counseling and listening are tools also available. The ability to listen to the person with a problem is often the best solution. Of course, simple guidance techniques may be developed. However, it should be stressed that caution is needed in "advising the patient" concerning problems.

Communication Between Workers

It has been said: "Where there is no communication, there is no solution." In other words, the problem must be relayed to someone who can solve it. Communication may ensure that a solution is reached, bringing together the problem and its solution. An example may be the patient who becomes ill in the night. She signals the nurse, who investigates by making observations, taking vital signs, and listening to the complaint of the patient. The nurse places an emergency call to the physician. The physician may order the patient to the hospital, make an emergency call, or prescribe from the symptoms relayed by the nurse. Should he prescribe, the pharmacist would be called upon to fill the prescription and deliver it. Finally, the nurse would prepare and administer it, then make continued observations as to the progress of the patient. By communication, she obtained the solution to the patient's problem.

Communication may effect the exchange of information. In the above illustration, the physician asked the nurse to relay the symptoms and vital signs which he, in turn, compared with the past medical history of the patient and his vast knowledge of physical abnormalities. Believing he had diagnosed, he prescribed emergency medication. This interchange of information between the physician was vital to the solution. It brought into play additional resources; again, in the above illustration, the physician called a local all-night pharmacy and asked for an emergency delivery.

Communication may focus attention on the problem, which may in turn help define it. A problem may not be clear until all the facts are gathered and evaluated. A clear understanding of the related facts is necessary for the best solution. Misleading information must be discarded. A free exchange of ideas must be possible. Both sides should learn the facts. Again, in our above illustration, the nurse should take all the vital signs of the patient and be prepared to make observations before she calls a physician. She must be prepared to receive and carry out his orders accurately. The solution must be consistent with the problem. Should the nurse relay the symptoms incorrectly—temperature, respiration, pulse, and blood-pressure—the action taken may not result in a solution. Finally, for the resolution of problems, a possible solution must be known. No amount of communication can make up for a lack of training and knowledge. For the resolution of the problem, the solution must be implemented. Calling the physician in this case is not enough; the right prescription is needed, and the right drug has to be properly administered.

Interdepartmental Relations

Unity within the whole organization of the nursing home is necessary for problem solving. Interdepartmentalization poses certain problems within itself which must be overcome. The line relation, generally, is up and down the chain of command. Consequently, the horizontal cooperation and communication between departments may be minimized. This tends to splinter the unity of functions. For example, the nursing service is dependent upon the laundry to keep adequate linen supplies; yet normal communication between the nursing department and the laundry is indirect.

The means of communication between departments must be implemented. The exchange of information between the various departments (at least between the supervisory personnel) is necessary. A friendly competition between the departments may be encouraged. A formal interdepartmental memo should be adopted. An occasional exchange of personnel may make workers more aware of the responsibilities and problems of related departments.

Communication between departments must be effective. In other words, it must be vitally related to their operation. Reliance on informal or "grapevine" information is not enough. The use of proper techniques of written communication will greatly strengthen cooperation.

The administrator can improve the relationship between departments in several ways. His best method is to unify the supervisory staff. He may magnify the position of a department head by scheduling activities that will bring together his supervisors. Given the opportunity to talk, think, and plan together, their cooperation is stimulated.

Another means is the training program. When the supervisors begin to learn together, there is an increased opportunity for harmony and consequently less likelihood for dissension.

Employee Morale

The importance of morale and its impact on problem solving cannot be too greatly stressed. Low morale makes for more problems in the nursing home, simply because those that crop up are not getting solved. *Morale is to the organization what attitude is to an individual.*

It is possible to improve morale; however, it takes time and will not be accomplished overnight. A three-fold plan for improving morale might be the following:

First, the supervisor: the administrator will set the pace. Pessimism from the top management will permeate the entire organization. He should study every negative thought and assess its value or detriment to the organization. Perhaps a convention, or a vacation, or even a long talk with a successful administrator in the area will inspire his thinking. This inspiration would be passed on to his supervisors. When they feel they are a team and are pulling together, then start tackling the problem of employee morale.

Next: eliminate the factors that defeat morale. This may require a reorganization of the departments, with replacement of some leadership. One chronic griper can keep the entire nursing home staff upset or uneasy. Some objectionable activities may have to be corrected. These are not necessarily moral but are rather practices that create tension, such as methods unacceptable to good nursing care. Some objectionable rules in the personnel policy may need to be changed.

Finally, plan activities to increase morale. Study every factor concerning employee attitudes and then offer something better. Any variety of employee activity, from social occasions to a recognition of merit may be utilized. The secret is to find programs that yield employee responses.

Factors that defeat morale are:
   Nonprogressive units of the organization.
   Lack of challenging work.
   Poor attitudes of leadership.
   Fear of reprisal.
   Unfair labor practices.
   Psychological factors such as unfriendliness, lack of pride.

Factors that increase organizational morale are:
Challenging work goals.
Successful accomplishments.
Recognition of achievement.
Rewards such as bonuses.
Better working conditions.
Higher wages.
Shorter hours.
Job security.

Absenteeism

Absenteeism is a result of human frailty. Even if there are employees who are punctual and never absent, they will be the exception; sooner or later they, too, will call in sick.

The causes of absenteeism are numerous, but fall into just a few categories: sickness and accidents; emotional and psychological factors, especially where home and family problems exist; problems related to nursing home staffing, and finally, the lack of dedication on the part of the employee. Sickness is predominent among some groups; at least, some find more reasons to call in ill than others. Accidents are unpredictable and usually must be accepted; however, there are people who are accident prone. Emotional and psychological problems make for an unstable worker. Unfair staffing assignments, incompatible workers, and long work periods without relief contribute to the problem. Finally, something should be said about the need for dedicated nursing personnel. Nursing home patient care, like hospital care, is unlike most other work. When a salesman is absent, fewer sales are made. When a factory worker is absent, fewer products are produced. When the nursing home aide is absent, however, there is no letup in the work. The patients still must be cared for, even if it requires someone working a double shift. The lack of dedicated, sacrificially motivated nursing home workers will cause the most frustrating experiences to the nursing home administrator

Any attempt to control absenteeism requires constant effort. It begins with the recruitment of new workers, their selection, and their orientation. Every attempt must be made to locate employees who will place service before self, who will make a sacrificial effort to be present, or who will never desert their duty station without proper replacement.

If the attitude of the management regards absenteeism not lightly and can be supported by accurate attendance records, firm written warnings, the ultimate discharge and replacement of chronic offenders is indicated. Supervisors should be made aware that their own attitude toward attendance and punctuality is reflected in the attitude of those under their direction.

Lowering the absentee rate is a possible by-product of the educational program: the better trained the worker, the more professional his approach to his responsibilities; when he is upgraded, his consideration for his job is also upgraded. The improvement of working conditions by better supervision, better environment, better organization of the work, is essential.

Finally, gaining the loyalty of the workers will help reduce absenteeism to the minimum level. Loyalty is based on respect, success, and psychology. Respect is akin to loyalty. It comes when the nursing home improves its image. Success will gain loyalty, because workers like to win. They work the harder for the successful nursing home. Finally, it must seem the best thing for the employee: go to work.

Labor Turnover

Labor turnover means the loss of employees for various reasons and their subsequent replacement. It is possible for the administrator to combat it, but to do so he will have to discover the cause and institute preventive methods.

When labor turnover is abnormally high, the administrator is likely to find that ineffectiveness of supervision is a cause. Properly set up personnel records will yield statistics pertinent to the problem of employee turnover, such as: the average seniority rating of all employees at a given time; how many new people have been added in any particular period; what type of worker or which department shows the highest rate of turnover.

There may be a lack of communication with the workers, or they may be poorly trained and improperly motivated. From the viewpoint of labor, the cause may be poor working conditions, the lack of incentive, or job security. Even personal factors, such as a dislike for the administrator or immediate supervisor, or the fact that employees feel that little appreciation is given their work are contributing causes. From an objective study of the causes, one may derive the true answer. The administrator may conduct interviews, analyze objectively all apparent reasons, look into any misunderstanding, or make an in-depth study of labor practices.

There are a number of immediate or short-range causes for labor turnover. High on the list will be working conditions; however, these may not be the deciding factors. The nature of supervision, misunderstanding, failure to get along with other workers, and lack of loyalty contribute greatly. There are also a number of long-range causes of labor turnover; important among these are nonprogressive methods and limited opportunities. However, unfair labor practices, a low range of pay, and low morale are also reasons.

Grievances

The "gripes" (grievances of employees) demand a fair hearing; for, when they are not answered, human relations within the nursing home suffer and problem solving ceases. *A grievance is a valid complaint about an alleged willful wrong or negligence toward an employee by management.*

The administrator would do well to provide some way for grievances to be heard. All too often the expression, "If I had only known," is made to the resigning employee. Develop a systematic plan for hearing grievances. Let it be clearly understood that supervisors will first hear a complaint and, if they cannot satisfy the employee, will pass it up the chain of command. It is good policy to write down the complaint for a permanent record of it and of the action taken. The idea of the industrial counselor may work in the nursing home. In this type of service a social worker or counselor is hired and given routine duties, during which he is available to discuss problems with the employees. A further variation is the employment of a chaplain who counsels patients as well as the employees.

An informal plan of hearing grievances may be developed; however, there is some feeling about its disadvantages. This plan is known as the "open-door" policy, where any supervisor or the administrator can hear grievances. It will be necessary for supervisors to have some training in the art of counseling and for the administrator to achieve a high degree of cooperation with them when this practice is allowed. In one sense, the administrator will always practice the "open-door" policy, since he will always be the target of some griper. However, he should discuss any complaint with the employee's immediate supervisor before he makes a settlement.

The recording of grievances is most important. It will provide a permanent record to facilitate further action and follow-up. Verbal requests also should be recorded and kept. Solving grievances is no small task. When a complaint arises, it should be evaluated with all haste. Not only should the supervisor or administrator keep working for a solution, but each should also make the employee aware of any progress. Supervisors usually can solve most problems; however, some will need to be submitted to a committee and, perhaps, to arbitration.

Transfer

From time to time, because of reorganization, a shifting work load, or for efficiency, it is necessary to transfer an employee from one position to another. Often this strains human relations between the administrator and the employee, plus those with whom he works.

Functional reasons may cause a transfer to be necessary. Supervision may be lax or ineffective in a department, and the administrator may feel a transfer, either in or out of the department, may solve the problem. A general reorganization may be needed the better to distribute the supervisory personnel, and some transfers may result.

Personal relationships often bring about the need for reorganization and the shifting of personnel. Jealousy between workers requires their separation. Sometimes cliques form that prevent a dynamic and progressive unit to function. At other times a successful supervisor who has strength of character may be needed to overcome a problem.

Certain problems related to transfer must be dealt with. The administrator should gain some insight into the possibility of problems developing as a result of transfer. Interdepartmental relations may suffer. "You robbed us," a supervisor may exclaim, and she may be right. One department has been strengthened at the expense of another. Intrapersonal relations may suffer. By weakening the group dynamics of a unit, the morale may suffer. Problems between workers may develop when an efficient and likeable worker is transferred out of a unit. The administrator may be wrong in his choice because there is always uncertainty in decision making. Often, one does not actually know if a transfer will work until it has been tried.

In making the transfer, the administrator should be aware that, if he gains as much information as possible and studies it carefully, it is more likely that he will act correctly. He needs the advice of the supervisory staff and should take steps to gain their cooperation. Often "trading out" may gain some cooperation. He needs to prepare the transferee and be aware of posttransfer problems.

Promotion

The promotion of a worker may be gratifying, yet related problems can and do crop up. The administrator should study carefully the full impact of a promotion. There are many reasons for promotion, not the least of which is its value to the nursing home staff. Since building a better staff is one of the major goals of the nursing home, the administrator is constantly trying to utilize the talents of his employees to better advantage. He finds advancement a means of rewarding the service of an employee. He may find that it improves personal relations between employees. However, the administrator should be aware that these reasons are secondary *to the primary reason for making a promotion: the employee has a greater potential in the new position.*

There are, of course, some inherent dangers in promotion. Not the least is the nonacceptance of a newly promoted employee by those he would then serve with. For every employee raised in rank, at least one other may feel he was "passed over" and was equally deserving. Jealousy arises and must then be dealt with. On occasion, the administrator may not have all the facts, or may be poorly advised as to the potential of an employee. It may be that a supervisor develops a personal liking for an employee and gives him glowing efficiency reports, which, when taken literally by the administrator, may prove disastrous.

Problems of personalities may come to the forefront after a promotion. "It went to his head" is a favorite comment. The balance of power may be upset within a department when one is advanced and another feels he is "down-graded." Disloyalty may result, and someone may even resign, further complicating the problem of replacing the one promoted.

The administrator should plan promotions well. There are a number of techniques to prepare for it. *First, make an accurate assessment of the potential of the one being promoted.* If the administrator is satisfied that the worker will be able to perform adequately, then he should prepare the staff. This should be done tactfully, however, by giving it some glamor. By always emphasizing the positive aspect, the related problems are de-emphasized. He may make the promotion competitive by the use of testing, by units of production, education, or seniority. Usually, the more objective and the less personal the means, the easier it is for others. Also, there is a right moment. Keyed to expansion, general reorganization, system of rewards, or in connection with certain concessions, a promotion may be fully accepted by all employees. The administrator should challenge employees to accept advancement as a part of progress and as a future goal.

Discipline

The discipline of employees is the effort by management to correct behavior, raise standards, and remedy breaches of working agreements. In the exercise of discipline, the administrator has several tools he may use. The establishment and public display of working norms is very impersonal yet effective. Educational efforts to correct attitudes is another group method. However, discipline is normally thought of as interpersonal and is usually accomplished between the individual supervisor and the individual employee. The simplest method is "talking it over" with the offending employee. This may be in the form of a simple admonition that voices disapproval or a positive calling the employee to account for actions. The latter is commonly referred to as "being called on the carpet."

The disciplinary action may be in the form of an official reprimand, one copy of which goes into the personnel files and another to the employee. The employee may be demoted, suspended, or otherwise denied certain privileges. It should be noted that certain privileges are inherent to a position, i.e., vacation, seniority, bonuses, pay above minimum wage, and certain other fringe benefits.

Should the disciplinary action warrant, the employee may be separated from employment in the nursing home. It is incumbent upon the administrator to keep records to substantiate his position, to render a fair and impartial decision, and to make every attempt to rehabilitate the worker.

A word should be said about the beginning of disciplinary action. Actually, there is a fine edge between discipline and supervision. The correcting of errors committed by the employee should begin immediately when detected. Even the smallest hint of discipline may be detected in the supervisors' suggestion that an employee repeat a certain operation. Without comment or personal accusation, the supervisor is insisting that the worker meet the working standards acceptable in the nursing home. In the case of the new employee, this is merely a part of training; however, in the case of a longtime trusted employee there should be no exception for meeting the same working standard. It is the inherent right of management to establish the standard expected of employees and to institute the means of developing the skills of the employees to meet these standards. In its final analysis, discipline is a corrective measure of the control process.

Separation

The most difficult task faced by the administrator is that of discharging an employee. Separation of employees falls into three general classes: voluntary on the part of the employee, nonvoluntary for reasons of the management, and as a disciplinary action for violations of the working agreement.

Voluntary resignation is usually for reasons of health or for accepting other employment. Occasionally, one may desire or be required to move to another locality, e.g., a nurse whose husband is transferred to another city. Nonvoluntary separation for reasons of the nursing home is likely to be for the sake of economy or efficiency. The nursing home in this case will be prepared to accept charge-backs on its unemployment insurance, which in turn may change the experience factor used to compute premiums.

A nonvoluntary separation for a violation of working standards is the most severe. Often it is based more on an opinion than on a clear-cut violation. Consequently, the administrator should compile a written case history that can be verified by supervisory personnel. The reasons may be wide and varied, but in every case there should be a documented violation of a working standard that the employee had been made thoroughly aware of his responsibility of maintaining.

In making the separation, the administrator and his supervisory staff have certain obligations. They should not be arrogant, punitive, or disrespectful. They should be aware that the employee may be hostile, may become emotional, and may never fully understand. The staff should be given a simple statement, with the reason presented completely objectively, for instance, "violation of working agreement concerning_____," taking care not to mention how the employee violated it. Silence is usually best. When opinions are offered by either the administrator or the supervisory staff, they may be completely misunderstood.

Prepare for the aftereffects of separation. Expect an unemployment claim and the possibility of an unfair labor practice claim. A copy of the proof of violation, a copy of warnings given the employee, and a copy of the dismissal notice should be filed. Any statements by supervisors should be filed also, i.e., efficiency ratings, complaints, etc.

The administrator should comply promptly with all nursing home obligations, such as terminal pay, release of personal property, and completion of prior commitments. In every instance, the administrator strives to protect the name of the nursing home.

Chapter 9

Creativity and Group Dynamics

Creativity and Imagination in Employees

There is great need for creativity and imagination in the nursing home employees. The task of serving the infirm and aged is gigantic in proportion to the number of available employees. If the administrator can improve the quality of service, he may be able to achieve the high standards and goals needed in nursing homes. When employees achieve worthwhile values of service, they will also find improved working conditions.

Creativity and imagination are functions of the mind. Each person stores his experiences, thoughts, knowledge, and beliefs in his mind. These come from many sources, such as work habits, reading, training, etc. The more experiences an employee is exposed to in the nursing home, the greater his resources. Mental resources are constantly updated by new experiences, thoughts, knowledge, etc. In other words, a person constantly adds to the reservoir. Subconsciously one evaluates new information to formulate new values. For example, an experience or new insight into a procedure or technique may replace an outdated concept. When faced with a problem, the employee draws upon these mental resources as they have been updated or re-evaluated. Thus, the process of comparison of the new situation with this reservoir of mental resources begins. Information is fed back for comparison. It is analyzed, compared, accepted, or rejected. Finally, a solution will result; but only if one persists in the search and is stimulated to succeed.

Some employees have greater creativity than others, but only because they have developed their ability to think. By developing a system of goals and values, they literally discipline themselves to accomplish feats which others may call imagination. It is possible to improve creativity and imagination. One may learn to establish reasonable goals and then diligently pursue them. By improving with practice and repetition, an employee may develop high standards of success for himself. Finally, the elevation of our ethics or values should give us the desire to improve.

Ethics and Improvement

In business, ethics could be termed "practices and working relationships that are concerned with right and wrong." It has its source in beliefs, morals, goals, and attitudes toward one's profession. Ethics is related to a philosophy of life, a term used to describe thoughts and conduct. More specifically, ethics is related to morals and spiritual conduct. Social concepts and culture may define ethics to some extent. In the end, however, what one believes is right and what one believes is wrong will embody one's ethics.

Ethics is related to goals, although this concept may be misleading. Goals, to be ethical, must have a set of values which in turn must be consistent with that which is right. When one elevates his standard of achievement and success, he also elevates his ethics.

Ethics is related to knowledge, although knowledge is not ethics. By asking, "Do we *know* this action to be honest? Do we *know* it to be fair?" it is immediately seen that ethics and knowledge have a certain relationship.

Ethics is related to one's attitude. "Am I *willing* to do the right thing? Am I *prejudiced*? Am I *aware* of the ethical value of the action?" These are some questions that relate both to ethics and to attitude.

Finally, ethics is related to one's beliefs. Essentially, the end does not justify the means. For example, a nurse cannot justify a mistreatment of a patient whose safety is endangered, except when the nurse has exhausted every possible means available to help the patient, for example, the use of restraint when another method would do just as well. A number of statements could be made to relate ethics to actions:

"An act is not right simply because one is not caught."
"What a person does not know *may* hurt him."
"You are your brother's keeper, especially when you work in a nursing home."

"You *will* harvest your injustice."
"Love *does* overcome."

Group Dynamics and Cognitive Improvement

A knowledgeable person is of great value in the operation of the nursing home because of the great variety of skills that are needed. To create an atmosphere of learning on the part of the workers is of high priority. Cognitive improvement is increasing our knowledge concerning a given procedure, operation, experience, or situation. It can be effected by the working unit, since a definite relationship exists between one's learning and the dynamic of the work group.

Involvement promotes learning. Being involved in patient care demands improvement, and the administrator will seek to effect a climate of learning in the work units. Role behavior in a group will implement learning. For example, a particular individual may assume the role of secretary for her particular working unit. She keeps records on the flower fund, posts notices, writes thank-you notes, etc. The group also places other demands on learning. People learn to work together, to adjust to changes, to compete, to cooperate, and to become aware of others.

A number of activities promote learning within the group, such as research and report, or even attendance and participation in group activities. Small-group discussions often facilitate learning, since this is the ideal unit for sharing information. On a more formal level, panels, forums, and discussion groups increase learning.

The administrator can promote learning with the use of several group activities. On-the-job training is a form of group learning, since learning is accomplished through observing and copying the performance of the students' peers. Conferences greatly promote learning by means of the mutual sharing of ideas. Study groups also increase learning, as do group projects.

Whatever the type of group learning, it is still the responsibility of the administrator to ensure that full and accurate information is presented to the students and that they demonstrate by their on-the-job performance a satisfactery degree of comprehension.

Group Dynamics and Attitudinal Improvement

By attitudinal improvement, we mean the development of values, opinions, beliefs, and thoughts. This, like ethics or professionalism, is important in the operation of the nursing home simple because employees primarily serve people. People, whether aged, infirm, or young, are generally sensitive to another's attitude. While the administrator is not directly dealing in the personality improvement of his employees, nevertheless, it is an important factor in serving the patient.

The group does effect changes in attitudes. There is a certain conformity in the group, brought about by subtle group pressures. The phrase, "When in Rome do as the Romans," is correct in picturing the individual within a new group. The group expects performance, progressiveness, and participation, which cannot help but affect one's attitude.

Adverse attitudes attributed to the group will affect the individual member to a degree. Picture the nursing home employee associated with a nonprogressive group. He is numbered with the other employees, whether he is a cause of their poor showing or not. Some adverse attitudes by the group may be:

Rejection by a clique. A new worker might not be given an opportunity to succeed because he could not break into the group.

Hostility. The group is always in trouble, because there is never any peace and harmony within its ranks.

Low morale. The overall viewpoint of the group is negative.

Defeatism. The group members expect to fail.

Better attitudes may permeate a group. There is a sense of success. Dynamic leadership develops, and the unit becomes progressive. The attributes of a progressive group may be described as follows:

A sense of success prevails. Having succeeded, the group strives to repeat its success.

Loyalty is exemplified. The reliability and punctuality of all workers in the group is expected.

Fairness is the rule. Labor practices are just, ethical, and fair to all.

Love prevails. Service oriented workers influence others to serve with a magnanimous spirit.

A number of group activities may be sponsored by the administrator to promote improvement of attitudes. These may include case studies, debates, brainstorming, forums, interviews, symposiums, or seminars. Of course, all the motivators, e.g., recognition, challenging goals, higher wages, etc., will help in the development of the group spirit.

Group Dynamics and Skill Improvement

When related to business, a skill is thought of as mastery of a particular operation, function, or procedure. There is some correlation between the group or working unit and the perfection of skills. In defining the relationship between the group and skill improvement, administrators will note several points. Usually, the group sets the standard in accordance with the challenge given. Thus the group will expect and accept a certain level of performance. Members then share in the overall achievement and perform specific roles within a group. It is precisely at the point of the individual's role within the group that conformity with group standards results. For example, a nursing unit takes in a new aide. It is not long before the aide "knows her place," that is, her role. Then begins the long process of achieving and maintaining her position. This is accomplished by her performance. She will seldom rise above the level of achievement accepted by the nursing unit.

There are several principles in learning a skill. It is ordinarily thought that individual learning predominates; however, there is a definite correlation between the working unit and the level of skill one will achieve. The student needs a goal in learning, and he often gains this from the working unit. He will need inspiration which, again, may come from the working unit. He will need information, which is supplied by his superiors and fellow workers, some of whom tell him how it is applied. He may need specific instructions in applying such knowledge, and again he can usually find help. The working unit thus becomes a laboratory for practice. Finally, the group will evaluate his skill. While it may do it politely, nevertheless, he will soon be aware of the level of his attainment.

It is possible for the administrator to utilize several learning activities to improve skills. These might be demonstrations, field trips, workshops, conferences, and seminars to implement group learning.

Group Sizes

The administrator should be aware of the effect the size of a group may have on the working interrelationships of his employees. *It is said that a group exists when two or more people are interacting in some relationship.* Group interaction is psychological in nature, that is, it deals with the thought process of the individual. While to a degree there are social, cultural, and physical implications in group interaction, one should be aware of the psychological functions of the group and its several members. Within every group there exist several relationships. There is group solidarity, group morale, group attraction, and individual roles of the group members. Solidarity means a sense of comradeship or brotherhood. Morale is the collective attitudes of the group. Group attraction means a feeling of esprit de corps. A number of identifiable roles, such as recorder, coordinator, elaborator, informer, etc., may be noted.

A definite relationship exists between the group and its size. *The number of relationships within a group increases, roughly, by the square of the number of the members in the group.* The actual formula is, "Relationships equal the number in the group times the number less one." The impact of the increase in relationships is evident in the increasing difficulty of supervision. Interactions are complicated as well. Effectiveness begins to decline with the increase, thus supervision and control diminish. Coordination is also more difficult.

The administrator should organize his supervision over the smallest number of employees that can accomplish the job goals. While opinions differ, it is generally agreed that one supervisor can manage well approximately six workers. This number would properly distribute the work, allow supervisory control, ensure that the more aggressive workers do not dominate others, and give fair consideration to personal relationships. This could mean that the ideal nursing unit will be one charge nurse with six nurse's aides. Of course, circumstances may require some variation of this ideal. It is logical that fewer supervisory personnel can be supervised by the administrator than line workers by a foreman. In addition, the working proximity of the workers to be supervised and the nature of production will need to be considered. Finally, the educational achievement of the workers may be considered.

Chapter *10*

Staff Meetings and Conference Leadership

Planning the Conference and Staff Meetings

Conferences are, or should be, an integral part of the nursing home organization. The staff meeting is in one sense a short conference. It has all the elements of a conference, including goals, the use of resources, leadership, instructional methods, and training techniques, i.e., training aids, evaluation, application, etc.

Every conference should have a definite purpose. When put in general terms, the aim may sound rather idealistic as, for example, "To offer the best nursing care possible." Further consideration makes it possible to narrow the goal to a specific, concrete objective and, in the process, make it more attainable, especially from the point of view of time. Then, using the same example, the aim might be stated as follows: "To train employees to give the best possible nursing care." Such a statement suggests types of practical action through which the conference can achieve its purpose. The chance of success of the conference is much greater when positive steps for implementing the chosen objective are indicated.

Planning the conference requires assembling the resources. After the goals have been defined in terms of both the overall aim and more specific short-range objectives, the conference leader selects the speakers, gathers materials, prepares displays, writes any materials not available, and provides training aids.

The conference is much more effective when a written agenda or program is distributed to the participants. Just a simple chronological statement of program personalities and the subjects to be covered is sufficient. Remember to include "who," "when," "where," "why," and "how." Be concise. Give an orderly statement of events. Avoid conflicts.

The length of the conference will be determined by the goal. Of course, staff meetings will usually be within an hour in length; however, the orientation of new employees could take from one day to one week. If the conference purpose is training, then plan it long enough to meet all training goals. Any conference should be short enough to maintain full interest, since monotony is the greatest enemy. The longer the conference, the more reason to break it into several short units.

Steps in Preparation for the Conference

The more thorough the preparation the less chance there will be of a disrupting factor during the conference. It is usually the little things that interrupt and sometimes kill the conference. The conference leader should make certain every possible detail is planned in advance.

In making the arrangements, high on the list is location. It may be the nursing home, a rented hall, or a local convention facility. Check the facility beforehand to see that all is in order. Check on its cleanliness and orderliness. Check the seating. Are there enough chairs for the expected attendance? Check the speakers's stand and the public address system. Will tables be needed for the display of materials? What about a chalk board? Or a tack board? There are a number of little things—chalk, eraser, pencils, thumbtacks, etc.— that make for sizable disruptions when not available. Consider it this way: if 20 employees who make $2.50 per hour are sitting idle at a staff meeting for 20 minutes while the administrator sends out for a chalk board, the money lost through valuable time wasted far exceeds the amount that proper preparation would have taken.

Check on comfort items such as heating and cooling, rest rooms, drinking fountain, communications, etc. Food service may be necessary, or refreshments in any event. Lodging has to be arranged during overnight conferences for the out-of-town speaker and guests. Training aids need to be secured, set up, and test run. These include projection aids, spotlights, audio equipment, etc.

Conference materials usually follow the program goals. Printed materials include the program, special instructions, reports, analyses, notes, etc. Brochures, pamphlets, leaflets, or handouts may need to be secured from organizations related to the program emphasis. For example, a labor conference should utilize materials secured from the Department of Labor. Additional resource materials might include books, workbooks, testing materials, displays, films, filmstrips, and slides.

Financial arrangement will need to be made. Where the nursing home is underwriting the cost, the administrator merely estimates the cost and makes budgetary allowance. However, for a conference where participants pay, some provision should be made for collecting the money and disbursing it for expenses.

Techniques of Conducting the Conference

The administrator needs experience and training in the art of conducting a conference. The successul use of conference techniques is learned and seldom comes naturally. In essence, leadership is the most important element. It sets the pace, keeps the meeting progressing, and brings it to a successful conclusion.

The first rule of conference leadership is getting started on time. Punctuality will set the discipline of the conference, which otherwise may be difficult to attain. Usually, an audience is polite and attentive if its expectations of the goal are met; but to leave the audience waiting is to leave them wondering about the importance of the goal.

The opening remarks are the keynote of the conference. Plan it well. Make opening statements positive and dynamic. Perhaps only a polite welcome and explanation is enough to set the pace. In any event, sell the conference in those first few moments. Imagine the impact of, "Hey, Joe, you got those papers . . . time to get going . . . you ready . . . hold on till we test this mike . . . I suppose you know why you're here. . . ." Better showmanship is called for if one is to become a professional nursing home administrator.

The conference leader should be in his best attire. While distractive dress should be avoided, nothing helps more than to appear before an audience in neat and stylish clothing.

Maintain a high level of conduct. Low and coarse humor may get a laugh, but it seldom makes a contribution to the conference goal. Simply expect the best and aim for depth in understanding. Why waste the time of valued employees who may not understand how one got so far afield of the purpose of the conference.

Keep the program moving. How ironical would it be for the conference leader to conduct a training session on organization and be unable to organize the study. "Follow the schedule" is the best advice for the conference leader. Remember how long it took to plan the schedule. Now consider if it can be replanned while the conference is in session. Usually this is an impossible task. Keep it moving and do not fall into disorder. Some conference leaders find it is well to plan extra material to keep in reserve, in the event something goes wrong. It may then be quickly substituted, as, for instance a film for the speaker who does not show, or an alternate method in case the film projector fails.

The master of ceremonies, often the conference leader, will make or break the success of the conference. He needs skill in speaking and leading. If he does not have these, he should learn them.

How to Vary the Program

Maintaining high interest is necessary for the success of any conference. In fact, learning is preceded by interest. A common expression, "lose the audience," is based on the educational concept of a pupil's interest being necessary for learning to take place. There are a number of ways the conference leader may use to acheve high interest. The best will be good teaching methods and techniques. When one notes that the best teachers are usually skilled in the use of a variety of methods, he will discover one of the secrets of public speaking. A variety of methods adaptable to the conference may include: lecture, symposium, panel of experts, question and answer, discussion, workshop, or demonstration.

All the above may be used singly or in various combinations. The conference leader can also give variety to his conference by the use of such aids as posters, charts, maps, tack boards, films, filmstrips, slides, overhead projector, and audio aids. Each has its place and distinct value in conference training.

The audience may need time for a break in the program. The "seventh-inning stretch" works well after an hour or so of sitting. A coffee break may go even better, and do not forget lunch.

The conference leader should be familiar with the use of parliamentary procedures when the audience participates, or when the meeting has some decision-making authority. For efficiency, for order, and to expedite meetings, certain rules of procedure have been adopted, and a good book on parliamentary procedures is of great help. For the larger conference, one of convention size, a parliamentarian may be engaged to advise the presiding officer on matters of procedure.

How to Make the Program Interesting

In the last discussion, ways to make the program varied were explored. In this section, consideration is given to making the specific parts of the program interesting. It is one thing to assign a panel in one period, a forum in another, and a lecture in the next. It is still necessary, however, to make each of them interesting. The materials and information presented must also be exciting. Who has not heard this criticism of a movie, "The photography was perfect, but the plot was lousy"? Thus, while the leader may use "showmanship," he has to see that every moment of the program is worthwhile and pertinent to the attainment of the conference goal.

Materials become more interesting if organized and presented in an orderly fashion. Having continuity from beginning to end of the program will, as in a novel, reach a climax, carrying the learner to the end of the conference. If the content of the presentation is planned well, an audience is the more receptive. Fresh personalities will enliven a conference, making it worthwhile to engage a prominent speaker. It may be either the best local personality available or a prominent authority. The administrator will find a reservoir of speakers in the business world, when the subject matter is directly related to that area.

Do not oversell the audience. An overwhelmed person is on the defensive, for he usually resists high-pressure tactics. Even giving too much information will sometimes defeat the program goal. Surprise the audience by coming up with new resources and materials. Even old materials can be freshened up to make them more acceptable. Look for fresh ideas, store them, and then spring them on the audience.

The conference leader should strive to establish rapport between himself and his audience. This is a sympathetic relationship which results in agreement or harmony. When this relationship has been established, it tends to carry the learning atmosphere toward the learning goals.

Evaluation of the Conference

The administrator and the conference leader greatly improve the prospects for the success of the conference when they conduct a postconference evaluation. Actually, there are three evaluations that could be beneficial. An immediate appraisal should be made. A formal critique may follow. A follow-up several days, weeks, or months after the conference is also helpful.

The immediate appraisal should be made while the conference is in progress. The administrator should make notes from time to time and, at the end of the program, take a moment for reflection, perhaps informally questioning several participants or leaders. A formal critique should then follow, as soon as it is feasible. Assemble the leadership and make a point-by-point survey of the entire program. Make the appraisal cover both successes and failures.

There are several methods of evaluation. The conference leader will use one or more of these to establish an achievement guide. There are certain effective appraisals that are readily discernible. Attendance is one. Then note the attention of the participants. Their comments will reflect their insight, while changes in attitudes may be apparent. Noticeable changes in work habits and production, after the conference, may reflect success. Written evidence that may be collected are statements or essays by the participants, information from questionnaires, and notes on interviews or observations made. Of course, work attendance records and correlated production records should be considered.

The administrator should become aware of change, and be able to appraise it. Noticeable change in the work habits of employees, i.e., less absenteeism, number of grievances, etc., may be considered for evaluation. Improvement in attitudes may also be discernible. A change in production would indicate a change in response and efficiency.

Success of the conference can be determined by comparing preconference attitudes, skills, and knowledge levels with their postconference levels. Perhaps one of the best methods of evaluation is to do a follow-up from three to six months later, in which a short conference is held covering the essentials of the first conference. Now, is the response still improved?

For Further Study

Selected Readings in Nursing Home Administration

Bonner, Hubert, *Group Dynamics*. New York: Ronald Press, 1959.

Chruden, Herbert J., and Sherman, Arthur W., Jr., *Personnel Management*. Cincinnati: South-Western Publishing Co., 1972.

Edge, Findley B., *Teaching for Results*. Nashville: Broadman Press, 1956.

Grant, E. L., *Statistical Quality Control*. New York: McGraw-Hill, 1946.

Jacobs, H. Lee, and Morris, Woodrow W., *Nursing and Retirement Home Administration*, Ames, Iowa: Iowa State University Press, 1966.

Kazmier, Leonard J., *Principles of Management*. New York: McGraw Hill, 1974.

Maltz, Maxwell, *Psycho-Cybernetics*. Englewood Cliffs, N.J.: Prentice-Hall, 1960.

Musselman, Vernon A., and Hughes, Eugene H., *Introduction to Modern Business*. Englewood Cliffs, N.J.: Prentice Hall, 1973.

Myers, Robert J./McCahan Foundation (Bryn Mawr, Penna.), *Medicare*. Homewood, Ill.: Richard D. Irwin, Inc., 1970.

Odiorne, George S., *Management by Objectives*. New York: Pitman Publishing Corp., 1968.

Yoder, Dale, *Personnel Management and Industrial Relations*. Englewood Cliffs, N.J.: Prentice-Hall, 1970.

PART TWO

Nursing Home Technology

The administrator will learn about the history and development of nursing homes; he should develop his own philosophy.

The administrator must provide for continuing medical attention, i.e., selection of the attending physician, continuity of care in transfer, emergency medical care, diagnostic services, dental care, restorative services, social services, and pharmaceutical services.

He will ensure staff cooperation with the attending physician by providing for the transmittal of doctor's orders, written and verbal, PRN (pro re nata) orders, progress notes, and medical examination and history reports.

His nursing staff shall include: supervisor of nurses, charge nurses, orderlies, aides, and ward clerks.

He will develop criteria for admission to include the need of the patient for nursing care, the type of care provided, criteria to determine noncovered levels of care, patient certification or recertification.

He will develop a transfer policy, discharge policy, and a policy to cover change in the patient's condition.

He will assist in the development of patient-care plans. He will establish means of collecting transfer information, self-care evaluation, social history, patient information, restorative information. Planning will include: safety precautions, adjustment to the nursing home, cooperation with the family, physical needs, and emotional needs.

He will ensure good medical record management through the systematic, secure, confidential, and legal collection and storage of records.

The administrator will develop a complete dietary service. His staff may include: dietitian or nutrition consultant, food service manager, cooks, helpers, dietary aides. He will make provision of preparing and serving a balanced diet and modified diets as prescribed, a food preference survey, substitutes, seconds, and reporting on eating habits. Food handling must be safe and sanitary.

The administrator will develop a plan of evacuation to include: priorities of action, designated exits, patient-carry methods, designated collection point, first-aid, and fire-fighting methods.

The administrator will develop safety practices to include provision for the handicapped patient, orientation to safety, emergency safety equipment, handrails, grab bars, nonskid flooring. He will encourage safety on the part of employees by continuous education, policies, practices, and safety equipment.

The administrator will develop sanitation and infection control, and facilities for isolation, disinfection, and sterilization. He will institute preventive methods in housekeeping by the use of germicides, proper mopping, refuse removal, pest control, and proper sewage disposal.

The laundry will be sanitary, properly ventilated, and safe. Linen, bedding, and patients' laundry will be properly cared for.

The administrator will be familiar with all aspects of gerontology, including the economic, housing, family units, community factors, retirement, education, cultural norms, social isolation, independent living.

The pharmaceutical services shall include consultation, security of drugs, safe storage, proper administration, record keeping.

The administrator shall be acquainted with some of the medical terminology.

Chapter 11

History and Philosophy
of the Nursing Home

The Forerunner of Nursing Homes

The history of the role of the aged is fascinating, since it parallels that of mankind in every culture. Ancient practices reveal certain concepts in the care of the aged and infirm. These concepts draw heavily on Hebrew culture, although there are others, including Babylonian, Egyptian, Greek, Roman, Persian, and Chinese.

The Jewish concepts are possibly the most fundamental, since they set patterns which before were not formalized. *The Hebrews honored their aged parents by giving their maturity a place of authority in their legal, social, and religious structures.* Because of the scarcity of written materials, the ancient Hebrew acquired, with age, a reservoir of knowledge and became the repository of tradition and lore. Hence the young sought their counsel and wisdom, gave them reverence and respect, and ultimately bestowed upon them the title of "Elder."

Another important concept, traceable to the Hebrew, is the responsibility of the children for caring for their aged parents. Others such as the Chinese, who lived in family communes, followed this practice; but it was the Hebrew nation that formalized it, wrote it into their law, made it religious tradition, and structured their society around it. They found that the concept of honoring the aged, with the children caring for them in their infirm and aged state, gave great unity to the family unit.

Christ elevated the Hebrew practice to one of love and compassion when he rebuked neglect of parents and commended those who honored them. He also gave us the first variation of this concept when he entrusted the care of his mother, not to his brothers and sister, but to the one who had the most compassion, the apostle John.

The medieval era arose out of the decline of the Greek and Roman cultures. With the breakdown of civilization, the aged were abused, cast aside, and generally neglected.

Religious orders filled the vacuum with the establishment of *"way-houses,"* refuges for the indigent elderly. The feudal system of the Middle Ages made some provision for the aged.

The *almshouse* became indirectly a forerunner of modern care for the aged. "Alms" meant gift, and came to be synonymous with a gift to a beggar. Thus, when the poor began to group themselves within a single residence, almshouse came to mean the dwelling of those who begged for their livelihood. It was eventually used for the indigent aged who lived on charity.

Rise of the Modern Nursing Home

Hospitals are traceable to the third century, as a formal, organized, and permanent institution. However, some care of the sick and infirm existed in all ancient practices of medicine. Modern nursing, as we know it, did not exist until the Crimean War (1853–1855), when hospitals were established to aid in the care of the sick and wounded. *Florence Nightingale* (1820–1910) is given credit for the establishment of the first modern nursing effort in the Crimea. For her efforts, the English gave her a grant of fifty thousand pounds sterling, which she used to found a nursing school. Because of her success, the English War Department established a system of hospitals.

In America credit is given to Clara Barton (1821–1912), organizer of the American Red Cross, for her efforts in nursing during the Civil War (1861–1865).

Influences of other institutions, such as the poor-farm, the flophouse, sanitoriums, etc., play a part in the history of the nursing home. The poor-farm concept arose when municipalities and communities began to "farm out" the responsibility for care of the poor—usually the elderly—to the highest bidder. Since the facility often had a rural setting, the term poor "farm" arose. The chronically ill and the indigent poor who needed hospitalization were likely the early candidates, thus giving a medical connotation.

Certain *custodial or domiciliary units* also pointed up the need for a nursing home. The indigent aged began to collect in hotels, apartments, and multiple-family homes as a result of the modern trend toward urbanization. The notorious flophouse of the slums came into being for the drunkard, the wino, and the poor. Veterans of early American wars fared only slightly better; they tended to turn their hospitals into domiciliary units. Eventually, the government began to make adequate provision for the veteran.

The resultant concept began to merge with that of the hospital. Early hospitals were largely domiciliary, associated with that common prejudice, "a place to die." Physicians only sparingly used hospital facilities for surgery. It was not until they changed their practices that change in the use of the hospital developed. When it appeared that hospitals would assume the responsibility for long-term care, physicians began utilizing operating facilities. Thus, long-term care patients began to be grouped together, or were separated from hospitals and placed in sanitoriums. The resultant facility was neither hospital nor domicile, neither sanitorium nor custodial unit. It needed further definition. However, it was not until this century that the licensing of a nursing home is recorded.

The modern nursing home is still undergoing a struggle for means by which to meet various needs. The present trend in the relationship between hospital and nursing home is evident. Originally, the hospital supplied medical needs, and the convalescent facility cared for long-term, chronic medical needs. In recent years, however, the domicile need has also merged with the medical need. Consequently, the nursing home is now faced with the necessity of providing care that begins with a purely domiciliary need and progresses as the person becomes chronically ill, to a purely medically oriented need. Thus the term, medical necessity, is being applied to determine the level of care. Because Medicare, Medicaid, private insurers, and the Veterans Administration all are interested in reimbursing for care based only on medical necessity, as opposed to custodial care, we are at present undergoing a period of definition. Reference is made to the *Extended Care Facility Manual Revision* (No. 24, September, 1970, U.S. Department of Health, Education, and Welfare, Social Security Administration) which, to clarify medical necessity, defines "Skilled Nursing Services" (ref. section 211.2):

A skilled nursing service is one which must be furnished by or under the direct supervision of licensed nursing personnel and under the general direction of a physician in order to assure the safety of the patient and achieve the medically desired result.

One component is the observation and assessment of the total needs of the patient. Another component is the planning, organization, and management of a treatment plan involving multiple services where specialized health care knowledge must be applied in order to attain the desired result. An additional component is the rendering of direct services to a patient where the ability to provide the services requires specialized training.

In subparagraphs the manual revision further specifies that skilled nursing care is to be on a continuing basis, when frequent skilled nursing services are required, and symptoms occurring or likely to occur indicate the modification of treatment or new medical procedures.

With this strict definition of "skilled nursing services," how does one define a lesser level of care? The initial thrust was "either-or," that is, either skilled or custodial. Recent facts have developed which indicate a progressive degree of need more nearly related to the opposite end of the spectrum: custodial care. If this is so, what of those whose need falls vaguely between the medical-necessity need and the custodial need? There is a whole series of supportive services that may be applied by nonmedical personnel, including routine medications, application of heat, care of the plaster cast, incontinence, skin care, bathing, lotions, maintenance of colostomy, simple dressing, exercises, and assistance in self-care. They can hardly fit on a continuing basis within a residential institution. The student will immediately notice the progressive needs of the patient:

Domestic: need for family and a home.
Residential: need for a place of abode.
Congregate: need to be near group services.
Custodial: need for assistance in activities of daily living.
Convalescent: need for assistance while recuperating from a short-term or long-term illness.
Intermediate nursing care: medically oriented care owing to chronic disease or long-term infirmities.
Skilled nursing care: medical care directed on 24-hour basis by professional nurses. Such care may involve multiple services where specialized health care knowledge must be applied. Restorative services are an integral part of medical rehabilitation.
Hospitalization: need of daily professional (physician and nurses) medical attendance in the treatment of acute illness, injury, or surgery.

Psychiatric hospitalization: treatment of mental illness.

It is difficult to separate the various needs and to relegate them to specific categories. Thus the nursing home and the hospital will complement each other and exist in close proximity as they share in the health-care endeavor.

The Philosophy of the Nursing Home

Just why the nursing home exists is a many-sided question, since it involves a medical concept, as mentioned above, a service motive, and a need for a place of residence. Philosophy will help to answer the problem of the definition of the nursing home.

The "service" motive comes as a part of culture. It is identifiable under several titles. The "brother's keeper" motive may be identified by a feeling of compassion for a neighbor or relative. It has its roots in religion, which devised it as a part of ethics. It has to do with the idea of the worth and sanctity of the individual, that life is sacred.

The "for the community good" concept is a social-political ideal, perhaps more social than political. There are those who are primarily community-minded, and may be described as being of this type.

The "serving mankind" concept is not bound to the social-political category but is more nearly related to the "need" concept. It breaks the bounds of family, community, and even country. It usually crosses lines of segregation by race, creed, or color. It is characterized by an individual's involvement in all of life, and it places high values on the worth of the individual. Some emphasis on relief of the suffering is given. However, "service" motives tend to be facility-oriented, that is institutionalized.

The "need" motive arises within the helpful individual in contrast to the "service" motive which originates primarily in the environment. It may be said that an individual projects himself into the "needs" of others and then attempts to supply them. The need motive is characterized by the recognition of human dignity, by the idea that the person is superior to the state, and the belief that life does have meaning. It is usually associated with the ideal of sharing. A selflessness or benevolency exists. It may be associated with the ideal of relieving suffering.

Dedication to God rates high as a motive in the Christian cultures. It is a principle of faith to the believer. For those having dedicated their lives to a higher calling, it is the summum bonum of life. They serve the needs of humanity as a means of sharing their faith.

The administrator should take the time to formulate his own philosophy of nursing home administration. He will note, as he deals with the government as a provider of services, a definite emphasis on the needs of the patient. For example, a utilization review for skilled nursing facilities is nothing more than reviewing the patient's need for care, reviewing the care he receives to determine if it meets his medical needs, and reviewing personnel and services to assure that the patient's needs are met. As the administrator serves and deals with the needs of the patients, he will become more and more personally involved and will find he needs a positive philosophy or belief to meet the challenge of his profession.

The administrator should write a statement to include his beliefs concerning the type of care, the person served, the individuals' needs, some exclusions, some ideals, and some of the purposes for service. The author has included his philosophy of nursing home administration:

> The nursing home has a dual role, both that of serving as a place of residence and of providing medical service.
>
> The nursing home resident may be aged, infirm, or convalescent from medical or surgical disorder.
>
> His need is basically to sustain life, health, spirit, and individuality.
>
> His need transcends race, religion, culture, and position.
>
> He does not need punishment, ridicule, criticism, or unethical treatment; he merely needs to reach optimal health and emotional stability. He needs to continue to be active in the pursuit of life, liberty, and spiritual dignity.
>
> He may need medication, rehabilitation, personal care, and assistance in hygiene. He may need counsel, encouragement, sympathy, and love.

Chapter *12*

Patient Orientation, Physician Relationships, and Medical Records

Introducing the Patient to the Nursing Home

It is the responsibility of the administrator to develop the procedures for admitting the nursing home patient. This was referred to in Part One, Chapter One in the discussion of policies. This is a discussion of the practical matters of actually admitting the patient and adjusting him or her to the nursing home. Some suggested forms will be shown merely to illustrate the complete requirements for documentation of a patient's stay within the home.

Prior to the patient's arrival, some preparation for introducing the patient to the nursing home may be expected. The preliminary interview with the patient and/or his relative or guardian affords the opportunities needed to begin the proper adjustment of the patient. There are questions to be answered, information to be secured, and agreements to be made. An admission agreement may be concluded after an interview. Care must be taken to review all home policies and conclude the full financial agreement. A nursing home statement of policy was discussed in the section of public relations, and a sample of a typical financial agreement was shown in our discussion of contracts in Part One. Admission requirements, such as the physical examination, arrangements for pharmaceuticals, certification by the physician (the medical history, examination, diagnosis, and his orders), counseling with the caseworker for Medicaid, and completion of the admission form—all these can be done prior to admission.

Receiving the patient is an important step in patient adjustment. The first impression, if it is cheerful, may make for a better patient attitude in the future. Care should be given to making the proper introductions and to relieving any apprehensions of the patient. Upon the patient's arrival, the administrator or assistant should be at the door or should meet the ambulance. This is a time to be prompt rather than to leave the patient waiting. Assign a nurse or aide to the patient and have her complete the admission adjustment, which includes completion of the patient admission record (see the sample on the following page).

Placement in the room should be complete and thorough. When showing the patient to the room, identify specifics, i.e., where the bathroom is, the closet, which bed, the dresser, chair, night stand, and any other items assigned for individual use. Anything belonging to another patient should be pointed out when the roommate is introduced. The patient should also be made aware of related facilities, such as safety features, handrails, grab bars, dayrooms, dining room, etc.

Adjusting the Patient

Adjusting the patient is of high priority in nursing home relations and efficiency. Future problems may be avoided with proper adjustment. The nursing home administrator should establish a thorough plan of dealing with the many factors affecting the adjustment. Essentially, adjustment begins prior to admission. By establishing a feeling of confidence with the patient and/or relative/guardian, a workable atmosphere of service may be created. The administrator and staff should be honest with their promises. Don't oversell, but be forthright and positive in any commitments. Having a clear understanding of policies makes it possible to discuss them fully; and it is wise to provide a written copy for further consideration. Having the patient visit the home prior to admission will answer many questions. It gives the person an opportunity to meet the staff, view the facility, and meet the other patients. It also gives the staff an opportunity to note the type of care needed.

The first day is an important one in the life of the patient. Care should be taken not to overwhelm him, since everything is new. If he is tired, let him rest. Too many details will overwhelm and confuse the aged, especially if feeble. Concentrate on the simple and essential matters at first. These may include demonstrating how to summon the

PATIENT ADMISSION RECORD

Patient _____ Date _____

Usual address _____ Medicare # _____

Referred by _____ Medicaid # _____

Date of birth _____ Age _____

Male_____ Female_____Race_____ Physician_____

Marital status   S____   M____   W____   D____ Physician_____

Previous occupation _____ Specialist_____

Birthplace _____ Dentist_____

Was the patient in the armed services? _____ Podiatrist_____

Dates of service _____ Optometrist _____

Order drugs from_____ Hospital _____

Member of what church_____ Cash_____

Diagnosis _____ Allergies _____

1. Name _____ Relationship _____

    Address _____ Phone _____

2. Name _____ Relationship _____

    Address _____ Phone _____

3. Funeral Home _____ Phone _____

    Address _____

Expenses will be paid by _____

ADMISSION WAIVER

The management of this home has agreed to exercise such reasonable care toward this person as his or her known condition may require; however, this home is in no sense an insurer of his or her safety or welfare and assumes no liability as such. The management of this home will not be responsible for any valuables or money left in the possession of this person while he or she is a resident.

Signed_____

nurse to secure help, acquainting the patient with the room, such as placement of personal belongings, explaining safety measures, and many other routine items.

Procedures for patient admission may be written as the example below:

WHEN A NEW PATIENT ARRIVES

Make the patient comfortable in the room.
Check medications and put in box in medicine cabinet.
Check Doctor's Order sheet and/or Transfer sheet.
Take all vital signs including weight if possible.
Open chart with first entry. Make cardex records.
Call doctor's office to notify the patient's arrival.
Check medicine with the doctor if signed orders are not received.
Check treatments and special orders.
Check for Diagnosis and Medical History.
Check for record of Physical Examination.
Make name plates for identification.
Make clothing list and mark clothing and valuables.
Notify dietary department, laundry, patient-activities director.
Make medication cards.

IN THE OFFICE

Complete the admission form and patient-admission agreement.
Obtain Consent for Care.
(Note: The admission form is usually done by administrative staff unless they are off duty, in which case the charge nurse MUST obtain it.)
Enter name in chronological record and assign case number.
Prepare permanent file.
Start financial records.
Notify Medicaid for assistance patients.

Magnify the meal service by determining preferences and special needs. It will mean much to the patient to discover that his desires and wishes are respected. The ultimate goal should be to release the patient to return to his home, even when there seems to be no possibility. Watch for emotional changes. Depression comes swiftly, and often without warning. If the patient is to make the proper adjustment, it is necessary that we help him avoid emotional upset. Simple teaching of the patient by the nursing staff may begin after admission as a means of helping the patient meet his needs.

Nursing Home and Physician Relationships

There are two primary relationships existing between the nursing home and the physician; one is legal and the other is ethical. The legal relationship is not necessarily a contractual one, but a relationship the nursing home assumes when providing care. Most state laws are written in a prohibiting vein. The physician is prohibited from practicing without proper training and license. The administrator is likewise prohibited, as is the nurse. The nurse must not only be trained and registered (licensed), but she is prohibited from infringing on the practice of the physician. Now, with the licensing of the nursing home administrator, this same type of relationship will exist between him and the physician. The physician shares, of course, the legal responsibility; but, like the nursing home administrator and the licensed/registered nurse, it is because he has been hired by the patient. The physician assumes no liability for acts of the nursing home. In the final sense, each person is responsible for his own acts.

There is an ethical interrelationship, also, which is very fundamental to the nursing care, as it involves the sacred trust that the home shares in the relief of suffering. It also involves the counsel that the learned physician may offer as to the involvement a nursing home assumes in the care of a patient. The administrator must never reflect upon the practice and reputation of the physician.

It is the responsibility of the nursing home to secure and follow the orders and advice of a licensed physician in the care of any patient. The policy of the home should require that the patient have a physical examination prior to admission. Normally, this is specified by a requirement of the licensing agency. The home will require written doctor's orders before giving a patient care, medications, or treatment. Transfer to a hospital will be on the orders of the physician. Verbal orders (telephone orders) will be signed by the licensed nurse taking the order and subsequently be submitted to the physician for countersignature within a specified time. All orders will be interpreted as written. PRN (pro re nata) for "as needed" allows the nurse to decide need only. Orders must be correlated to automatic stop orders established for a specific type of pharmaceuticals. Medication errors are to be reported to the physician immediately.

The policy of the home will require regular physician's visits for each patient, the maximum length of time between visits being set to comply with state and contractual requirements. In addition, the home should arrange for emergency attendance by a licensed physician other than the patient's attending physician. Should the attending physician not be available, it will be understood that the second physician may be called in an emergency. A transfer agreement with a local hospital should be executed. It is the privilege of the attending physician to recommend a private duty nurse in case of acute illness. The nursing home may render assistance in securing a private duty nurse and set patient-care standards for them, but they are independent contractors with the patient.

Another legal consideration will be the confidential nature of the clinical information concerning each patient. It is generally considered "privileged" by legal bodies and must not be revealed except by the expressly written permission by the one whom it concerns, so that it may be used for legal purposes, e.g., insurance claims, Medicaid classification of level of care, etc.

The nursing home may choose to use an organized medical staff, with rules and regulations which govern the care given by the physician and nursing staff to the patients in the home. In this event, the cooperation of the physicians in organizing and exercising the functions of the medical staff will be necessary. It has been suggested that the nursing home should hire a medical director who will assume this responsibility.

Medical Records

The keeping of good records is an essential business procedure that must not be overlooked. The administrator should survey every medical need and every medical service to see that it is appropriately recorded. Certain records pertain to various responsibilities. The student will ultimately, as he assumes the responsibility of management of the nursing home, collect, correlate, and use those records he feels is necessary to good management, legal documentation, and efficiency. The purpose of medical records is to assure the continuity of care of the patients in addition to the afore-stated usage.

A medical records librarian is employed in the larger nursing home, while a consulting medical records librarian may be used in the smaller home. This person's primary responsibility is to manage the collection, correlation, usage, and storage of records. The administrator will delegate the necessary authority to the medical records librarian through established policies and procedures.

Records needed at the time of admission are: medical history, physical examination, diagnosis, medical treatment initially required, recommendations of the social worker, admission, consent for care, and financial.

The admission record is essentially a record for identification and should include: the patient's name, usual address, age, sex, marital status, birth, occupation, birthplace, mother, father, military service, religion, Medicare and Medicaid numbers, emergency address, emergency phone number of responsible party, next of kin, attending physician, and any other necessary information.

Records to be completed at the time of discharge include: the transfer record to hospital/other facility/patient's home, release of responsibility when patient leaves against medical advice, request for release of medications, closing of financial agreement, release of valuables, plus recommendations by social worker. The transfer record may contain medical recommendations.

The closing of records imposes the following requirement: to close records within a specified period including a summary by the physician of discharge, diagnosis and prognosis; to store records permanently (a minimum of five years in the absence of state requirements), to see that some records (admission, discharge, and death) are preserved in the facility perpetually and are not destroyed, and to see that permanent records or stored records are transferred to any new owner.

The administrator should develop a great respect for records. The business market provides many fine record systems, or the administrator may devise his own. In fact, this is to be encouraged in some areas. While a number of records may be combined, it is difficult to be thorough when this is carried too far. Also, some system of maintaining the confidential nature of medical records should be devised. The security of records is the responsibility of the management.

For purposes of the control and cataloging of medical records, a serial number system may be used. In simple terms, each record is assigned a number as it is established. When used in connection with microfilm, the retrieval time for records in storage is minimized. This may be equally true for box storage of outdated records. The administrator may wish to assign each patient a case number and correlate all records for a specific patient according to this case number. Some examples of patient records appear on the following pages.

INCIDENT REPORT

Patient_____Date_____Time_____

Description of incident. (Include circumstances under which the incident occurred: Where did it occur? What was extent of injuries?)

_____
_____
_____
_____

Describe treatment given (Include first aid, state whether physician was called, what were his orders, whether patient was sent to hospital):

_____
_____
_____
_____
_____

If fatal, coroner's or physician's verdict:

_____
_____
_____

Witnesses to the incident:

_____
_____
_____

Physician notified _____Time_____
Relative notified _____Time_____
Supervisor notified_____Time_____

Signed by _____Title _____

PATIENT TRANSFER RECORD

Patient's name _____ Date _____

Birth Date_____ Sex_____ Medicare # _____

Marital Status   S____   M____   W____   D____   Religion _____

Nearest Relative _____ Relationship _____

Address _____ Phone _____

Facility transferred to_____

Address _____ Phone _____

Attending physician_____ Phone _____

Address _____

Diagnosis _____

Medications at time of transfer   Treatments

_____   _____

_____   _____

_____   _____

_____   _____

_____   _____

_____   _____

_____   _____

_____   _____

_____   _____

Mental status: Alert_____   Forgetful_____   Confused_____

Ambulatory: Yes____   No____   With assistance____   Bedfast_____

Diet _____ Appetite_____

Elimination: Bowel control_____   Bladder control_____

Remarks and pertinent information (brief description of condition)

_____

_____

_____

_____

Signed _____Title_____

Daily Clinical Records

On a continuing basis, the administrator will establish systems for keeping nurses' daily notes, routine clinical records, and the physician's orders and progress notes. There is a variety of record forms, but the nursing home will wish to correlate all records. The American Nursing Home Association, in cooperation with the Reynolds and Reynolds Company, Celina, Ohio, developed a standard record system for nursing homes. The administrator may wish to use such a standard system or devise and print his locally.

A list of the types of records required on a daily basis includes: the updating of identifying information; physician's orders concerning medication, treatments, diet, and medical procedures; physician's progress notes, including periodic medical examination, observations, and recommendations; nurses' notes, including medication, treatment, vital signs, and observations of the patient's progress and condition; nursing care plan; laboratory reports; incident reports; progress notes of paraprofessional personnel, i.e., dentist, physical therapist, occupational therapist, psychiatrist, and consultants; and director's plans and progress for social activities.

For records to be authentic, they must be complete, including the time, date, patient's name, type of medical attention given, and appropriate signature in ink. The signing of records includes the physician, the nurse, the administrator, and other paramedical personnel. It is noteworthy that an individual may be required to verify his signature; therefore, he should make it legible. He should sign only records of his own actions.

The correcting of records must be done according to legal precedent. The most acceptable has been to draw a line through the error and write the correction above it. The person making the correction should then initial and date the correction.

There is a pattern of certain medical records which must be correlated. This sequence is: observations and medical symptoms are relayed to the attending physician, who makes a diagnosis, for which he then prescribes drugs and/or treatment. The nurse administers what the physician has prescribed and then continues to make observations and detect symptoms of improvement in the condition of the patient. The new observations are relayed to the physician, who may in turn revise his diagnosis and treatment which require new orders. This cycle may be repeated many times for the long-term illness. The important factor is that observations, diagnosis, and treatment shall be in agreement. This factor will demonstrate the effectiveness of medical care, and medical records should reflect this key factor.

Another record that helps the nursing staff to correlate the total care of the patient is the Patient Care Plan developed under the direction of the supervisor of nurses. This is essentially a summary of all patient needs and the nursing actions necessary to meet those needs. This record is usually set up on a cardex system. It may take one of two styles, each of which has merit. The first type is a chronological summary of all entries. In this, the entries are dated and entered consecutively. Each entry will state the nursing or patient care problem and the action to be taken. Recorded at the top of the cardex is identifying information and the long-term goal.

The second type of a patient-care plan is a comprehensive listing of problems and patient-care needs with suggested actions. After the customary identifying data, several general areas of needs are identified and space is allowed for the plan of correction of each. Although each area is identified, it does not preclude making more specific entries as to the need of the individual patient. General areas of need include: safety precautions, living adjustments, assistance in physical needs, emotional needs, family involvement, and patient teaching. It is easy to see that this type tends to suggest entries that may be made.

In both plans, periodic updating is necessary to make the use of the record effective. It is suggested that a period be established, i.e., each week, month, or quarter, for the updating and revision of the plan.

Social and Miscellaneous Records

While social and incidental records are technically not medical, in a nursing home all records concerning a patient are treated as having a medical-social relationship, except purely administrative records, i.e., financial. Social activity records have a complementary relationship with medical records.

A social history should be kept. It may be accumulated and compiled by a social worker. Even if the nursing home does not employ a professional social worker, a staff member could be designated to accomplish these records.

The initial social history should contain entries concerning: previous occupation, cultural background, educational achievement, interests, hobbies, and other pertinent information. Additional notes concerning adjustment to group living, responses, problems, attitudes, and interests, are made from time to time. The social record is correlated with the medical records. The Medicaid caseworker assists in compiling the history of old-age assistance to recipient patients. The administrator may wish to include within this record system a record of social activities.

The social activities director should make notes of the various activities which each patient attends and transfer this information to the permanent record of each patient. Medicaid and Medicare require the director to develop a plan of activities for each patient. The plan is to be within the goals of the overall plan of care developed by the supervisor of nurses for each patient. Periodic revision of the plan of activities is suggested, with notes, attendance records, and other data recorded to document progress in meeting the plan.

A record of clothing and possessions should be kept. Upon admission, a complete record is made, signed by the representative of the nursing home and countersigned by the patient and/or relative/guardian. This record should be updated with any addition or disposal of items. It shows clothing, valuables, luggage, and any other items. A copy of the initial survey is furnished the patient, and the other copy remains with the patient's records.

Incident records should be kept. A report is made for each incident affecting the patient, whether or not bodily injury resulted. It includes a report of either injury or abuse of the patient. Since this is a legal matter that may be used to document the absence of negligence by the home, it should be thorough and complete. It will be specific as to the time, place, circumstances, and persons involved. It will include actions taken after the incident, including notification of physician and next of kin, the treatment given, transfer to a hospital, etc. Witnesses should be listed. It is signed by the supervisor, one copy going to the administrator and one remaining with the patient's clinical charts. It should be noted that some administrators may prefer to receive the only copy of this record because of the legal ramifications. In this case, he would first check his state regulations and act accordingly.

The information recorded in an incident report should be totally objective. That is, no opinions are written into it. Take, for example, the following statement:

"I heard Mrs. M. crying for help but did not think it was my responsibility to go see about her; however, the continued crying grated on my nerves, because the person assigned to give her nursing care simply would not go to her aid. When I found her, she had slipped on a wet spot the janitor had failed to mop up. She was seriously hurt with a broken leg. I immediately picked her up, taking care to watch her broken leg and put her on the bed. It was then that she died. I am glad that I got her off the hard cold floor first."

It is obvious that several opinions were written into this statement, as well as some damaging evidence of negligence by the person making the report. In its proper perspective, a properly trained aide would have made a more objective report. It might read:

"I heard Mrs. M. cry for help and went immediately to her room, where I found her lying on the floor about three feet from the foot of the bed. I immediately signaled for the charge nurse and stayed with Mrs. M. until she came. I did not move the patient. The charge nurse examined her and requested she still not be moved until she called the doctor. He ordered her to the hospital. Ambulance attendants removed her from the floor and transported her to the hospital; she was reported to have internal injuries."

The administrator should endeavor to train his employees in the proper handling and reporting of emergencies.

Chapter 13

Nutrition and Modified Diets

Dietary Facilities

The dietary facilities of the nursing home appear in several areas, depending upon the size and arrangement of the nursing home. No matter how varied the facilities are, a number of common provisions are made.

Provision must be made for the proper storage of foods. Since requirements by contractual agencies or the licensing agency usually specify the minimum amount to be on hand at any given time, the size needed for proper storage can be determined. The home will need storage for perishables, frozen foods, staples, ice, milk in bulk, and smaller supplies.

A systematic provision for receiving foodstuff, one that is correlated with planned ordering, should be provided. Temporary storage at the receiving point will be made until stocks can be put on the shelves. Larger homes may have a system of preportioning foodstuff before placing on the shelves.

Provision for food preparation allows for cooking and baking, and care of perishables and liquids. The arrangement will depend upon the size of the facility and the number of meals prepared daily. Whether it is a central kitchen or a small decentralized kitchen, using mostly prepackaged preparations and frozen portions, will affect the arrangement.

Provision for serving includes a system for assembling and preparing the trays, use of carts or other means of transporting trays, means of keeping foods warm or cool, and a system of identifying special diets.

The dining room should be systematically arranged, aesthetically designed, and socially appealing to the patients. Tables should be attractive, high enough for wheelchair patients, and small enough to allow selective companionship. Chairs should be stable, easily cleaned, and comfortable. Nursing home patients usually like a chair with arms.

Provision for cleanup includes a way of retrieving dishes and trays, a dishwashing system, a pot washing system, and means of cleaning and sanitizing the entire dietary facility. Most authorities recommend sanitizing dishes at 170 °F to 180 °F. In connection with cleanup, dishes and utensils are put away in the space reserved for them.

Employees working with food must be provided with rest room facilities for washing their hands and storing personal possessions. A means of disposing of garbage and refuse has to be set up. Some control measures, including the recording and filing of menus, are needed to maintain the dietary system in compliance with local regulations and those of the Food and Drug Administration. Also, it is necessary for dietary aides to supervise and report on eating habits of patients. This report is then sent to the charge nurse, who enters it in the patients' clinical charts.

Finally, it is the responsibility of the administrator to develop and publish the dietary policy of the nursing home. This may be done with the cooperation of the dietitian or nutrition consultant. It is recommended that they be reviewed and revised annually and, when a change of policy is necessary, that they be amended.

The following is a typical statement of dietary policy.

DIETARY POLICY

The food service manager with the regular consultation of a registered dietitian is responsible for the total food service. This manager will participate in conferences with the administrator, the director of nursing, and others responsible for patient care.

A head cook, relief cook, breakfast cook, and kitchen helpers are under the supervision of the food service manager. There is at least one person on duty in the kitchen at all times from 6:00 A.M. to 6:00 P.M., seven days a week. All employees shall participate in selected in-service education programs. Work schedules and duty assignment are to be kept posted.

Three meals are served daily at regular times with not more than 14 hours between the night meal and breakfast. Snacks are served regularly before bedtime, at midafternoon, and at midmorning.

The menus are planned in advance by the food service manager, in cooperation with the dietitian, to include a four-week cycle and these must meet the dietary allowances of the Food and Nutrition Board of the National Research Council. The menus are posted in the kitchen. Any substitutions made are to be noted on the menus and are to be of foods of an equal nutritional value. The menus as served are kept on file for at least thirty days.

Food will be purchased in sufficient amounts to ensure a supply of staple food for one week and a supply of perishable food for at least two days. These foods are stored off the floor and at proper temperature.

The patient's food preferences are served in a form the individual patient can eat without difficulty. Food is kept at proper temperatures before serving.

Table service is encouraged for all patients who are able to come to the dining room. A tray for each patient is marked or flagged with a color-coded diet card to ensure reaching the correct individual. Sturdy tray holders and over-bed tables are provided for patients who do not come to the dining room. Food service attendants report the eating habits of the patients to the food service manager, who will send a compiled report to the charge nurse for entry into the clinical charts.

Modified diets are served as ordered by the physician. It is the responsibility of the dietitian or nutrition consultant to advise as to the preparation and food exchange for such modified diets. A good recommended diet manual will be kept with the records of the food service.

It is suggested that the food service manager maintain a file of menus, cookbooks, portions, and ingredients. It is further suggested that the pantry shelves be marked to indicate types of staples normally stored. A pantry checklist will facilitate ordering.

Sanitary procedures are used to ensure proper sterilization of dishes and utensils. Compliance with local and state health regulation for food service and eating establishments will be maintained.

Dietary Staff

Staffing the dietary facility with trained, competent help is no small task because of the demand placed upon the food service. Even the smallest facility prepares meals, annually, numbering in the tens of thousands. The fact that the kitchen must be open seven days a week, the year round, is exceeded only by the demand on the nursing service.

Place the kitchen and related dietary facilities under the direction of a registered dietitian. If the facility is not large enough to afford a dietitian full-time, then engage a nutrition consultant (a registered dietitian) to assist the food service manager.

The food service manager, if not the dietitian, will be totally responsible for the supervision of the dietary department. She will be considered the head of the dietary department and will participate on the supervisory level. With her, there will be one or more cooks who will be directly responsible to her. These may be specialists, such as a breakfast cook, dinner cook, baker, salad maker, etc. The number varies with the need.

The dishwashing and clean-up staff will function as a unit but be responsible to the head of the dietary department. The dining room attendants will likewise function as a unit and be responsible to the food service manager. Both dining room and clean-up units may have a foreman, when the number warrants it. Room service is usually handled by the nurses' aides after the trays are delivered to the various distribution points.

The dietary staff has several specific requirements. Periodic health check-ups are required, and the daily health maintenance of staff members must be met. Hygienic food handling is required. There is no other single source of infection that can be so disastrous as the food service.

Training is required to maintain the high standards of a successful food service. The study of special diets, nutrition, food handling, food poisoning, and patient relations are a few items of the special curriculum for dietary personnel.

Daily work assignments are essential to the efficient operation of the food service and will vary from facility to facility. The job description will indicate the total responsibility of staff members; however, the food service manager will develop and post daily work assignments. An example for one of the cooks might be:

Reports ready to work at 9:00 A.M.
Makes preliminary preparation for noon meal.
Prepares meal, including special diets.
Supervises serving of meal.
Stores all leftover food; plans for its use.

Supervises and inspects clean-up.
Break.
Checks pantry and supplies.
Makes preliminary preparation for evening meal.
Assists evening cook in preparation of meal.
Lets evening cook supervise serving.
Checks out at 5:00 P.M.

The administrator will work with the food service manager to see that adequate duty assignments are written and that a procedure manual is prepared and in use for all tasks within the food service.

Some assignments are made not daily but weekly. These will be posted just as is the daily assignment. The food service manager will study work loads and schedule for periodic revision. Note the following example:

Day:	Duty assignment:	Person responsible:
Monday	Straighten pantry; requisition	Mrs. A.
Tuesday	Clean filters, refrigerator	Mrs. B.
Wednesday	Clean shelves	Mrs. C.
Thursday	Clean stove	Mrs. A
Friday	Clean ice machine, freezer	Mrs. B.
Saturday	Wax dining room floor	Custodian

To this list of duty assignments may be added a number of tasks that a particular food service manager may identify and assign to various employees. It is also necessary for the manager to conduct periodically performance checks on these assignments. The times for certain duties may be designated or left flexible.

Food Preparation and Serving

The scope of this text will not permit a course in nutrition, merely the listing of the essential elements required. The administrator should take the training opportunities offered by the dietitian or others.

The menu is the cycle established for food offerings. It generally follows the three-meals-per-day plan but could be expanded to five per day. The menu will usually repeat itself in two to four weeks and will be revised, seasonally, to take advantage of seasonal foods and eating habits. Once the menu has been established, care should be taken to see that it is followed, that substitutions offered are of equal nutritive value, and the changes are recorded.

Special consideration in preparation should be taken to see that measuring is accurate, that there is proper refrigeration of perishables and that a minimum of food handling is done. Prepackaged and prepared quantities, such as frozen portions, may be more efficient. Foods should be covered at all times for sanitation.

Special consideration of seasoning should be given according to the type of patients the nursing home is serving. It is generally thought that aged persons have only 25% of their taste buds functioning, thus making the natural flavor a goal of the food service. Consideration of the special diets required will make seasoning more difficult.

Special safeguards for handling food should be established. Immediate removal of food spillage should be practiced, as well as thorough cleansing and sanitation. The use of hairnets for women should be required. The administrator should not allow the use of cracked china, improper containers, poor refrigeration, or careless practices of employees. A proper and safe rodent and pest control system should be established.

A word about portions and offerings is in order. Since the home is primarily engaged in rehabilitation of the patient, care should be taken that every patient has an adequate meal. Allowance for seconds and substitute offerings will need to be made. Allowance for substitutes because of religious beliefs is sometimes necessary.

Basic Nutrition and General Diet Menu

The administrator should provide, for the dietary department, several resource books on food preparation, special diets, and serving techniques. The Austin Dietary Council of the Austin Area Hospital Council, Austin, Texas, combined resources and published a diet manual peculiar to its own local needs. The Dietetic Service Staff, Ruby P. Puckett, R.D., Director, Shands Teaching Hospital and Clinic, University of Florida, Gainesville, Florida publishes a *Guide to Normal Nutrition and Diet Modification Manual,* which represents an excellent regional effort. Other good manuals are the *Mayo Clinic Diet Manual,* W. B. Saunders Co., Philadelphia, and *Food Service Manual,* American Hospital Association. An excellent planning book for the cook is *Nursing Home Menu Planning–Food Purchasing, Management* by Brother Herman E. Zaccarelli, C.S.C., and Mrs. Josephine Maggiore, R.D., Cahners Books, Boston. This book will help the dietitian/cook to plan for the systematic purchase of foodstuff and the preparation of a well-balanced diet. It contains a number of aids, but its chief value is in the section, "Menus for 52 Weeks."

The basic foods are considered to be milk, meat, fruits, vegetables, breads, all of which should be offered daily. However, the aged differ from younger persons in their general requirements of nutrition. Because of tissue saturation, the protein requirement is much higher the older a person becomes. Eating meat is sometimes difficult for the aged, so care should be taken to chop or grind it for them. The need for vitamins and minerals increases. The use of fortified foods is to be encouraged. Caloric needs usually decrease because of the slowdown in activity.

The food nutrients are listed as the vitamin and mineral groups. The vitamin groups include A, B, B₁, C, D, and K. The mineral groups include calcium, phosphorus, iron, iodine, copper, and sodium.

In achieving a good food service for the elderly, a number of factors are important. Proper nutrition is important. To overcome the effects of weakened body systems, eating becomes all important. Consider the weakened, rarefied bones, the saturated cells, the thinning of the skin, the atrophy of tissue, the loss of circulation, and you soon note the jeopardy in which the average elderly person lives. Allow for the poor eating habits of the aged. Their differences, their peculiarities, the need for chopped and strained foods, their incessant hunger when meals are late, and dozens of other problems, make for an unusual food service.

Special Diets

It is frequently necessary to prescribe for a patient a special diet, because of some imbalance in the physical condition of the patient. Generally speaking, there must be a balanced number of calories eaten with the the amount of energy loss or calories used up by the body. Any loss in body matter or liquid must be replaced. In addition, some diseases are aggravated by certain elements in the diet, and these must be restricted. Thus the physician will prescribe a modified diet.

Diets may be modified in a number of ways. Increasing the liquid content is the most common. Restricting sodium content is another. Sometimes irritating foods or heavy residue foods will not be offered. One may restrict fat or gluten, control calories, or lower mineral content. Some patients may need a high protein diet, and others may not. Some of the more frequently prescribed modified diets are as listed below.

Diabetic diet. This is a very complicated diet-control procedure in which a basic metabolism rate is maintained by the
control of carbohydrates and insulin. It has the dual purpose of
restricting the intake of both sugar and calories.

Low sodium diet. Usually prescribed as #1, #2, #3, etc. Low
salt is not the same diet as low sodium.

Low residue. Cellulose or roughage is removed.

Low fat. To restrict lipids, lower cholesterol.

Soft diet. Often, because of postoperative physical handicaps, or chronic infirmities, it is necessary to serve foods of soft
consistency.

Liquid diet. Foods are sometimes prepared in a semiliquid
form because of tube-feeding, swallowing difficulties, or need for
large amounts of liquid.

The administrator and the dietitian, in cooperation with the
supervising nurse, develop a system of modified diets. First the diet is
prescribed by the physician. A diet sheet should then be prepared for
the cook. Some notation system should be developed to ensure that
the correct patient receives his prescribed diet.

Food As Related to the Patient's Well-Being

The diet is a means of encouraging the patient toward greater satisfaction and happiness and of combating some of the emotional and
physical problems accompanying nursing home living. Some of the
related emotional factors that present themselves in institutional living
are relocation, loneliness, and new diet. These may bring on problems
such as food phobias.

A number of physical problems will make the problem of diet
more difficult. Some patients have an inability to masticate their food
properly. Others are confined to their room and must eat alone. Still
others may resent the rigid serving schedule, having eaten at home
when they felt hungry. With the loss of up to 75% of their taste buds,
the loss of dexterity of the hands, and the restrictions in their diet,
many elderly have a difficult time adjusting.

The administrator must train his staff to realize the difficulties and
make some effort to surmount them. There are a number of things that
can be done. A survey to determine individual food preferences can be
made, and food can be prepared to overcome eating difficulties. The
meal should never be hurried; congenial companions should eat
together, so that the meal may become a satisfying social experience.

The use of lightweight dinner service may be helpful. With some encouragement, most elderly eventually will accept the meal schedule.

The dietitian will want to offer the widest variety of foods possible. She should strive to make the tray colorful and to make the food offerings appetizing. Break up the serving routine from time to time by having a patio picnic or special holiday offerings. Nothing will gain wider acceptance than having the patient's family invited to dinner. With some study and planning, the dietitian may cater to the patients' requests.

A supplementary diet between meals will break up what may be a long monotonous day. Often the patient is lonely, and the tray service by a cheerful attendent will be the only bright spot all day. A bedtime snack or the five-meal-a-day plan may help to create a completely new atmosphere in the nursing home.

Chapter *14*

Safety, Sanitation, and Housekeeping

Safety, Disaster, and Evacuation

Safety should become a way of life for the staff of the nursing home. It is an obligation to make the facility safe for the patient, to practice safe work habits, and to continue to upgrade safety. Even the location of the nursing home near fire protection is important.

Disasters never come with warning; they just happen. It is the obligation of the administrator to plan carefully what actions will be taken if disaster strikes. Disaster takes many forms, for each of which there should be a plan of action. Fire is the most common and will constitute our primary concern. However, windstorm, explosion, riot, or contagion may strike. For any disaster, the staff must be trained continually in the proper procedures.

The administrator should be aware of the psychology of reaction to disaster. There is usually some inability to act, an inability to think or reason, lack of time for decision, and an almost complete reliance on action by rote methods or training. In planning for safety after disaster, one should predict as nearly as possible the probable results, i.e., smoke, loss of light, fear, panic, etc. Priority should be given to averting loss of life and the summoning of help.

Disaster planning has certain basic elements. *Plan to gain the maximum warning, in time to avoid loss.* In such planning, mechanical devices are better than human reactions and may be a simple heat-activated sensor, a smoke detector, or a fully automatic sprinker system that will not only sense the fire and give an alarm but will in addition give off a preventive spray of water in the danger area.

Plan for priority of action. Investigate, sound the alarm, remove the patient, notify the office, and fight the fire are actions to be taken. The administrator must establish the correct priority of actions and then train the employees to react in this sequence.

The foremost question is whether an emergency actually exists; therefore a quick investigation is the first priority. Pulling the nearest manual alarm would seem to be the next priority. However, two things may be done as a part of investigation: remove any patient in immediate danger and close the door to contain the fire. But quickly—don't let these actions detract from sounding that alarm because you will need help. One should get the attention of someone to handle another priority: confirming the fire with the office and calling the fire department, if the alarm system is not directly connected with it. Now another priority: reduce the fire with emergency fire-fighting equipment, the extinguishers. Another priority emerges in that general evacuation may be necessary. Don't worry, since others are now arriving and can handle this. Keep fighting the fire until the fire department arrives; they are less than five minutes away.

Planning for a complete evacuation according to specific methods is the final priority. The evacuation shall be through specified exits to designated collection points, using proper patient-carry methods. Because of the adoption of the National Life Safety Code, most nursing homes (especially those that provide care for bedfast patients) have been arranged to allow the patients' beds to be rolled through the bedroom door into an unobstructed corridor and then through any fire exit. Normally, fire exits are specified and marked according to fire regulations. The employees should be made aware that the presence of fire hose strung through the corridors will nullify the evacuation of the patient's bed, unless they are prepared to lift it over the hose. There has also been some reconsideration of the type of fire extinguisher (Type A is designated for trash and rubbish, type BC is for grease and oil, and type ABC is an all-purpose dry chemical extinguisher for type A fires, type B fires, and type C electrical fires). While an ABC extinguisher might seem logical, some fire marshals recommend only pressurized water for the patients' living areas. In any event, the fire extinguisher must have the approval of the local fire marshal. The evacuation plan must also be approved.

The completed disaster plan is then written, posted, studied by the employees, and practiced regularly, at least 12 times a year. It is noteworthy that nursing home employees are now expected to demonstrate their knowledge and skill in executing the nursing home disaster plan.

Multi-storied facilities will develop a basic plan with a subdivision for each section or floor. To this basic plan may be added such additional information as patient-carry methods, first aid, first aid firefighting measures, instructions on alarm systems, and additional evacuation information necessary to complete a plan for a particular home. One necessary part of each plan is a diagram of each section of the nursing home with avenues of escape clearly marked through approved exits. The Life Safety Code, National Fire Protection Association (Boston, 1967 edition) asserts that panic among persons fleeing an emergency will usually not develop as long as they are moving away from the point of danger through a clearly marked passage that is unobstructed and leads to safety. We include a basic plan which may be used for a specific section:

DISASTER PLAN IN CASE OF FIRE

Investigate quickly the circumstances of emergency, remove any patient from immediate danger, and close the door to contain the fire, then:

Pull the alarm at the nearest alarm box. Send the next person at hand to the office to confirm the fire and notify the fire department.

Fight the fire with extinguishers to reduce it. When the person reporting to the office returns, let him get a second extinguisher.

General evacuation is begun by the next arrivals. Lead the ambulatory patients first to the safety of another fire section. Use patient-carry methods for moving most bed patients and move the remainder in their beds.

Emergency measures: See that fire doors between sections are closed and remain closed. The designated collection point in the event of total evacuation of the building is:

Location of fire extinguishers.
Notify the following persons.
General information.

The employees of the nursing home must be familiar with its first-aid fire-fighting and emergency equipment, which includes fire extinguishers, alarm systems, sprinkler systems, and patient-evacuation aids. Cooperation with the local fire department and a planned training program provide fundamental preparation for coping with fire emergencies. An excellent demonstration seminar could be conducted concerning the four basic types of patient-carry methods, as indicated below:

Pack strap carry method: Place the patient on your back, draping his arms over your shoulder, letting his feet drag.

Hip carry method: Carry patient horizontally across your back and hips.

Extremity carry method: Two people carry the patient, one taking the arms and shoulders, the other the legs.

Swing carry method: Two people carry the patient between them, dragging his feet.

Planning to reduce fire hazards should include: supervision of smoking by the patient, protection for the wandering patient, safety rails, oxygen safety practices, regular inspections. The hazards of oxygen are perhaps the most frightening. However, the therapeutic value of this life-giving substance far outweighs such dangers because, with careful handling, proper administration, and constant education, it may be used safely.

One of the characteristics of oxygen is that, while it does not itself burn, it combines with other flammables to raise the temperature very rapidly. Some flammables in the presence of oxygen ignite spontaneously, for example, oil in most forms, grease, ether, some alcohols, dust and electrical equipment not sealed against arcing. When a substance itself contains heat, such as lighted cigarets, heating pads, flashlights, electric razors, or open flame, oxygen will cause flash fires of intense heat.

It is for the reasons cited that the administrator must formulate safety rules and regulations for the handling, storage, and administration of oxygen. It is suggested that storage be limited within the building, that oxygen be under restricted conditions when stored, e.g., cylinders chained to stable mounts, ventilation in closets, mercury switches, and warning signs.

Safety Check List

The following check list was prepared for instructional use by the Department of Nursing Home Administration, McLennan Community College, Waco, Texas. The material is adapted from the *Building and Construction Manual* published by the Texas State Department of

Health, Nursing and Convalescent Home Division, Howard Allen, Director. This department has adopted the 1967 edition of the Life Safety Code as their minimum standard. This check list will reflect these standards.

NURSING HOME SAFETY CHECK LIST

ALARM SYSTEM: Installed as required?____; Electrically supervised?____; Manually operated?____; Visible warning device?____; Coded as to section?____; Manual pull station in each fire section?____; Maximum travel to sending station is 200 feet?____; Tested weekly?____; Arrangement to notify fire department?____.

BEDROOMS: Doors to means of egress?____; Doors not through other rooms?____; Attendants have keys to locked rooms?____; No basement bedrooms?____; Are beds on casters?____ Are nonmovable beds occupied by self-care patients?____.

CAPACITY OF THE NURSING HOME: One person to each 120 square feet in sleeping quarters?____One person to each 240 square feet in treatment area?____; Private rooms of at least 100 square feet?____; Multiple occupancy bedrooms of at least 80 square feet per person?____.

CHUTES FOR LINENS, TRASH, RUBBISH: Are safeguards provided?____; Is chute not directly connected to flue or firechamber?____; Does it have self-closing doors?____; Protected by one-hour fire resistive construction?____; Or automatic sprinkler?____; Is fire detection provided?____; Is it vented to the outside?____.

CONSTRUCTION: Does new construction conform to all requirements of the Life Safety Code?____; Does the conversion of structures to nursing home conform to requirement of the code?____; If the nursing home existed before adoption of the code, have modifications been made according to the authority having jurisdiction?____; Were these modifications of equal safety?____; If one-story, does it have one-hour fire resistive contruction?____; If two-story, or higher, does it have two-hour fire resistive contruction?____; Are occupancies other than nursing home separated by two-hour fire resistive construction?____.

CORRIDORS: Newly constructed to be eight-foot widths?____; Existing construction at least 48 inches in width?____; Are dead-end corridors limited to 30 feet in length?____.

DOORS: Are bedroom doors of the swinging type?____; Is direction of swing in the direction of egress when serving 50 or more persons?____; Is bedroom door width 44 inches in the clear?____; 40 inches in the clear for existing construction?____; Are doors not subject to use by bedroom occupants at least 28 inches in width?____; Are bedroom doors constructed of 1-3/4 inch bonded solid core wood?____; If locked, is the lock accessible on corridor side?____; Does an attendent have the key?____; Are fire doors and smoke doors self-closing?____; Are they held open electrically?____; Is hold device activated by the alarm system?____; Are doors to the stairway enclosure normally closed?____.

DRAPERIES, CURTAINS, ROOM DIVIDERS: Are they of fire retardant materials?____.

EGRESS OR AVENUE OF ESCAPE: Are all avenues of escape unobstructed?____; Free and unlocked?____; Arranged for distinct pathways?____; Well marked?____; Illuminated by at least 1.0 candlepower?____; Powered by an acceptable electrical company?____; Illuminated in emergencies?____.

ELEVATORS: Are they properly installed according to Life Safety Code?____; Are they counted only as supplemental exits?____; Do the doors work properly?____; Have a fireman's switch and safety control been installed?____.

EQUIPMENT: Has air-conditioning, heating, and other equipment been properly installed?____; Is it operated with safety?____; Is it maintained promptly and regularly?____; Are portable space heaters not allowed?____; Are open gas flame heaters not allowed?____; Is combustion air for heaters taken from the outside?____; Fumes vented to outside?____; Is fire protection of one-hour construction or automatic sprinkler provided?____; Does the authority having jurisdiction require both one-hour construction and automatic sprinklers?____.

EVACUATION PLAN: Does the nursing home have an approved, written evacuation plan?____; Is the plan made available to all employees?____; Does the nursing home administration provide instruction?____; Is simulated evacuation practiced regularly?____; (See Fire Drills.)

EXITS: Do you understand that exit means a continuous path of egress to ground level, outside a building?____; That access is considered part of the exit?____; That exits counted include only doors, stairs, ramps, and horizontal openings?____; That discharge area is also considered part of the exit?____; Is exit access protected by one-hour construction up to three stories?____; Two-hour construction for four or more stories?____; Do all exits have self-closing doors?____; Is the capacity of exits in the nursing home computed at 30 persons per 22 inch unit of travel space?____; Is this capacity computed at 20 persons per unit over stairs?____; Are exits illuminated at 1.0 foot-candle?____; Are the exit paths well marked by exit signs?____; Do the signs have constant internal illumination of at least 5.0 foot-candles?____; Are the letters at least 4½ inches high?____; If the signs are externally lighted, are letters at least 6 inches high?____; Are at least two exits provided for each fire area?____; Is one either a door or stairs?____; Is the travel distance from the patient's door to exit door no more then 100 feet?____; Is the maximum travel distance from any point limited to 150 feet?____; Have these distances been increased 50 feet with the installation of an automatic sprinkler system?____; Do you know that existing construction can have a maximum travel distance of 150 feet?____.

FIRE EXTINGUISHERS: Do you have manual extinguishers?____ Are they CO_2?____; Dry chemical?____; Pressurized water?____; Has the authority having jurisdiction required automatic fire extinguishers in hazardous areas in lieu of an automatic sprinkler system?____.

FIRE DRILLS: Do you have at least 12 drills pe. year?____; Do you have them on each of the three shifts?____; Are all employees expected to participate?____; Do you have drills at unexpected times?____; Does the drill simulate sounding the alarm?____; Actual emergencies?____; Do you major on evacuation rather than fire-fighting?____.

FURNISHINGS: Are furnishings of fire-retardant materials?____; Are drapes?____; Are cubicle curtains?____; Are carpets?____; If some furnishings are not of fire-retardant materials, are they not highly flammable?____; Or do not produce high, acrid smoke?____; Do furnishings not obstruct exits and avenues of egress?____.

GUARDRAILS: Are guardrails in use on balconies, horizontal openings?____; Are they 42 inches high?____; Is there no more than a 10-inch clearance above the floor?____.

HANDRAILS: Are handrails placed in corridors or other community passages to afford independence to the handicapped?____; Are they mounted 30 to 34 inches above the floor?____; Is there 1½ inches clearance from the wall?____; Will they support 200 pounds deadweight?____.

HAZARDOUS MATERIALS: Are hazardous materials clearly separated from patient areas?____; Are they stored in a vented room?____; With self-closing door?____; With one-hour fire-resistive construction?____; Are avenues of egress away from storage area?____; Are they clearly marked as hazardous materials?____.

HEATING: Has the heating and air-conditioning room been constructed of one-hour fire-resistive construction?____; Is there ventilation from the outside?____; Is smoke-venting led directly to the outside?____; Is the heating room properly sprinkled?____.

HORIZONTAL EXITS: Are horizontal exits at least 44 inches wide?____; Are they protected with one-hour fire-resistive constuction?____.

LIGHTS, EMERGENCY: Is emergency lighting of at least one hour duration provided?____; Does it come on automatically?____ Is there no more than a 10-second delay before coming on the line?____.

OCCUPANCY: Do you restrict occupancy to those under your control?____; Do you have additional educational activities?____; Do you offer 24-hour patient care?____; To four or more persons?____; Who are incapacitated?____; Who need the assistance of another person?____; When occupancy for other purposes than nursing care is allowed, is the activity separated by two-hour fire-resistive construction?____.

PANIC HARDWARE: Is the panic bar at least ⅔ of the width of the door?____; Is it mounted 30 to 44 inches above the floor?____; Will it open with 15 pounds body pressure?____; Is it approved when required?____.

RAMPS: Are they at least 44 inches wide?____; No more than 1 inch rise to 12 inches run?____; Is the vertical travel no more than six feet?____; Is proper construction used?____.

SMOKING: Is smoking regulated?____; Is it prohibited near oxygen and combustibles by "No Smoking" signs?____; Is smoking prohibited for patients who are not responsible for their actions?____; Are fire-proof ashtrays provided in smoking areas?____; Do trash cans in smoking areas have self-closing lids?____.

SPRINKLERS: Are they required by the authority having jusrisdiction?____; Are they exempted by reason of one-hour fire-resistive construction?____; When required, are they automatic?____; With proper supply of water?____; With a water-flow system?____; Is the system periodically tested?____; Was the system approved for installation?____; Is it properly maintained?____; When a fully automatic sprinkler system is not required, is at least a partial system required for hazardous areas?____; Is the kitchen protected?____; Heater rooms?____; Laundry?____; Soiled linen storage?____; Maintenance area?____; Hazardous materials storage?____.

SMOKESTOP PARTITIONS: Are two fire sections provided on each floor?____; Are corridors limited to 150 feet in each fire section?____;

Are smoke-stop partitions of one-hour-fire-resistive construction?____;
Is the only passage through smoke-stop partitions by way of smoke
doors?____.

STAIRWAY WELLS: Are stairway wells of one-hour noncombustible construction?____; Do they have self-closing doors?____; Are the
doors normally kept closed?____; Are stairways well marked?____.

VERTICAL OPENINGS: Are vertical openings of one-hour noncombustible construction?____; Do they have self-closing doors?____;
Are the doors normally kept closed?____.

WINDOWS: Are windows in smoke-stop partitions of wire-
glass?____; Limited to 1296 square inches?____; Installed in approved
metal frames?____; Do bedroom windows open on to the outside?____; Do they have an operable section?____.

The check list is an adaption of minimum requirements for safety.
Some of the requirements are by the authority having jurisdiction,
which may mean the local ordinance, the state regulation, or the
federal statute. For example, the 1967 edition of the Life Safety Code
does not require automatic sprinkler systems but a later edition does.
The former edition presupposes that the authority having jurisdiction
may require a sprinkler system.

Sanitation Principles

A good administrator is keenly aware of the relationship between filth,
infection, and disease. Filth may be caused by anyone who makes no
provision to prevent it; he may simply contribute to the conditions that
allow filth to exist, or fail to exercise proper control measures.

*Like disease, filth has certain symptoms: odors, accumulated
rubbish, unsanitary methods, evidence of dirt and grime, poor building
maintenance, and cross-contamination.* Specimens may be taken and
cultures incubated to detect bacteria. Most health inspectors are
looking for these evidences. Disease, if given proper incubation
conditions (warmth, moisture, lack of disturbance, and time) will
usually develop.

*Prevention of the spread of filth and infection may be done in three
different ways: eliminate the microorganism that causes the disease,
eliminate the conditions for incubation, or disrupt the time cycle which
allows the bacteria to incubate.*

Sanitation, or infection control, may be so designed as to prevent
the spread of disease. There are three basic methods which are normally used. The first is sterilization by heat, incineration, or boiling,

which destroys the pathogen, the agent that causes disease. The second method is to disinfect through chemical application. This method does not destroy the pathogen except in the case of complete chemical saturation with the powerful chemical disinfectants. Normally, the germ-killing power of a disinfectant is rated in comparison with carbolic acid. Thus, if the germ-killing power of an agent is rated as a coefficient of 10, it is ten times as powerful as carbolic acid. The third method is to remove the condition that permits the bacteria to grow. This is normally done with soaps, cleansers, and detergents, all of which can remove the dirt and filth that allows incubation of germs. Proper ventilation will further facilitate sanitation.

There are other preventive methods that the nursing home may adopt, such as containing potential contamination within a specified area. For example, the linen room should be considered a "clean area" and the staff trained to keep out infection-causing conditions. The same principle should be applied to the handling of trash, soiled laundry, contaminated materials, etc. There must be a hand-washing requirement for all personnel after handling contaminated materials. Laundry services must be organized and performed so as to prevent the spread of disease. Storage of contaminated materials and waste in plastic bags in a separate area will isolate contamination. A central source of sterile supplies and materials will allow greater control. Finally, the application of sanitation principles to the entire housekeeping process will keep contamination from starting within the facility.

PROCEDURE FOR PATIENT ISOLATION

Objectives: To prevent direct or indirect conveyance of an infectious agent in the event of a patient suffering from a communicable disease.

Equipment needed: Extra bedside stand, table, garbage can, basins, thermometer, paper towels, paper bags, polyethelene liners, waste baskets, I.V. standard, aqueus zepharin 1:1000 with antirust, laundry bags, gowns, caps, and masks.

Set-up procedures: All personnel will be informed. Notify the family and the patient of procedure and regulation. Identify the isolation room with ISOLATION sign. Place the extra bedside supply table outside the door and fill it with gowns, laundry bag, bags, liners, paper towels, caps and masks. Aqueous zepharin

will be placed near supply cabinet. A table with a basin of a-
queous solution will be placed near door, inside room. The
garbage can will be lined with polyethelene liner and placed near
basins. It should be covered. Place a wastebasket near by and
paper towels on the table. A small open bag should be placed
near patient's head of bed. Make the laundry bags available to use
in linen changes. They will be distinctly marked with red stripes.

Entering for direct patient contact: Take gown, cap, mask
from outside supply cabinet, and attire self. Enter room and close
the door, explaining procedure to patient. Check other isolation
procedures, such as Care of Linens, Dishes, etc.

Departing the isolation room: Wash hands first with aqueous
zepharin and dry hands with paper towel, which is disposed in
wastebasket. Remove gown, roll contaminated side in and place in
dirty linen (soiled) or dirty linen (unsoiled). Wash hands second
time, dry with paper towel, and dispose in wastebasket. Open
door, exit, and close door. Wash a third time, as you normally
would, in the utility room.

The above procedure will illustrate the exact detail needed to
explain certain measures of sanitation, such as isolation. Additional
subjects to be reduced to definite procedures are:

Care of dishes and disinfection of food.
Care of linen in isolation techniques.
Disposal of waste.
Disposal of excreta.
Care of examining and surgical supply equipment.
Taking temperature, pulse, respiration.
Taking blood pressure.
Collecting specimens.
Assisting with examination and treatments.
Transporting patient from unit:
    via stretcher
    via wheelchair.

The above meets only one area of hygiene for which the administrator will see that procedures are written, incorporated into duty
assignments, used in training of personnel, and supervised. Sanitation procedures will need to be developed for all departments, including nursing, dietary, laundry, housekeeping, and ancillary services.

Microbiology

The proper knowledge and respect for the causes of disease will help the administrator to establish provisions for the prevention and control of it. He and his staff have a direct responsibility to establish policies and practices that will prevent its spread.

Effort should be made to ensure the safety of both nursing home employees and patients. While the patients are treated by the prescription of the attending physician, first-aid measures should be established. A good first-aid kit, poison antidote charts, and education to combat the spread of infection are but a few of the methods. It should be noted that some food poisonings, e.g., salmonella and botulism, are most severe, and antitoxins are not effective except in the early stages. Frequent health examinations required of all employees will also be effective.

There are a number of causes of disease. Animal parasites are the largest group. Among the one-celled animal parasites are the amoebae, which cause dysentery; sporozoa, which cause malaria; and flagellates, which cause sleeping sickness. There are a number of multicelled animal parasites, such as the pinworm, hookworm, and tapeworm.

Several plant parasites are common, such as the one-celled bacteria called staphylococci, streptococci, diplococci, bacilli, and spirilla. In addition, we have fungus parasites.

There are a number of pathogens of microorganisms which can cause disease, such as a virus. Pneumonia and nerve-damaging pathogens are in this group.

In addition malnutrition is treated as a disease. Some physical or chemical agents, such as lead poisoning or chemical poisoning, cause disease.

The administrator must ensure provision for the control and prevention of the spread of disease (sometimes called contagion, which may become an epidemic, or is spread over a vast area as a pandemic, or be confined within a locality as an endemic). To ensure its control in the services, the administrator must develop policies and procedures such as hand-washing procedures, cleaning mops, isolation maintenance, the customary use of cubicle curtains, methods of examination and treatment, maintenance of the sterile supply etc. In addition, the autoclave may be important for proper sterilization techniques.

The Housekeeping Staff

There is a very important relationship between the housekeeping staff, sanitation, and the patients' well-being. The nursing will be brighter, more cheerful, and much more pleasant when the housekeeping is efficient and thorough. However, the personnel should be cordial and cooperative, both with the patients and with the nursing personnel. Generally, there are three types of positions, beginning with the executive housekeeper. Working with the executive housekeeper are the maids and the custodian or janitor.

The executive housekeeper supervises the total housekeeping program. He or she may have one or more subordinates, usually called maids or janitors, and will make the daily job assignments, conduct in-service training, and purchase or requisition supplies. She will plan decorations and furniture arrangement, in cooperation with other supervisory personnel, and will maintain the supply closet. Among her supervisory duties will be the promotion of safety and sanitation standards.

The maid may be called simply a housekeeper; her counterpart is the janitor. There is usually some distinction in the type of work she does in the nursing home. Generally, she is responsible for cleaning the baths, showers, utility room, closet, patient's rooms, furniture and equipment. She is also responsible for dusting, some mopping, and making some special furniture arrangements and decorations. She should report and requisition supplies and repairs.

The custodian's or janitor's duties parallel those of the maid. While there is some tendency to give the janitor the heavier duties, for example, mopping and floor care, it should be pointed out that new laws concerning equal rights and equal pay for women may have some bearing on the distribution of the workload. Generally, a custodian is responsible for general cleaning and disinfecting, floor care, window care, trash disposal, and minor maintenance. Special details, e.g., fogging, safety, arrangement of furniture, etc., may be added to his duties. He also should be alert in reporting needed repairs and requisitioning supplies. If he receives a pay differentiated from that of the maid, it should be either a heavier job assignment, and or for greater skills, e.g., maintenance requirements, not because of sex or tradition.

The housekeeping personnel also are responsible for taking training. In fact, perhaps a more comprehensive program of training should be inaugurated for housekeeping personnel, because of the nature of their work, which affects the patient's well-being and safety, public relations, and all the facets of the nursing service.

Equipment for Effective Housekeeping

Organizing the equipment for housekeeping is essential. The administrator or executive housekeeper plans each detail and assembles the necessary equipment to ensure the best possible housekeeping program.

The maid's cart should contain at least the following:

clean mop, 14 oz. to 16 oz;
mop bucket with wringer;
dust mop and dustpan;
cleaning rags;
dusting sprays;
polishing rags, furniture polish;
cleansers and disinfectants;
soap, tissue, supplies.

The janitor's equipment includes:

vacuum cleaner;
clean mop, 16 oz. to 20 oz.;
mop bucket with wringer;
floor machine, 15-inch minimum;
scrub and polishing brushes for floor machine;
wax applicator;
cleansers, disinfectants;
hand tools for minor repairs;
dry floor mop with treatment spray.

Special equipment that will be needed:

trash containers;
fogging equipment;
carpet shampooing equipment;
wall-washing devices;
window cleaning devices;
hand truck for moving equipment;
ladders.

Repair facilities that may be maintained:

> small repair shop or area;
> small power tools;
> hand tools;
> painting equipment.

Storage needed for housekeeping:
> janitor's closet with service sink;
> maid's closet;
> housekeeping supply closet;
> space for unused equipment.

The administrator or executive housekeeper should establish a procurement policy for supplies and repairs. A purchasing agent should be designated, perhaps the assistant to the administrator, and a system of ordering developed. It may be by periodic ordering and/or requisition. Some type of purchase order may be used. Assign a receiving agent who will receive and inventory purchases. He will also see that goods are properly stored.

Administering Housekeeping Duties

Undoubtedly, the greatest skills the executive housekeeper needs are those used in scheduling and supervising the many housekeeping duties. There are several methods of scheduling, and they may be used in various combinations.

Duties may be assigned by area. By this method, the home is divided by areas; duties are assigned to be done at certain times. For example, employee A is assigned to clean the West wing, employee B is to clean the East wing, etc. Simply stated, a number of rooms of proportionate size are grouped into a single assignment. Some housekeepers may prefer the functional approach, i.e., assigning one person to mopping, another to dusting, etc. Of course, the assignments are made to a particular person.

The executive housekeeper should evaluate each cleaning duty and assign a sequence for cleaning. Some cleaning is done daily, i.e., dust mopping, bathroom disinfecting, etc. Other cleaning tasks may be done on a bi-weekly or weekly basis. Such tasks would probably be assigned on a personal basis. Some cleaning tasks can be done on a monthly or seasonal basis, such as waxing, window-washing, etc.

The executive housekeeper should prepare the master duty schedule and post it, perhaps near the time clock. In order for it to be equitable and efficient, a job-and-time study for each task could be made. The job analysis has been previously discussed and should be referred to. In any event, each duty will have a procedure written for it, published, and made available to the housekeeping staff.

Constant evaluation of housekeeping is necessary. Periodic inspections will list needs to be corrected. This review of the quality of work should be done by the supervisory staff, with the executive housekeeper inspecting on a regular basis, perhaps daily, while the administrator will inspect less often, but regularly. Such evaluation could be coupled with a training program for improvement. Of course, direct supervision of housekeeping employees will be necessary to maintain a high standard.

Building and Grounds Maintenance

The condition of the facility, its ease of cleaning, and the most efficient use of it will be aided by a program of constant maintenance of the building and grounds. Such a program is commonly called preventive maintenance.

Structural maintenance requires upkeep of the basic facility. For ease of evaluation, for gaining the maximum efficiency, and attaining the best cost-for-usage factor in budgeting and operation, a program of preventive maintenance should be adopted. Such a program contains the regular reporting of maintenance needs by all the personnel, minor upkeep by the custodian, regular 3-day, 30-day, 90-day, and 180-day inspections. A few items may be inspected yearly. Major equipment manuals will specify the frequency of maintenance. Some major repairs can be incorporated into remodeling programs or an enlargement of the facility. Continuous maintenance has proved the most satisfactory in most industries. Nursing homes, because of the high usage factor, need more upkeep, and many items should not be held up for an expected remodeling or major improvement program.

It is possible to group maintenance into three catagories, each having distinct problems of maintenance. These are:

The basic structure:
>the roof, eaves, and gutters;
>all wall surfaces, inside and out;
>doors, windows, and all other openings;
>the ceilings, inside and on porches;

all floors, porches;
the substructure, foundation, crawl space;
stairs, elevators.

Equipment and furnishings:
air-conditioning and heating systems;
electrical system;
plumbing and fixtures;
machinery;
office equipment;
nursing equipment;
household furnishings.

Exterior and grounds:
lawn, shrubbery, gardens, etc.;
outdoor facilities, patios, walks, porches;
fences, sprinklers, hydrants;
trash and garbage disposal, incinerator.

The two types of general maintenance, continuous preventative maintenance, and periodic maintenance are accomplished in the nursing home by two types of personnel, the regular staff and contracted services. Normally, any home, no matter what the size, uses a combination of the two; it is merely a question of how often each will be used. If qualified personnel are not available, or if it is economically impractical to keep a specialist, such as an electrician, on the staff, this service is contracted. The type of repair dictates when contracting is required. Contractual maintenance usually is needed for electrical, plumbing, radio or television, nurses' call system, air-conditioning, refrigeration, machinery, automatic sprinkler systems, emergency lighting systems, and fire-alarm systems. The rule is never to violate a local ordinance and code, a state regulation, or a contractual agreement. Local codes often specify a licensed journeyman repair certain systems, e.g., electrical, plumbing, and fire protection.

Maintenance personnel, i.e., the custodian, janitor, or maintenance engineer, may do most of the normal upkeep, which includes painting and minor upkeep of machinery.

Laundry Facilities and Staff

A key facility in every home is the laundry. In a true sense, the nursing home functions only as well as its linen service. There is hardly a place in the entire household that the laundry service does not affect.

Even the office is dusted with laundered dustcloths. Of course, the nursing service uses vast quantities of linens, enough that the licensing agency requires a supply of at least three times the normal occupancy.

The laundry department is normally a line-organization functioning as a separate department. It may be supervised by the head laundress. In some homes, the laundry is placed under the supervision of the housekeeping department. In such a case, a foreman of the laundry would likely be appointed.

The laundry manager, or laundress, is directly responsible for operating the laundry. She, or he, should develop efficiency in laundry processing, a fair and equitable method of making job assignments, and a schedule for the various functions of the laundry process.

The laundry system includes a method of collecting and storing soiled linens. Closed and separate containers are recommended to ensure infection control. The storage room will be so located as to insure no cross-contamination of the clean supply. It should be ventilated with forced air, separately from the house ventilation, with the airflow from clean to dirty area. This is the opposite direction as the process flows. The storage of linens will be coordinated with the procedures of the nursing staff, so that the temporary storage and transporting of soiled linens do not spread infection and odors.

A method of transporting the soiled linen must be developed, one that will prevent the spread of infection. The process of washing soiled linens begins with sorting, goes through washing with soap and bleach for disinfection, and a fabric softener. Bleach is usually not recommended when no-press linens and fabrics are washed. Drying and ironing are the next step, followed by a method of folding that ensures uniformity. Stacking with a single edge outward on the shelf will help nurses to count out the correct number desired. When the patient's clothes are included, a separate system should be established, with some method of control to ensure that each individual's laundry is done and returned promptly, in good condition. This includes a marking system. Finally, some minor mending could be done.

A job description for the laundress should be written and furnished to each person employed in this capacity. By the nature of the process, it will need to be correlated closely with a procedure manual, which should be written for each function within the laundry duty assignments.

Job description: Laundress

The laundress shall be responsible for the storage of soiled linens in the utility room and their removal to the laundry room for processing.

Clothes shall be properly sorted and kept within the area designed for processing soiled linen in the laundry room. Never mix soiled linens with clean linens, nor use containers designated for clean linens to store soiled linens.

Laundering the clothes is done after proper sorting, as follows: bed linens, towels and wash cloths, belts, and patient wearing apparel. Wearing apparel is to be laundered separately, usually in the small washers. It is sorted as to color of clothing and/or type of clothing.

The formula for washing is posted on the washer. Adhere strictly to this formula, since we have developed it to meet the needs of the mineral content of the water, the need for disinfection, the length of washing cycles, softening, and scouring to cut the last traces of soap.

Soaking clothes, to remove spots and stains, may be necessary.

Drying will be in the dryer. Adhere strictly to the procedure for drying, as posted on the front of the dryer. The lint trap must be cleaned each day.

Folding will be hospital style. Stacking is with the single edge outward.

Linen will be returned and stored in the linen room. Care will be taken to keep the linen free of contamination.

Personal clothing will be returned to the patient's closet or dresser. Care should be taken to see that all items are marked and returned to the proper person. Any item found out of place is returned to its proper storage immediately.

Discarding clothing: Laundry personnel shall not assume this responsibility. Consult the supervising nurse.

Maintenance of equipment: Clean the laundry before leaving for the day. Clean the floors; put up all containers; clean the washers and dryers; remove trash for disposal. Turn off the iron, leave one light burning, and empty the lint trap of the dryer. Note any repairs needed, check for supplies, and leave requests at the office.

Housekeeping As Related to the Total Program

Housekeeping is related to the public relations of the home. Patients and relatives will readily make known their impressions of the home. If they find it generally dirty and unkempt, this is their impression. Eventually, someone will ask them about the home, and they will reveal their feelings about it. Guests and the general public form their own opinions. They will carry this impression in their minds until one day it is called for. Professionals also recommend on the basis of their impressions. The general condition of the home, its appearance or cleanliness, affect their impression.

Housekeeping is related to a patient's well-being. Disease and infection may be prevented by good housekeeping and maintenance. A dirty, trashy, unkempt facility is depressing to the patients. Melancholy may result, and the entire rehabilitation program may be cut short. Cross-contamination may result from poor housekeeping, and contagion may rage. Safety practices, such as proper storage of oxygen, supervised smoking, etc, are an integral part of patient's well-being.

The housekeeping department is essentially the link between all departments with a common goal: infection control, and hygiene. The nursing department must correlate its total work with the housekeeping department. In fact, housekeeping is an integral part of nursing. However, the licensing agency will not permit a promiscuous mixing of nursing and housekeeping functions. A single individual may perform both duties; but her job description and duty assignment must clearly show this, and the time she performs each duty must be so scheduled. In addition, the sequence of the performing duties must not be cross-contaminating, i.e., doing contaminating housekeeping duties, and then patient care, without bathing and changing uniforms before each duty. The administrator may find it better to separate housekeeping duties from the nursing duties by assigning different personnel to each function.

The dietary department also relies on the housekeeping department. However, it is good practice to separate the nursing-department housekeeping from that of the dietary department. This will ensure no possibility of cross-contamination between the patients' rooms and the dining room.

Housekeeping is closely related to safety. The prevention of slipping, by good floor care, the removal of obstructions, the replacement of light bulbs for adequate illumination, the removal of rubbish and trash for fire prevention—are all necessary for safety.

Adequate housekeeping helps to ensure a constant program of maintenance, if upkeep is constantly evaluated and reported by conscientious housekeepers.

Chapter *15*

Gerontology and Geriatrics

The Study of Gerontology

There are two words commonly used concerning the aged: gerontology and geriatrics. There is a difference between the two, although it is actually a matter of the scope of each. Gerontology is the study of the aging, encompassing every social, cultural, and physical aspect. Geriatrics concerns that specialty of medicine, the care of the aging. We take two words from the ancient Greeks, who referred to the aged as *geras*, or "old." Adding this, we have taken a second ancient Greek word, *logos*, and have given it the meaning, "study." Thus we say gerontology when we refer to the study of the aging.

A number of physical changes take place in the elderly as the aging process develops. These are studied under geriatrics. By taking the term *geras* and adding the Greek word, *iatrikos*, or "cure," we get the modern word, geriatrics.

Gerontology deals with the general study of the aging. In the United States, there is today a remarkable increase in the number of elderly persons. The age of 65 has been adopted as determining the initial phase of retirement. Subsequently, most statistical data concerning the aging refers to those 65 and above.

Beginning in 1860, the percentage of population, 65 and over, was a mere 2.6; by 1900, it had risen to 4.1; by 1970 it had risen to 9.5; and by 1974 it exceeded 10.0. With 10% of population aged 65 and above, over 20,000,000 Americans are in this age range. The control of disease and the increasing of the life span have given rise to this growth. The male at birth has a life expectancy of opproximately 67 years, while a female can expect to live to 75 years of age. Such a life expectancy would be less if a person were nonwhite, and slightly higher if he lived in a rural instead of an urban area.

Housing for the aged is critical. With neighborhood changes, such as those caused by urbanization, many elderly are caught between housing blight and shifting construction demands. The progressive shift from the family care of the elderly to institutional care has left many with an existance with little care at all. In many cases, the family unit cannot care for the infirm, and for psychological or economic reasons, the elderly may not choose institutional living.

Housing for the elderly is now a specialized field. Most persons do not choose the ultimate home with age in mind; it is the family they are raising that is considered first. Thus, persons grow old in homes that were never designed with the aged in mind, and they grow old living with stairs, high porches, large yards to care for, and countless other problems. In addition, the neighborhood slowly moves away, the neighboring house becomes apartments for young couples or the poor with large families of children. Noise, harassment, and ostracism may occur. These problems have brought many older persons to consider moving to the retirement home. Some have moved to rural areas, to a lakeside, or to a southern state. Some have taken to mobile living in trailer parks or in motor homes.

Studies reveal that retirement housing should have several conveniences. It should promise independence as long as is practical. It should be near certain services: fire safety, medical care, shopping, and recreation. There needs to be means of transportation. The size of the houses or apartment should not overburden the aged occupants, or some common means of upkeep, and maintenance should be available. Finally, the elderly should be near their own kind, but not to the extent of segregating them from other age groups, especially children.

One possible move is toward congregate living, in which a group of residents share common conveniences, e.g., food service, recreation, education, etc. In this concept, residential dwelling for the elderly might be a high-rise apartment with safety features for the aged, or cottages grouped in a select area near which the needed services were available.

Economics are of vital concern to the elderly, because his income is usually fixed or declining. Inflation erodes its purchasing power, and he finds himself being forced closer to the poverty level. In recent years, the federal and state governments have joined forces to improve the position of the elderly. For example, local governments have given additional exemption from taxes to those over 65 and have made low-rent housing available. The federal government has used several basic programs to benefit the elderly.The Social Security Act, of course, has had old-age benefits available since 1935. To this program there have been added Medicare, Medicaid, and in 1974 Supplemental Security Income, to which need is related. The Older Americans Act sponsors many programs which benefit select groups. When combined with local cooperation, such programs have attacked the need for trans-portation, for shopping services, for visitor services, housekeepers, and a multitude of other needs. By tying the benefits of Social Security to an escalator clause which grants a rise in the cost of living to be-neficiaries, the purchasing power of the Social Security check is not being eroded by inflation. Another special consideration is the status of the pension of American workers. In 1974 legislation was passed which protects the workers pension from forfeiture clauses. The Veterans Administration has increased pensions, and the military services have done likewise.

The cultural concepts of the aging contribute to the dilemma. America places an accent on youth and productivity; therefore, it expects the elderly to retire to leisure and nonproductivity to make way for younger persons. Pension restrictions also help to force the elderly into nonproductivity and out of the wage-earners class. Thomas A. Rich and Alden S. Gilmore have developed a programed manual en-titled, *Basic Concepts of Aging*, which is available from the Superintendent of Documents, U.S. Government Printing Office, Washington, D.C. This manual is an excellent aid for the administrator who wishes to develop a basic knowledge of the principles of gerontology.

Our study of gerontology could carry us into many fields for information concerning the aged; however, the health-care field is of primary concern. Through the years, the elderly have been unable to afford adequate care, and have treated themselves whenever possible. It is estimated, however, that fewer than 25% of the aged are free of health problems. Of those 65 and above, 5.7% live in institutions such as nursing homes.

The Study of Geriatrics

The study of the aged includes a study of the physical changes they undergo in their passage through time. A number of physical changes take place to cause one to age. The tissue gradually changes to become dry and nonelastic because of a slowing of cell division and fatty infiltration. Listed below are many other changes one may expect.

> The aged experience less resistance to disease.
> They must have long recuperation from illness.
> They experience a gradual loss of strength.
> A decrease in chest expansion causes improper breathing.
> Rarefied bones result in easy breaks.
> The loss of circulation brings senility.
> Foreign matter and fluids may accumulate in the lungs.
> Most vital organs are overworked.
> The hands and feet may seem perpetually cold.
> Some changes in mental capacity may result.
> The eyes gradually fail.
> Hearing may deteriorate.
> The teeth have decayed.

The changes the elderly experience have a definite relationship to nursing care needs for the elderly. In fact, nursing the aged is quite different from nursing younger persons, for a number of reasons. The administrator and his nursing staff must learn to take certain precautions in the care offered the elderly.

> Be cautious about infection.
> Expect the patient to rest more.
> Expect little physical exertion.
> Watch for signs of pneumonia.
> Expect a cold to turn to pneumonia.
> Expect fluids to collect in the lungs.
> Protect patients against falling.
> Turn and rub bed patients regularly to prevent bedsores.
> Intensify safety precautions.
> Expect some respiratory difficulties to develop.
> Watch for dizziness, fainting, loss of equilibrium.
> Note frequent changes in the vital signs.
> Note lapses of memory.
> Note a loss of a sense of time.

The nursing home administrator should begin an intensive study of gerontology and geriatrics. Both the Gerontological Society, Inc., and the American Geriatrics Society will supply reading materials. In addition, there are seven centers on aging in geographical areas throughout the U.S. One such is the Center on Aging, North Texas State University, Denton, Texas. These centers specialize in research and higher education in the field of gerontology. They also offer special seminars and short courses for the administrator and his nursing staff.

Emotional Factors in Geriatrics

The emotional life of the aged person is subject to great stress, especially if he becomes chronically ill. Behavior patterns develop that cause others to apply words such as "senile," "feeble," "foolish," etc. This is often the result of a simple lack of an understanding of the personality changes that may result from growing old. While it is true that the elderly may grow emotional, their new condition usually has its basic cause in a physical deficiency. They need the same love, sympathy, concern, and compassion that any person needs. When they become patients in the nursing home, certain emotional changes are evidenced in physical symptoms; others are shown as psychological effects.

> There are changes in rest habits.
> The loss of taste buds changes eating habits.
> There is an emotional reaction to group living.
> The aged may experience a loss of pride.
> The aged may lose their sense of worth.
> Some lose their sense of modesty.
> Many change their habits of hygiene.
> There may be general nervousness.
> Hypertension may develop.
> Melancholy may develop.
> The elderly may become withdrawn.
> Attitude is related to recovery from illness.
> Nearly all will be impatient at times.

Sometimes the emotional difficulties may become psychotic. While these symptoms do not necessarily indicate a psychotic state, they are signs of more difficult emotional states. Such indications are suspiciousness, fear, anxiety, hostility, hallucinations, delusions, depression, hysteria, and a persecution complex.

Senility is perhaps the most misunderstood of all the conditions that may beset the elderly. Because of the general ignorance of the cause and effect of senility, and the erroneous supposition that most older persons face it, the administrator should learn its cause and symptoms. Senility is often taken for mental illness. While it is true that senility exhibits some of the same signs as mental illness, there is a distinct difference.

The basic cause of senility is the restriction of the circulation of blood to the brain. There are two distinct types, arteriosclerosis and cerebrosclerosis; the symptoms are the same: loss of the ability to reason, loss of the ability to store a new experience in the mind, loss of the sense of time, and loss of memory. The student of nursing home administration will need to develop skill in dealing with such specific behavior problems as result.

Retirement

Retirement means to withdraw or turn to leisure as a primary occupation. Society thinks of retirement as a reward, as making room for the younger person in labor, because a person is "too old to work."

To the worker, retirement may mean loss of prestige, loss of an occupation, loss of relationships, loss of reference groups, and is the most traumatic experience of old age. There are three periods of adjustment to retirement: contemplating retirement while still employed; a period of adopting to a new routine; and a period of physical dependence on others. The most severe is the initial period of adjustment to actual retirement. Preretirement may have been the most productive stage; however, as the major factors of family building are accomplished, preretirement develops into a time of more social involvement.

The nursing home is primarily concerned with the later periods of retirement and with patient care. This is not to say that some concern will be given to the general retirement of employees. It is in the latter stages of retirement that the person's need shifts to physical care. The administrator should be aware that other needs do not diminish simply because of incapacity. The need for sociability still remains; the emotional needs are not lessened; the need for continuity or regular participation in activities, in productivity, or complex involvement does not change. The need for status and self-esteem is as great as in youth. The learning capacity is as great as ever, except for physical handicaps and psychological barriers.

Chapter 16

Pharmacology and

Medical Terminology

Policies and Procedures of Drug Administration

Drug administration begins with the physician's order, continues through the procurement and storage of the medicine, and finally, ends when properly administered and recorded. To this is added another duty, which is discontinuing medicine and legally disposing of any that remains. The physician's orders are to be specific as to the patient, the drug, the dosage, the times of administration and discontinuation. His order is to be written and placed in the record of the patient at the time of administering the drug. In the case of class A narcotics (pharmaceuticals are also classified under the Drug Abuse and Controlled Substance Act, narcotics of the class "A" type are classified as Type II), the nurse will never administer a dose without a specific written order in the patient's clinical chart. In the case of certain drugs, a verbal order or telephone order may be permitted. However, the professional nurse taking the order must immediately reduce it to writing, sign it, and get the countersignature of the physician within a specified time, usually 48 hours to 72 hours.

Procurement of drugs is known as the dispensing process. Dispensing is always by a licensed pharmacist, according to what the physician prescribes. The pharmacy may be within the nursing home or it may be a local pharmacy; in either case, it is licensed to dispense pharmaceuticals, and subject to control of the state board of pharmacy.

Upon receipt, drugs are checked against the orders, and then properly stored until time to be administered to the patient. The storage system must be designed to provide: space for each patient's medications, refrigeration of certain drugs, separate storage of nonlegend drugs in bulk, separate storage of controlled drugs, separate storage of drugs for external use only, and the proper security of all stored drugs.

The provision for security includes locking and keeping locked all drugs except during the actual time of administering them. Controlled drugs, those subject to the Drug Abuse and Controlled Substance Act (DACA), are to be double locked in a cabinet within a cabinet. It is recommended that the medication room be locked, also, when it is not occupied by the medication nurse. Other control measures to be instituted are listed below:

Professionals only shall administer drugs. Some states allow a nonlicensed medication aide who has training or has completed a state-approved course to administer drugs on the night shift from 11:00 P.M. to 7:00 A.M.

Medication errors shall be reported immediately to the doctor prescribing the drug. An incident report should also be made.

Each nurse prepares, administers, and records the prescribed doses on her shift only. This precludes a nurse setting up medications for the next shift.

There shall be a complete recording of drugs administered.

Maintain a separate narcotic and controlled substance record. This is a perpetual inventory with the remaining balance kept current.

Make a narcotic count at the change of each shift. While this is time consuming, there is no other legal method. A permanent record should be kept of the transfer of responsibility.

Establish automatic stop-orders. The physician's orders, the manufacturers control number, or state established stop-orders for different pharmaceuticals in the absence of a specific physician's order will be the guidelines for this requirement.

When a patient dies, his medicine dies with him. His medicine is also considered discontinued.

Discontinued pharmaceuticals will be stored and disposed of in accordance with state pharmacy regulations.

The Consulting Pharmacist in the Nursing Home

The consulting pharmacist fills the need for consultation concerning the use of pharmaceuticals in the nursing home when a registered pharmacist is not available on a daily basis. His services are contracted for on a regular basis, perhaps the minimum of one day per month. A routine is established, and an understanding reached about his being available for emergency consultation.

The services rendered by the consulting pharmacist include specific pharmaceutical problems considered and answered, procedures for handling medications, education, and counseling on community relations. A program of consultation would probably include a preliminary interview with the supervising nurse when problems for discussion and procedures to be reviewed would be noted. Educational needs should be decided with the cooperation of the administrator or his authorized training leader. A review of the medication nurses' procedures also needs to be made.

The consulting pharmacist may then make a routine inspection of the medication storage, including the controlled-substance storage cabinet and its record book. He should spot-check several of the patient's medication boxes, check through the nonlegend drugs and those "for external use only," and recommend corrections to the storage procedure if any are necessary. He will examine doses, and finally, do a routine check of pharmaceutical and medical supplies.

The consulting pharmacist is a good source of information for a short course on handling drugs. Such a curriculum might include:

> Basic terminology, drugs, side effects.
> Drug labeling.
> New drugs, their names, uses, side effects.
> Food and drug legislation.
> Dispensing methods.
> Ethics in drug administration.
> Hygiene in drug administration.
> Legal requirements, Drug Abuse and Controlled Substance Act.
> State and local regulation.

The pharmacist can help the nursing staff stay abreast of new procedures and equipment. He may also be able to institute efficiency procedures, safety measures, and ethical standards.

He should record each visit in a permanent file. His report should include the time and hours of his visit. A short report is made of the results of his review; recommendations are listed. The administrator will wish to review this report as he does all reports of consultants.

Medical Terms

The administrator should develop the ability to use correctly terminology related to the body functions and systems. Below are several lists of technical words and phrases which are given here merely to help acquaint him with the type of terms he frequently will hear used by the professionals in the medical field. *It must be stressed that in no way should it be considered that a study of these lists can make one an instant expert.* They only make it possible to listen more intelligently and to research information more readily in the proper, authoritative reference sources.

For an authoritative definition, the student administrator should purchase a good medical dictionary such as *Taber's Cyclopedic Medical Dictionary*, Clarence Wilbur Taber, F. A. Davis Company, Philadelphia.

BODY FUNCTIONS AND SYSTEMS
The skeletal system
    Skull
    Vertebral column
    Thorax
    Upper extremities
    Lower extremities
The muscular system
The respiratory system
    Nostrils
    Larynx, pharynx
    Trachea
    Bronchi
    Lungs
The circulatory system
    Heart
    Arteries
    Veins
    Capillaries
The nervous system
    Central nervous system
    Brain
    Spinal cord
    Peripheral nervous system
    Sense organs

Eyes
Ears
Tongue
Nose
Skin
The digestive system
Mouth
Esophagus
Stomach
Small intestine, colon
Large intestine
Rectum
The urinary system
Kidneys
Ureter
Bladder
Urethra
The reproductive system
Ovaries
Uterus
Vagina
Breasts
Testes
Ducts
Penis
The skin cells, tissue
The endocrine glands

COMMON DISEASES AND DISORDERS OF THE ELDERLY
Diseases attacking cells: Pathology
Cancer
Carcinoma
Disorders of the skeletal system: Orthopedics
Bone injuries
Congenital growth deformities
Osteomyelitis
Arthritis
Rheumatoid arthritis
Diseases or condition of the muscular system
Dystrophy

Atrophy
Diseases of the respiratory system: Thoracics, Allergies
Asthma
Emphysema
Tuberculosis
Pneumonia
Diseases of the circulatory system: Cardiology, Hematology
Thrombophlebitis
Thrombosis leading to stroke
Occlusion (blood clot)
Embolism (moving clot)
Coronary thrombus
Infarction (when blood supply ceases)
Myocardial
Pulmonary
Congestive heart failure or disease
Cardiovascular accident
Aneurysm
Hemorrhage
Arteriosclerosis
Cerebrosclerosis
Diseases of the nervous system: Neurology
Cerebral vascular accident
Paralysis
Hemiplegia
Paraplegia
Quadriplegia
Multiple sclerosis
Epilepsy
Parkinson's disease
Diseases of the digestive system: Internal Medicine
Ulcers
Diverticulitis
Hepatitis
Gallstones
Gastrointestinal
Diabetes
Malnutrition
Incontinence
Pyorrhea

Diseases of the urinary system: Urology, Genitourinary
    Uremic poisoning
    Bladder infection
    Kidney stone
Diseases of the reproductive system: Genitourinary, Gynecology
    Prostatitis
    Hysterectomy
Diseases of the skin: Dermatology
Diseases of the excretory system: Proctology
    Hemorrhoids
    Incontinence
Diseases of the blood: Hematology
    Jaundice
    Leukemia
Diseases of the ear: Otology
Diseases of the eye: Ophthalmology
Diseases of the glandular system: Endocrinology
Diseases of the female: Gynecology
Illness of the mind: Psychiatry
Diseases of the aged: Geriatrics
Diseases of the feet: Podiatry, Chiropody
Diseases of the teeth: Dentistry, Orthodontics

FORMS OF TREATMENT
Treatment of disease by natural methods: Physiatrics
Treatment of disease by manipulative correction: Osteopathy
Fitting of glasses: Optometry
Fitting of hearing aids: Audiology
X ray: Radiology
Operation: Surgery
Reduction of ability to feel pain: Anesthesiology
Cobalt treatment: Isotopes
Bedside treatment: Clinical medicine
Experimental medicine: Research
Group medicine: Clinics
Nonsurgical treatment: Internal medicine
Physical medicine: Physiotherapy
Preventive medicine
Psychosomatic medicine, mental disorders: Psychiatry

REHABILITATION SPECIALTIES
Physical therapy
Occupational therapy
Speech therapy
Recreational therapy
Social work
Peripatology
Inhalation therapy
Prosthesis

SYMPTOMS COMMON TO THE ELDERLY
Amblyopia
Anorexia
Apathy
Apprehension
Atrophy
Clonus
Coma
Confusion
Cyanosis
Degeneration
Depression
Distention
Dribbling
Dyspnea
Dysuria
Euphoria
Edema
Fainting
Fever
Flaccidity
Hallucination
Hematura
Hyperactivity
Hyperesthesia
Nausea
Nervousness
Oliguria
Orthopnea
Paralysis

Paresthesia
Retention
Skin color
Slurred speech
Stupor
Turbidity
Unconsciousness
Vital signs:
    Temperature
    Pulse
    Respiration
    Blood pressure

ABBREVIATIONS OF MEDICAL AND NURSING TERMS

aa	equal
Abd.	abdomen
Adm.	admission
a. c.	before meals
Ad lib.	as desired
A/G.	albumin globulin ratio
A.M.	Morning
A. S.	Ear
A.S.A.	Acetylsalicylic acid
A.S.H.D.	arteriosclerotic heart disease
amt.	amount
amp.	ampule
aq.	water
ax.	axillary
B. E.	barium enema
b.i.d.	twice a day
BP	blood pressure
BRP	bathroom privileges
C.	centigrade
Ca.	carcinoma
caps.	capsules
Cath.	catheter
c̄	with
CBC	complete blood count
cc.	cubic centimeter
cm.	centimeter

chem.	chemistry
CO_2	carbon dioxide
comp.	compound
C.N.S.	central nervous system
C.S.F.	cerebrospinal fluid
CVA	cerebral vascular accident
D.	right
Diff.	differential blood count
Diab.	diabetic
Diag.	diagnosis
Dil.	dilute
Disc.	discontinue
Disch.	discharge
dr.	dram
Dr.	Doctor
EEG	electroencephalogram
et	and
exam.	examination
Fe	iron
fl.	fluid
Fr.	fracture
FUO	fever of unknown origin
G.I.	gastrointestinal
G.B.	gallbadder
Gm.	gram
gr.	grain
gtt.	drop
H, hr.	hour
h.s.	at bedtime
hypo	hypodermically
I.M.	intramuscular
inf.	infusion
I.V.	intravenous
K	potassium
K.U.B.	kidney-ureter-bladder
l	liter
lab.	laboratory
Lat.	lateral
lb.	pound
liq.	liquid

LLQ	left lower quadrant
LUQ	left upper quadrant
m.	minimum
Mcgm	microgram
mg.	milligram
min.	minute
ml.	milliliter
mm.	millimeter
MN	midnight
N	noon
no.	number
noxt.	at night
NPO	nothing per mouth
N.&V.	nausea & vomiting
pt.	pint
O.R.	Operating room
O.T.	occupational therapy
oz.	ounce
P.	pulse
p.c.	after meals
per	by, through
P.M.	afternoon
P.O.	phone order
p.o.	by way of mouth
p.r.n.	as needed
P.T.	physical therapy
prog.	prognosis
Pro. T.	Prothrombin time
Q.h	every hour
q.d.	every day
q.i.d.	four times a day
Q.n.	every night
Q.2h.	every two hours
Q.3h.	every three hours
Q.4h.	every four hours
q.o.d.	every other day
Q.s.	quantity sufficient
R.B.C.	red blood cells
Rh pos	Rhesus factor positive
RLQ	right lower quadrant

Rx.	prescription
s̄	without
Sc	subcutaneously
Sig.	let it be marked
so.	solution
solv.	dissolve
S.O.B.	shortness of breath
s.o.s.	one dose if necessary
spec.	specimen
spts.	spirits
S.S.	soap solution
ss	half
stat.	immediately
subcu.	subcutaneous
Surg	surgery
tab	tablet
T.	temperature
T.A.T.	tetanus antitoxin
T.B.	tuberculosis
t.i.d.	three times a day
tinct.	tincture
U.	unit
ung.	ointment
U.R.I.	upper respiratory infection
U.S.P.	United States Pharmacopoeia
vol. %	volume
V.O.	verbal order
W.B.C.	white blood cell/count
wh. ch.	wheel chair
wt.	weight

DRUGS FREQUENTLY PRESCRIBED

Antihistamines: Benedryl, Clor-Trimeton, Dimetane, Naldecon, Periactin, Phenergan, Pyribenzamine, Tomaril

Anti-infectives:

Antithelmintics: Povan

Antibiotics, Tetracyclines: Achrocidin, Achromycin, Tetrex APC, Declomycin, Panalba, Terramycin

Antibiotics, Penicillins: Bicillin, Compocillin V, Penicillin G, Polycillin, Syncillin, Tegopen

Antibiotics, Erythromycins: Erythrocin, Pediamycin, Hosone, Hosone-sulfas

Antibiotics, miscellaneous: Chloromycetin, Lincocin, Tao

Antibiotics, Neomycins: Cortisporin, Nepolycin, Neosporin

Antibiotics, Nystatins: Mycolog, Wycostatin, Declostatin, Terrastatin

Sulfonamides: Gentanol, Gantrisin, Madribon, Trisulfamanic Furadantin, Mandelamine, Pyridium

Antinauseants: Antivert, Dramamine, Tigan

Autonomic drugs: Combid, Donnatal, Probanthine, Robaxal

Cardiovascular drugs: Lanoxin, Diupres, Hydropres, Raudixin, Resperine, Serpasil, Ser-Ap-Es, Aridin, Nitroglycerin, Peritrate

Central nervous system drugs:

Analgesics, narcotic: Codeine, Emprin Compound with codeine, Fiorinal with codeine, Phenaphin with codeine, Demerol, Percodan

Analgesics, nonnarcotic: Darvon, Darvon compound, Darvon compound 65, Equagesic, Norgesic, Sinutab, Tylenol

Analgesics, antirheumatics: Butazolidin, Indocin, Tandearil

Anticonvulsants: Dilantin, Phenobarbital

Respiratory and cerebral stimulants: Aventyl, Desoxyn, Dexamyl, Dexedrine, Elavil, Ritalin, Tofranil

Sedatives and Hypnotics: Butison, Carbrital, Doriden, Fiorinal, Nembutal, Noctec, Noludar, Placidyl, Seconal, Tyinal

Ataraxics, tranquilizers: Atarax-Vistaril, Compazine, Equanil, Miltown, Librium, Librax, Mellaril, Stelazine, Thorazine, Valium

Electrolytic, caloric and water balance:

Diuretics: Diuril, Dyrenium, Esidrex-Hydrodiuril, Tygroton, Renese

Antiobesity: Biphetamine, Eskatrol, Preludin, Pre-Sate, Tenuate

Enzymes: Ananase

Ear, nose, and throat drugs:

Expectorants and cough sedatives: Actifed, Ambenyl Expectorant, Benylin Expectorant, Dimetane Expectorant, Dimetapp Extentabs, Hycodan, Novahistine DH or Expectorant, Ornade, Penergan Expectorant, Pobitussin, Sudafed, Triminic, Tussionex, Tuss-Ornade

Nasal decongestants: Afrin, Neosynephrine, Ovitrin

Ear: Auralgan

Gastrointestinal: Donnagel PG, Lomotil, Maalox, Paregoric

Hematinics: Fecosol, Trinsicon, Coumadin

Hormones:
  Adrenals: Aristocor-Kenalog, Celestone, Cordran Decagesic, Medrol, Neo-Cortef, Neo-Decadron, Prednisone, Synalar, Viororm-Hydrocortisone
  Antidiabetic: Orinase
  Estrogens: Premarin
  Hypothyroid: Cytomel, Proloid-Thyroid, Synthroid
Spasmolytics: Tedral

Chapter *17*

Physical Therapy
and Rehabilitation

Facilities and Equipment for Therapy

Every nursing home has some space devoted to the rehabilitation of the patients, since the basic goal of restoring them to their optimum potential demands this provision. How extensive this facility is will depend on a number of requirements, including those of the licensing agency and contractual agencies, such as Medicare, Medicaid, Veteran's Administration, and more recently CHAMPUS. It may depend on the type of patient being cared for; naturally, a custodial type of facility will have more need of recreational facilities and less need for a physical therapy room. However, every nursing home should plan for the rehabilitation of the patients. The scope of such a program includes physical therapy, occupational therapy, restorative services, speech therapy, audiology, sight preservation, podiatry, and recreational therapy. Some would include spiritual therapy within this plan.

When the facility maintains a therapy room, it should be equipped so as to develop and restore the muscular-skeletal deficiencies in patients, devices to relieve pain, i.e., heat, massage, hydrotherapy, etc., and devices to preserve maximum performance.

For other patients, the facility should make some provision for proper bed-positioning of the bedfast patient by the use of, for example, footboards, hydraulic lift for ambulation, exercise devices, etc.

219

There are a number of physical difficulties the therapist assists in correcting. Those relating to the muscular-skeletal system, of course, are the most numerous. Arthritis is the great enemy of the aged, causing considerable pain and discomfort. Devices used in treatment for the relief of pain, which sometimes are called physical medicine, such as the moist-heat pack or whirlpool (hydrotherapy), are needed. For the hemoplegic who has suffered brain damage and the loss of the use of one side of his body, a number of devices may be used. The paraplegic, whose spinal cord has deteriorated, will naturally need wheelchair therapy. Victims of fractures, amputations, and other skeletal deformities will need special devices and training in their use.

Those having difficulties with sight, speech, and hearing will need other types of therapy. Specialists have developed methods of assisting in adjustment to or correction of many of these handicaps. Finally, the social and emotional problems of the patients will need to be dealt with by occupational and recreational therapy.

Principles of Physical Therapy

Because physical therapy is the basic type of restorative service that the nursing home staff has to offer, it is very important that the administrator learn to respect the principles underlying it. His entire nursing goal is, essentially, related to it.

The practice of physical therapy is a science. Normally, it requires a college degree with a one-year internship, and is recognized nationally by the American Registry of Physical Therapists. One is ordinarily licensed or registered in his own state. *The physical therapist assists the physician in evaluation of the patient* through the use of prognostic muscle, nerve, joint, and functional tests. The physical therapist, upon orders of the physician, helps to maintain the maximum ability of the patient. He may train, or retrain, the daily living habits of the patient. He may train the movements necessary for walking, dressing, etc. On the other hand, he may use or train the patient in the use of artificial limbs when prescribed by the physician. He may further help to develop substitute skills, substitute movements, or the use of a substitute device. Finally, the physical therapist helps to relieve pain. He has a number of skills at his command, including the use of whirlpool, massage, heat, water treatment, ultrasound, and others.

Therapy is directly related to the patient's recovery, since it is a part of the total program of restoration. The plan for rehabilitation is developed under the supervision of the physician, but includes the nursing actions, social needs, and the need for physical therapy. Physical therapy is not an end within itself. It should be coordinated with other types of therapy, such as occupational therapy, recreational therapy, and other restorative measures. Anything less than a total effort toward rehabilitation of the patient by the entire health team should be unacceptable. The ultimate aim is to restore the patient to an active, normal life.

Restorative Services

Rehabilitation, as we have said, is the process of overcoming a functional, physical, or mental deficiency. Complementary with the physical therapist is the occupational therapist. *Occupational therapy* encourages the patient to contribute to his own recovery by directed activities. The activities may be some type of handcraft; however, crafts are selected merely because of the flexibility of application. They are easily adapted to the nursing home environment and may be directed individually, in a shop situation, or by classes. There is, however, a long list of skills the occupational therapist may use to encourage the patient to apply his own rehabilitation. Closely related is the *remotivation* process, which attempts to make the patient aware of reality and environment, and has a use in the rehabilitation of mental deficiencies. The Veteran's Administration has made extensive use of remotivation in psychiatric care. More recently, this fine governmental organization has developed a process known as *reality orientation*. While they are not the originators of the process, they have given it widespread use in their own geriatric units. Nursing home administrators have found it adaptable to the regressive mental state of senile, withdrawn, or depressive patients. It finds its strength in the constant endeavor of nursing personnel to make the patient aware of the reality of time, including day, week, month, and year; not letting the patient forget specifically where he is; and knowing those persons around him, including other patients and personnel.

Speech therapy is directed at removing speech deficiencies. For the stroke patient who suffers aphasia—inability to use words—speech therapy may be recommended by the physician. Occasionally, because of surgery, a patient will need speech restoration.

There are a number of other types of restorative services the patient may need. *Podiatry* treats foot disorders. *Audiology* and *otology* work with hearing deficiencies. *Inhalation therapy* deals with the respiratory system. *Sight preservation* and *peripatology* deal with handicapped conditions owing to deficiencies of the eyes. Peripatology teaches ambulation to those who have difficulty because of failing eyesight. Sight preservation teaches methods of protecting and preserving sight. *Recreational therapy* is directed toward the social activities of the patients. *Psychological treatment* is a form of therapy although its practice is limited in nursing homes because of the fact that the licensing agencies usually do not permit it. However, there are experimental homes at present in both California and Florida plus certain other states that find about 50% of the elderly confined in mental institutions can be cared for in a nursing home.

In developing a plan for rehabilitation, the physician initiates the evaluation of the patient's needs and potential. Consideration would be given to his physical needs, his emotional or behavioral needs, his social needs, and his functional deficiencies. Then a team is assembled which includes the physician, the nursing staff, therapists, social workers, the minister, and other paramedical specialists, i.e., dentist. Once the plan is in progress, it should be reviewed periodically, and necessary revisions made until the patient has reached his optimum potential.

For Further Study

Selected Readings in Nursing Home Technology

Crooks, Lois A. (ed.), *Long-Term Care Facility Administration, Case Study Manual.* Washington, D.C.: U.S. Department of Health, Education, and Welfare.

McQuillan, Florence L., *Fundamentals of Nursing Home Administration*, 2nd ed. Philadelphia; W. B. Saunders Co., 1974.

Memmler, Ruth Lundeen, *The Human Body in Health and Disease.* Philadelphia: J. B. Lippincott, 1970.

Organizing Health Records. Chicago: American Medical Record Association.

Physicians' Desk Reference. Oradell, N.J.: Medical Economics, Inc.

Rapier, Dorothy Kelley; Koch, Marianna Jones; Moran, Lois Pearson; Geronsin, J. R.; Cady, Elwyn L., Jr.; and Jensen, Deborah MacLurg, *Practical Nursing.* St. Louis; C. V. Mosby, 1962.

Shafer, Kathleen Newton; Sawyer, Janet R.; McCluskey, Audrey M.; and Beck, Edna Lifgren, *Medical Surgical Nursing.* St. Louis: C. V. Mosby, 1971.

Taber, Clarence Wilbur, *Taber's Cyclopedic Medical Dictionary.* Philadelphia: F. A. Davis Co., 1973.

Zaccarelli, Brother Herman E., C.S.C., and Maggiore, Josephine, R.D., *Nursing Home Menu Planning — Food Purchasing, Management.* Boston: Cahners Books, 1972.

PART THREE

Personal and Auxiliary Relationships in the Nursing Home

The administrator will be aware of such outside factors as marketing, advertising, public relations, governmental regulation and control, health care facilities, medical societies, hospitals, pharmacies, educational facilities, religious organizations, recreational facilities, and volunteers.

The administrator shall be aware of alternatives to nursing care: visiting nurse, housekeeper service, foster care, meals-on-wheels, and day care.

The administrator shall make use of Administration on Aging, Older Americans Act, Small Business Administration, Mental Health Act, Legal Aid Society, Federal Housing Administration, and others.

He will be familiar with voluntary associations including: Nursing Home Associations, Hospital Association, Medical Association, Accreditation Associations, National Fire Protection Association, Blue Cross Blue Shield Medical-Surgical Associations, and the American Red Cross.

The administrator will improve communications, understanding instruction, the clear meaning of assignments, message construction, message reception, prevention of message distortion. He will improve channels of communication, using oral communication for person-to-person effectiveness, and written communication for basic directives. He will improve his reading ability and memory.

The facility shall be designed and located properly to include offices, recreation facilities, dining room, kitchen, utility, janitor's closet, and shop services. The nursing unit will include the nursing station, medication storage and preparation, examination isolation, sterile supply, patients' bedrooms, baths, lavatory, restroom, and provision for safety and privacy. Additional facilities include the barber shop, beauty shop, laundry, maintenance, and storage.

The structural design shall include provision for lighting, heating, ventilation, air-conditioning, electrical supply, including an emergency system, patient-call system, plumbing, elevators, stairs, corridors, and safety factors such as exits, sprinklers, heat detection, and alarms.

The design of the exterior includes walks, lawns, patios, outdoor recreation, parking, and driveways.

The administrator and his staff will strive for the patient's self-discipline, and self-groverning councils.

The administrator, his staff, and his social worker shall use counseling and discussion for problem solving. They shall promote personal dignity of the patients by treating them as mature adults, granting freedom of choice, giving privacy in personal care, allowing visitors, free communication, and ensuring kind, compassionate, and loving care.

The administrator and his staff may help, but not treat, psychiatric needs. They will recognize the senile patient, the neurotic, the stroke patient, and the mentally ill, including those detrimental to themselves and others.

The administrator will develop restorative services, including physical therapy, occupational therapy, speech therapy, and recreational activities in keeping with the patients' needs, interests, and abilities. Religious activities will be available.

Chapter *18*

Public Relations

Factors In Creating the Public Image

The reputation of the nursing home is what one might call its public image. Not only must it be right, but it must *seem right* to the general public. There is a difference. A nursing home may be immaculate, give excellent service, yet have a poor image with the general public because of an unpleasant past experience. Many factors make up or contribute to the image of the nursing home.

People contribute to the reputation of the nursing home. Every person who is remotely associated with the home may make a contribution. Certainly, the relatives and patients form opinions and find many opportunities to reveal these opinions to the general public. The employees are another vital link to the outside. They daily demonstrate the home's character and personality, and the home is judged accordingly. Their talk, their honesty, their attitudes, their own general appearances speak constantly for or against the nursing home. The professional people who attend the patients in the nursing home may show willingness or unwillingness to recommend it on a basis of performance and policy. The vendors who deliver supplies are spokesmen for a nursing home's atmosphere. The visitors tell others about their impressions of the nursing home's services. Finally, the inspectors and regulatory personnel know perfectly well what the nursing home's image and reputation deserve to be.

The appearances of a nursing home make a large difference in developing its image. Every facility presents its first impression as the visitor makes his initial visit. From the viewpoint of psychology, this is the most lasting impression. In addition, there is what psychologists call an aesthetic impression concerning a facility. It may be one of wonder, pleasure, or surprise, on the positive note, but if it is described in the visitor's mind as a "dump," as a filthy place, etc., the impression is negative. The general condition of the facility at any given moment will be the basis for an individual to form an opinion. The condition of the patients and their attitudes may contribute to this opinion. The administrator must make an intensive effort to develop the best aesthetic, first impression for those who visit his nursing home.

The image of a particular nursing home could be formed by asking a number of questions, and then by giving an honest and objective appraisal of the answers. Such a list of questions may include:

> What do the patients think of the care given?
> What do the relatives say about services?
> Do vendors speak well of the home?
> Do the professionals recommend the home?
> Does the home get good reports in the news?
> Is the home continually cited for health violations?

The Administrator and Public Relations

The administrator is the key to good public relations. He will either accept this fact and make a determined and continued effort to create a good image, or he will soon find himself overwhelmed by a poor one.

The administrator should continually strive to perfect his organization. His personnel selection, supervision, delegation of authority, and work practices have great effect on the public opinion of his home. The patient-care, whether it is "loving care" or "little care," is under his control; he can improve it and thereby improve the home's reputation. Employee relations are another key factor, the one that may be the first noticed by the public. As long as harmony prevails, little notice is given, and public opinion is formed more on impressions and appearances. However, let labor trouble develop, and the whole community soon knows about it. Finally, his business ethics are the responsibility of the administrator: his fairness, justness, and promptness affect the impression made by the home.

The administrator should always attempt to project the best image. Just as he will be judged on his own appearances while he is in the community conducting business, his home will also be judged.

Eliminating factors detrimental to the reputation of the nursing home is the task of the administrator. This is not to say that he is to whitewash a poor image, but that he is to solve the problems that may be causing it. When criticism comes, as it usually will, he should give a straight answer and correct the misconceptions. Criticism is to be expected; however, it does not have to be unfavorable if he can correct a poor appearance by adding cheer to the patient-care, cleaning up the facility, and generally eliminating factors likely to arouse criticism.

The administrator should never miss an opportunity to improve his relations with the public. His participation in community activities and his invitations to the public to special events at the home will help. He can enter into a well-planned publicity campaign to focus attention upon the services offered by the home.

The Employees and Public Relations

The employees are the first line of public relations for the nursing home. They are the salesmen of the public image. Since they are in direct contact with the patients, visitors, relatives, professionals, and vendors—any one coming into the nursing home—they can strengthen its reputation. The administrator should be aware that employees also make news. Constantly, they are in the spotlight of publicity because of achievements, funerals, weddings, divorces, traffic violations, and so forth. Because of their association with the nursing home, their public image is closely akin to that of the home.

The administrator should recognize the public-relations value of his employees and train them to project the best image. He may start with a series of discussions or seminars, perhaps at the staff meetings or in-service training. He begins with the essentials of public relations, progresses to problem solving, then enlists his staff in a talking campaign to sell their friends, relatives, and associates.

Should an employee not prove loyal, it is not desirable to have him remain on the nursing home staff. Perhaps the worst public relations are rendered by a disgruntled employee. If he cannot be convinced of the integrity of the service, and if he maintains a negative attitude, the nursing home would be much better off without such a person. The employees need to be convinced of the importance of public relations. An educational program, a recognition program, and an active campaign to enlist the employees in public relations should be established.

The administrator should establish a definite curriculum of public relations as a part of in-service training and should encourage the employees to participate in definite projects to boost the image of the home, as for example, an open house. The administrator should send his people into the community with the message of the nursing home, for instance, as a representative of the United Fund drive, or as a guest at a formal luncheon. An alert administrator is constantly looking for ways the employees can project a good public image of the nursing home.

The Patients and Public Relations

The patient is the greatest public relations asset of the nursing home. In a true sense, the patient is the product of the nursing services. What he is or what he is encouraged to become, whether friend or not a friend, will be a witness to the quality of the nursing services.

The patient is constantly telling what he thinks about the nursing services. He talks to visitors, to his relatives, to his doctor, to any who will listen. He may telephone, write a letter, or just talk. He may never say a word, and yet his appearance will speak for him. His hygiene, his clothing, his bed, his room, his meals, or his attitude is identified with his presence in the nursing home.

The patient cannot be silenced. It is illegal to do so. The licensing agency forbids censorship; however, the administrator will not wish to silence a patient, for ethical reasons. Rather, the administrator will want to listen to the patient to hear what he is trying to say. The criticism may be valid and will alert the administrator to the need for corrective measures. Many times, the act of listening convinces the patient of the management's sincerity and gains his cooperation. Of course, some patients are biased in their opinion, but they may also be won with the patience and understanding of the administrator and his staff.

It should be the aim of the administrator to make every patient a friend. While it may seem beneficial to direct a potential resident to the bedside of a patient who could be expected to commend the nursing service, in the long run it will be far preferable to allow anyone free access to converse with any patient, being confident the nursing home will be commended. The administrator will maintain a constant program of upgrading, in order to cultivate the patients, to gain their understanding, and to maintain a high quality of service.

Publicity Release

Every administrator should learn to write a good news release. The techniques are largely learned, as are letter writing, good grammar, and good communication. A news release consists of reports of the home, the patients, the visitors, activities, accomplishments, etc. Normally, the editor's principles decide the newsworthiness of submitted material. The first thing he will recognize is a seeker of free advertising. News is not advertising. What is news, then?

News concerns people, and that which is immediate, prominent, outstanding, and factual. News from the nursing home to the public should be something that will be of interest to the community, such as the 100th birthday of a resident. It may concern the visit of a prominent citizen, or it may be some interesting action, such as the opening of a new wing to the nursing home. It could be when the administrator or employee is appointed to an important position in the community. Numbers or volume have meaning to the public, for instance, the admission of the one-thousandth patient.

In submitting an article for publication, there are several basic principles. Send your article directly to the editor. Type it double-spaced on plain white paper 8½ inches by 11 inches. In the upper left corner of each page, type: name, address, and phone number of the person submitting the article. In the upper right corner type: name of publication and below it the release date. If it is available immediately, say so, and the editor may use it as soon after receipt as he chooses.

Writing the article should not be too difficult. Remember, pack the lead paragraph with the elementary details. Explain these details in subsequent paragraphs by telling the story step by step. Every article will tell: "Who?" "When?" "Where?" "What?" and "Why?" The editor will write the headline and edit the article. He normally cuts the article from the bottom up, so place the less significant information last. The editor will cut an article to fit the space available, not because he disapproves of what it says.

Pictures may be submitted in much the same manner as the article. A short caption giving the facts and the names and addresses of each person in the picture should be attached; however, do not use a paper clip. It is well to employ a professional photographer. Never publish a patient's picture without his permission.

One word of encouragement: You can get your news printed. Those who keep sending the editor copy are the administrators who get their nursing homes in the news. Many editors are eager to have your news.

Advertising

The administrator controls the advertising released by the nursing home. From time to time he will wish to place a display ad in the local newspaper. It should be factual and dignified. Never oversell or make claims not in keeping with the service being offered. As the nursing home profession advances, there will develop a trend to become more modest in the advertising, as has been the practice of other health-related professions. However, there will always be need for strategic nursing home advertising.

Newspaper advertising is usually in the form of what is known as display advertising. The display advertising department of the newspaper will assist in the layout or arrangement; however, any art work is the responsibility of the customer. The cost of engravings may also be charged to the advertiser. Since advertising is sold on a column-inch basis—one column in width (usually two inches) and one inch deep—the cost can easily be estimated. An advertising firm can be hired on a contract basis to do all the layout, art work, photos, and reservation of space.

A good ad is not crowded, need not be large, yet is large enough to get the message across. Normally, one idea is sufficient for each ad. If you have two messages, buy more space and change your appeal at a later time for the second message. Also, repeat the ad just enough to be sure the public has got the message. The best pattern of advertising is to schedule periodic ads of a modest-to-large size. Between their appearances, schedule small signature ads to keep your name before the public. A signature ad contains the name of the nursing home, address, telephone number, and perhaps a line-drawing of the facility. Some signature ads contain a slogan or pithy statement.

Brochures

Each nursing home should print a neat, well-arranged brochure or folder stating its operating policy. It may contain pictures, and should have pertinent information on admission policy, ownership, location, etc. It is advisable to seek professional help in this publication. The distribution will be to the patients, to the general public, to relatives, to mail inquiries, to potential applicants, and a file copy to the licensing agency.

Normally, the brochure is required by state and federal regulations. It may be found under the requirement that the administrator will publish a general statement of his operating policy and make it available to the general public and the patients and their relative/ guardians. This policy statement will reflect all the requirements imposed on the patient for admission, such as rules and restrictions. It will reflect equality for minority groups. It will be in accordance with all laws regulating the nursing home. It should also describe the type of service offered, the facilities, and the type of patients accepted.

This normally becomes a basic publicity piece to be used in advertising the nursing home. It may be supplemented with other leaflets and brochures to further describe services available in the nursing home. The administrator may select some other types of novelty advertising, which may include pencils, matchbooks, calendars, post cards, signs, and souvenirs. Such advertising must be selected with care so as to reflect dignity on the home.

Radio and Television

Radio and television stations exist through the revenue made from the sale of advertising. While it is true that some time is devoted to public interest, the administrator should think of the stations as an advertising medium. Time is sold at commercial rates. Some of the time is considered prime time and will be more expensive because of the larger audience expected. Also, because of the uniqueness of the medium, professional help in preparing this type of advertising is necessary. Your local station employs specialists in their advertising departments to help in this area.

The administrator may select instead an advertising agency. An agency can usually get you more for your money, but its charges are likely to be greater. Of course, if the administrator places only an occasional announcement, he may wish to deal directly with the station. When submitting pictures for television, he should consider two types: 8 ″ x 10 ″ glossy prints and 16 mm film clips. Artwork may also be submitted. It is better to use a professional to make the picture, the film clip, and the artwork; sometimes the television station will offer assistance here. Copy submitted with the pictorial data will need to be edited to match the time purchased. Again, the station will assist in this. The use of television advertising will vary with the nursing home. Perhaps the administrator will hold open house and tie advertising in with this event. Usually, during the initial opening of a new facility, saturation advertising will be needed.

In submitting radio advertising, the administrator will follow the same procedures as for television, except that there is no need of pictures. Simply purchase the time—normally a sequence of several announcements of a predetermined length, and at strategic times during the day and week—and then prepare the copy. The station will usually take care of this step as a part of the fee. The sponsorship of a regular program should be considered. This, of course, will involve much more money because of production costs.

Community Relations

The nursing home is an integral part of the community. It may play the role of the sole health-related facility in the rural community; in the larger city, it is considered a part of the service-oriented health organization. The nursing home must relate itself to the larger community by supporting community needs. It may join one or more of the trade organizations, or cooperate in the support of others. It may be a resource point for educational enterprises or become a focal point of service activities. Even governmental agencies will sometimes utilize the nursing home for polling, sampling, or even experimenting. Without attempting to explain the nature of the following organizations, a listing of several of each type is given below.

Trade organizations include the Chamber of Commerce, Better Business Bureau, Nursing Home Association, etc.

Service organizations include the United Fund, Cancer Society, Heart Foundation, Red Cross, Legal Aid Society.

Fraternal organizations may include Rotary, Civitan, Kiwanis, Masonic lodges, etc.

Educational organizations include the Parent-Teachers Association, local school service leagues, college leagues, etc.

Churches will have missionary activities, service groups, Bible class projects, etc.

Governmental agencies may include the Office on Aging, Mental Health and Mental Retardation, Community centers, Legal Aid, etc.

Special Activities and Events

The administrator should constantly be planning special events to further his public relations. There are many types of activities he may sponsor; however, his ability to organize is as important as the choice of activity. The first step is to decide what is most appropriate to meet the need. The genesis of the idea may come from the staff meeting, a special meeting of supervisors, an advisory committee of service volunteers, the trustees, the administrator, or annual tradition. Then it is necessary to set objectives, to enlist help, and consolidate plans.

A coordinator of activities should be appointed. Certainly, the function determines who is placed in charge. Employee functions normally are sponsored by the employees themselves, while others draw on the volunteers. Of course, important annual affairs, such as an open house, would be directed by the administrator, or his assistant with additional help from the employees or from the volunteers. In some things, even the patients may be of assistance.

Once plans have been devised, a date is set and publicity released. Depending on the size of the venture, committees are appointed, such as program, decoration, equipment, furnishings, publicity, receiving, etc.

It is important that any special nursing home undertaking be coordinated with the dietary department, the nursing department, and with the patients and/or relatives.

There are numerous projects that may be considered. There are those such as an open house, parties, clubs, drafts, dedication services; religious occasions such as mass, communion, worship, prayer meeting, hymn singing; special events such as festivals, picnics, field trips, concerts, plays, variety shows; educational events such as study courses, dental clinics. The administrator will wisely monitor the programs so that he can insure a balance in the type offered.

Elevating the Nursing Home Profession

There is a growing need for the standards of the nursing home to gain the full respect of the public. Until the administrator can conduct his business as professional instead of practicing the traditional paternalistic management of the past, he will never render optimum service. The fears of the public in regard to nursing homes are gradually being erased, yet they still exist. Prejudices about the elderly need to be eliminated.

A survey of nursing home administrators in 1970 in the state of Texas revealed that only 16% had attained a college degree. A mere 2% had the master of arts degree or higher. Approximately 50% had only a high school diploma or an equivalency. This compares equally with several other states. When one considers the administrator's frequent contact with physicians, social workers, dentists, podiatrists, therapists, registered nurses, or pharmacists, all of whom have professional standing through educational achievement, it is no wonder that, with his lack of professional background, such disparagement of the nursing home administrator exists. He is called upon to handle complicated data, technical matter, professional communication, and to work with skilled and professional personnel. Because of recent licensing laws, the administrator now finds himself in the position of a fully health-related professional, a role that demands that he educate himself.

Because of Medicare and Medicaid, any states wishing to participate in these programs have been required to enact licensure laws as a condition for receiving matching funds. In the state of Texas, the law which requires licensing is known as Senate Bill 388. The bill required provisional licensing by July 1, 1970, and regular licensing by July 1, 1972 for anyone "who administers, manages, supervises, or is in general administrative charge of a nursing home, irrespective of whether such individual has an ownership interest in such home or whether or not his functions and duties are shared with one or more persons." Thus by law minimum standards have been established.

Voluntary Organizations

A number of voluntary organizations exist primarily for the purpose of upgrading the nursing home administrator, the nursing home, or the health services which he offers. We list these:

American Association of Homes for the Aged. This is a voluntary organization of nonprofit nursing homes, custodial or retirement centers, and homes for the aged. Most states have supporting organizations.

American Hospital Association. A voluntary organization for upgrading the professional standards of hospitals.

American Medical Association. The physician who attends the patients joins this organization.

American Health Care Association. The nursing home with its administrator may belong to this voluntary organization. It seeks to upgrade the standards of the nursing home industry. Both nonprofit and profit nursing homes, custodial homes, and personal care facilities may join its membership. All states have supporting organizations.

American College of Nursing Home Administrators. For voluntary accreditation of nursing home administrators. Ranks are: nominee, member and fellow. This organization has been found to be the professional organization of nursing home administrators having legal standing.

American Red Cross. Organization dedicated to the relief of the suffering, which offers supportive services to the nursing home.

Joint Commission on Accreditation of Hospitals. A voluntary association to accredit hospitals and nursing homes.

National Association of Boards of Examiners for Nursing Home Administrators. A voluntary association of official state license board members, former members, advisory committees, and associate members. This organization publishes an examination used in licensing nursing home administrators.

Chapter *19*

Business Communication

The Process of Communication

Communication is a factor of persuasion in imparting information and in providing entertainment. The administrator needs proper communication in the course of conducting the business of the nursing home. His understanding and use of communication will greatly aid his work.

All communication begins with a *source*, such as an idea, intention, purpose, etc. To be classed as communication, it must be expressed as a message. The process starts with formulating ideas, gathering information, and forming them into a logical, orderly, and understandable message. This is known technically as *translation*. It is one thing for an administrator to intend to do something; it is yet another for him adequately to formulate his plan.

The message is then *encoded* by the use of symbols, the voice, words, numbers, etc., into a form that may be transmitted.

To complete the process of communication, the encoded message must be delivered—this is usually referred to as *transmission*—and on being received, it is *decoded or* retranslated.

Using the above principles, there follows a simple pattern of communication: *source, translation, encoding, transmission, decoding, and reception.* This is the pattern of all communication, whether person to person, person to an audience, letter writer to recipient, or even unspoken communication, i.e., gestures, cultural, or psychological transmission.

The Psychology of Understanding

The administrator needs to know something about the psychology of understanding. *Do his employees understand his instructions? Do they get the message he intended?* Are they reading other meanings into his instruction? Can they comprehend what he has said? The best plan is doomed if communication fails. Think how disastrous it would be if a vital doctor's order went unheeded, or an open house celebration were unattended for failure to reach the public with the invitation.

In studying the process of thinking, one notes that the mind usually follows certain patterns or mental processes. It first attempts to identify, then it begins to classify, and finally it relates to known information. While these are interchangeable processes, anything perceived follows one or more of these psychological concepts.

The process of thinking may also be analyzed according to certain learning concepts. Starting with the *stimulus*, thinking progresses through a process known as *perception*. In simpler terms, a person becomes aware that something is stimulating him to think. Thus the stimulus may be thought of as the external source, while perception is the internal source. Stimulus, for example, may be a source of heat, while perception may be thought of as feeling something hot. From perception, thinking continues to *interpretation*, and then to *response*. As an example, one feels the heat and interprets its meaning to be that of a burning hand; therefore he responds by jerking his hand away from the source of heat.

When these principles of understanding are applied to the process of communication, the example is simplified. The message of a burned hand comes through "loud and clear." All communication is not, however, clearly understood for a number of reasons. The administrator may not be skilled in formulating a message. The receiver of the message may apply his own peculiar understanding. It could then become a matter of *semantics*: the study of the meaning of words. Usually, the receiver of a message will do four things to a message. He may apply *denotative meaning* to the message, which may be compared to a dictionary meaning. However, he will begin to structure meaning much as one forms a sentence. He may say, "This is an action to be performed today." Occasionally, he will evaluate the message in the light of past communication and begin to think of it in this context, and then say, "It should be done tomorrow." Finally, he may apply connotative meaning and say, "I don't think the boss wants this done at all."

In summary, we say that we must perceive and comprehend a message, then respond to it for it to qualify as communication. However, the recipient may apply his own ideas to the meaning of the message and give us problems in semantics. He may apply denotative meaning, something everyone agrees with; he may structure the meaning to formulate action; he may compare the meaning with other meanings; he may apply connotative meaning. Thus, understanding is affected by many things: emotion, interaction or feedback, culture, social structure, and even judgment. Personal bias or prejudice also restricts communication.

Avenues of Formal Communication

Communication may be classified as formal or informal. By formal, we mean it is intentional, planned, definite, and explicit. In other words, it is transmitted through a normal channel established to promote the business of the nursing home.

Communication methods may be written, oral, symbolic, or pictorial. Written communication is normally thought of as memos and messages between management and personnel, or between outside sources and employees. It may include letters, reports, books, pamphlets, brochures, newspapers, statements of policy, job descriptions, etc. As the administrator develops his supervisory policies, delegates authority, correlates the work, and exercises constant control of the organization, he uses written communication. In many instances, oral communication may be preferable because of the constant flow of orders, announcements, and reports. Pictorial communication is the use of sketches, posters, paintings, or cartoons to transmit a message. Symbolic communication is the use of computer language, code, graphs, statistics, or symbols. One more type, sometimes called "silent communication," is said to exist. This is like the empathy a speaker develops with his audience, an unspoken communication between companions, or the transmission of culture from one age to another.

Formal communication implies a prearranged channel for the transmission of messages. It may also prescribe the formulation of messages and their receipt. For example, certain forms, reports, letters, etc., are required. Upon receipt, the initials of the one for whom the message was intended are required. Requiring signed doctors' notes or nurses' progress notes, etc., is an example. In developing communication, the administrator will note three areas for definite consideration. He first will establish a positive means of communication between levels of management. Orders flow from the superior to the subordinates; thus a formal duty assignment has to be made. Next, he will plan a definite means of communication between departments, intercommunication must be established. Such an arrangement facilitates, for example, one shift giving a report to the oncoming shift. Finally, the administrator will make sure every person and every audience is included in planning communication. Whether it be the employee, the patient, or the general public, the administrator needs to plan some channel of communication to reach them.

The Grapevine—Informal Communication

Informal communication may be distinguished from formal communication by the difference in intent and purpose of message transference. There is no system, normally, to informal communication, thus the title "grapevine." The idea of informal communication is a paradox. Formal methods are utilized, i.e., writing, speaking, etc.; however, there is always a distinction of purpose and motive. Informal communication serves its own peculiar purpose, as "gossip," "news," "inside information," a sporadic or intermittent flow of information. A message may come piecemeal over several channels.

The messages of informal communication lack uniformity. The basic idea is that whatever is communicated informally will usually be without order, comparable to the labyrinth or an actual grapevine. It is usually secretive, unauthorized, and should be compared to gossip. It may be compared to the statement, "I overheard the boss saying . . ." It will always be of a secondhand nature and reflect connotative judgment. The information may sound authentic, but it usually is not. The deliverer of a piece of information will sometimes preface his remarks with "I have it on good authority . . . ." The source may not be authoritative, may be inaccurate, may be merely preliminary, and is seldom complete. Why, then, should the administrator consider the use of informal communication to be of any value in his nursing home?

The first answer is the fact of its existence. As a by-product of personal relations, it exists as a part of unconscious behavior. Every person has a desire to communicate; in the process, learning may take place through the natural interaction of people, or the reflection of attitudes, or it may be a means of relieving tension and anxiety. The second answer is that it cannot be eliminated, therefore, the administrator should learn to utilize it. How then, can it be utilized?

The administrator may use informal communication to test reactions by subtly leaking some information in order to analyze the feedback. Is the reaction favorable? Unfavorable? The administrator may use it to raise the hopes and expectations of his staff. An anticipated change could be revealed before the planning is complete, to inspire the employees. The administrator uses informal communication to gauge attitudes. After a formal presentation at a staff meeting, it is the informal interaction of the employees that clarifies the full meaning of what was said. Sometimes the administrator may prefer that his viewpoint be made known informally. A formal warning to an employee may break his spirit, while the encouragement of a sympathetic employee, who may say, "The administrator will not accept this," should not.

Written Communication

The use of written communication is an ever present fact of doing business. It is estimated that written communication is now doubling every five years, while only a generation ago the rate was every ten years. Thus the magnitude of the utilization of written materials is becoming overwhelming. The nursing home is no different from other businesses; in fact, some administrators may recall when a nursing home kept no clinical charts, except when a person became ill. Today, documentation is required of every nursing action. In the administrative office, the use of written communication is just as great.

Perhaps the most beneficial education available to the administrator in the area of communication is letter writing. College departments usually call it, "Business Communication," or "Business English."

The administrator must become adept in message construction. The man who said, "If I had time, I would write a shorter letter," recognized the value of being brief and to the point, and that it takes thought, concentration, and skill. Like a news article, a message should be natural, informative, factual, and well arranged. Give the essentials in the first paragraph and the explanations in the latter paragraphs. Avoid repetition and redundancy. Essentially, be brief and concise.

Letter writing is one of the most important skills of communications. The administrator should be able to compose a proper letter, complete with all its parts in the proper arrangement. *The parts of the letter are: letterhead, date, inside address, attention line, salutation, subject line, body of the letter, closing signature, signature line, reference, enclosure, and "cc" line.*

The second most important skill is the writing of reports. *The parts of a formal report are: title, table of contents, introduction, body, conclusion, recommendations, summary, and supplemental information.*

The maintenance of records is also an essential part of administration and business communication. For material to be of value as a record, the format should be legible, understandable, and complete enough to be useful. The administrator should learn to arrange the flow of written material into a useful pattern. All too often records are of no use because of improper compilation or storage, and failure to retrieve them for further use.

The normal channels of written communication are: mail, telegram, telefax, pneumatic tube, microfilm, film, transparencies, and printed materials. Signs, posters, and other display material may be included. Publications, i.e., newspapers, magazines, books, also are a part of the vast area of communication. There are no real criteria for selecting the method of transmission except to consider the original purpose, the need, the cost, and the availability of services. In every case, however, *the administrator will consider the permanency of the record, its confidential nature, its legal requirements, and its use as a management tool. Some items such as statements of policy, procedures, job descriptions, etc. need permanency to avoid misunderstanding;* thus, written communication is necessary.

Oral Communication

The process of oral communication follows the same steps as written communication, with the exception that the source or message is vocalized and the reception auditory, which creates a distinction in translation and retranslation. In one sense, there is no translation, merely interpretation. However, oral communication, like all other processes, involves the transference of meaning. The speaker is the originator of the message, and the audience is the receiver of his communication. While the channel may be speech, we may also convert speech to electrical impulses and transmit it electronically.

One important factor of oral communication is the interaction between speaker and audience, i.e., stimuli, response, and interaction. These factors are not present in other communications, unless one were to consider that they are present but with a delay factor. In oral communication, the stimuli are both the message and the ability of the speaker effectively to convey his message. In audience-speaker communication, the response is both immediate and apparent; in written communication interaction is delayed and perhaps never publicly manifested. In some types of oral communication, such as television and radio, there is little or no interaction. In other words, the speaker does not know whether he is getting his message across to his audience as in direct person-to-person discussion and public speaking.

Person-to-person communication is best for the transference of an idea. Written communication is better for permanency and documentation of the message. In public speaking, the small group is far better than the large audience. Of course, in the time of mass communications, we must utilize improved means of conveying our message. A nursing home may have a patient-call system to include voice communication between the patient's room and the nurses' station. It may use a public address system, a telephone system, and be connected with the cable television circuit. It may schedule periodic announcements over radio and television. For the enjoyment of the patients, taped or recorded music may be played. Some churches prepare tapes of their services, which are then played back to members confined in the nursing home.

One of the major responsibilities of the administrator is speaking publicly. It may be at a staff-meeting, before the civic club, or at the annual meeting of the board of directors. He will need to learn to prepare a message or speech, using the basics of all communication, good grammar, sentence structure, and organization. In preparing a speech, first make the basic assumption or topic of the message; state it in one sentence, if possible. Next, collect the basic facts and figures to be dealt with. Then select supporting materials such as examples, comparisons, authorities, illustrations. Finally, arrange the material in outline form, starting with the introduction, proceeding to the main statements with their supporting statements, and finally to the conclusion.

Barriers to Communication

Information distortion is possibly the largest single hazard to consider in message construction. In fact, the administrator initiates communication for the purpose of overcoming distortion. There are basically two schools of thought concerning communication: some say the goal is to effect change, while others say the goal is to convey differences. These may sound like two statements meaning the same thing, but there is a subtle difference. The first may be illustrated by the administrator who conveys an order, expecting obedience by the subordinate. An example of the second is the administrator who uses tools of communications to inspire the workers to evaluate work habits, note deficiencies, or variations from the accepted norm, and make improvement.

The administrator may fail to be understood by his subordinates for many reasons, but most likely is his failure to state clearly his message. Imagine the publicity release which says,

Semiprivate rooms for ladies and gentlemen with private baths.

He obviously means the rooms are with private baths and are to be occupied by ladies *or* gentlemen. However, this is not what he has said. A subordinate will not react properly to an ambiguous message.

Overcoming failure in communication is a matter of study, reevaluation, and practice. When the administrator is aware his communication is not effective, he should rephrase it. When he is confident he is not at fault, he should evaluate how he is transmitting his messages. Would another method be more effective? Would a secondary method strengthen his communication? Has he been conveying policy changes orally?

Message distortion can be traced to a number of reasons: faulty information, wrong wording, typographical errors, poor expression, lack of clarity, poor retention, or inattention. The administrator could learn from the printer the value of proofreading; from the dictionary, how to spell, and from practice, how to write. Of course, a renewed study of English grammar and business communications will help.

Message distortion may not be entirely the fault of the originator of a message. The receiver of a message may not take sufficient time to impress the details on his memory; thus he may "forget." He may even procrastinate, toss it aside for "future reference." Finally, some messages fail to get to the proper recipient. How a recipient understands the meaning of the message has been previously discussed.

In some cases, the organizational structure may restrict communications. The problem of departmentalization places the supervisors apart from one another in the organization. The decentralization of decision-making authority will make it imperative that methods of communication be uniform and efficient. Clear lines of communication, explicit policy, precise directives, etc., ensure unity.

Developing Better Communication

Communications within and without the nursing home must be effective. Every administrator differs in his habits of communication, but everyone will need to develop the best possible system of communication. Communication bears a definite relationship to the organizational goals of the nursing home. If goals cannot be transmitted clearly, effectively, and without distortion, the organizational pattern, plans, and activities will break down.

Integrity in communications is a predominent factor. It is easy to convey the wrong message. For example, a nurse may agree with the supervising nurse as to a certain standard of work, but may convey a lesser or even different standard to the aides. She may feel the message lacks usefulness or validity. She may not have the proper time to implement the message. At times, a nurse may be bypassed in the chain-of-command and not be aware of a change in the procedure or policy. A nurse may deliberately distort a message for a personal reason, such as protecting her own interests. These are factors that cause problems and misunderstanding, and result in poor service.

Accuracy in the information flow is most important. Always assemble the correct data, proofread it, and select the best method to assemble it for transmission to its intended recipient. Accuracy in transmission can also be improved. Transcribing from rough draft to letter, from dictation to report, or from copy to stencil are but three areas in which to go astray. When printing, a proofed copy, legibly reproduced and well-arranged, is important to accuracy and readability.

The administrator may also need to improve his message reception. There are countless communications flowing across his desk, which must be appraised and acted upon. He should develop methods of appraisal, analysis, and response. A follow-up of message reception will overcome loss of contact, and prompt evaluation pays dividends.

Consider the areas within the nursing home that must be kept at peak efficiency and that depend upon an effective message flow. The staff meeting, in which duties are delegated to responsible supervisors, or the change of shift in the nursing department are but two key areas. Some method of feedback and evaluation will greatly enhance the effectiveness of communication.

Reading Improvement for Better Communication

Improvement of reading habits offers perhaps the best opportunity for improvement of communication. Faster reading by the staff will make additional time available for patient care. Better reading will make for greater efficiency. Tests show the fast reader to be superior in comprehension, perception, and recall.

The administrator should test himself as to his need for reading improvement. The test is very simple, merely a measure of reading speed by timing, but there is more than speed to reading efficiently. An understanding of what is read, an ability to recall the material, and ability to interpret or relate the material are but three factors of reading skill. Look for physical causes of poor reading habits: vision is very important and should be checked periodically; the environment may hinder reading, i.e., poor lighting, an uncomfortable chair, a noisy office, etc.

A program of reading improvement will result in faster perception and better comprehension. Perception concerns the amount of material or the number of words the eye may perceive in a single fixation. Some persons may perceive only a single syllable or a single word at each fixation of the eye. Others may perceive several words or even several lines of printing at one fixation of the eye. Perception may be speeded up with practice. However, to be effective, it must be coupled with increased comprehension. Comprehension is related to the degree of understanding of the ideas embodied in the written material and also may be improved with practice. To speed up perception, one should work for speed and try for less eye movement. He should make a definite attempt to grasp the ideas of the words more quickly, so as to increase comprehension. Some reading improvement systems utilize a mechanical pacer in which the eye is challenged to cover more lines in less time. One obstacle to perception is vocalizing the words while reading. Also, a stumbling block is the lack of knowledge as to the meaning of words. Vocabulary study improves the power of comprehension. Such techniques as reviewing before reading, concentration, and recalling will greatly help to improve one's reading ability.

Memory Improvement for Better Communication

Since the administrator is required to remember details from several areas of knowledge, any way of improving his memory is an advantage.

Types of memory may vary. There is the *incidental memory*, which stores random ideas, concepts, and perceptions. Everyone has incidental memory and will use it to some degree. In fact, on-the-job training makes use of many randomly acquired ideas to meet the job requirement, rather than systematic presentation. Some have an *in-*

tentional memory, in which desired data, statistics, numbers, facts, etc., are stored. Some have an *associative memory* for related structures, ideas, concepts, etc. One may have a better *visual memory* for objects, pictures, graphics, and concrete structuring. A few persons may develop a *specialized memory*. They have a system, a habit of remembering, or the natural ability to remember better than others. The administrator may improve his memory if he can remember to try to improve it!

Someone has said the best way to memorize is to memorize. This is facetious, but true. One could qualify this statement to show some of the ways to improve memory. The oldest method is that of association; that is, relating what is desired to be remembered with something familiar. Another way is to structure ideas into familiar or similar groupings. One may remember some unusual aspect to which he can tie what he wishes to retain in his mind. Many years ago a series of nonsense syllables was developed, to which one would tie the facts to be remembered. Repetition is undoubtedly the best aid to memory, e.g., "Hello, Mr. Jones? Mr. Jones, I. . . . etc." Overlearning for emphasis will often crowd out and reduce an interference in learning; in the same way the interference of a more recent memory tends to crowd out important details of past memories. The administrator should practice memory improvement by making it a pleasant avocation.

Restriction on memory includes overcrowding, lack of confidence, failure to utilize, falsification, disorganization, poor association, and exaggeration. One may not memorize simply because he has thoroughly convinced himself that he cannot. Usually, poor organization and poor association result in confusion in remembering.

Chapter 20

Employee-Employer Relationships

A Historical Look at Labor-Management Relations

Labor-management relationships have been traced to the beginning of civilization, from the ancient Euphrates valley which spawned the Egyptians, the Babylonians, the Persians, the Greeks, and the Romans. One of our earliest references is in the Hammurabi code dating to the seventeenth century B.C. The code is of a legal nature but deals with the rights of the worker. These ancient laws were discovered in 1901, at Susa, by Jacques de Morgan. It is noteworthy that Babylonian culture in the time of Hammurabi was largely urban, but it developed an intricate irrigation system through cooperative labor efforts. Evidence of this vast irrigation system was recently confirmed by aerial photography. Some of our information concerning the Egyptians comes to us through the discovery of ancient papyri and some from the Bible, which refers to the sojourn of the Hebrews in Egypt. In the book of Genesis, the story of Joseph tells of the position of "chief of butlers," "chief of bakers," and "overseer;" Egyptian documents confirm these supervisory positions. In later Hebrew history, we have the development of the Levitical Law, which offered labor protection from the unjust overseer. Jesus refers to the position of "steward," and his statement, "The laborer is worthy of his hire," is often quoted.

In later years of ancient history, the Romans and Greeks devised a system for defining the rights of labor and management. While the Romans are generally known for their use of forced labor, the Greeks are credited with the development of administrative procedures. During the Middle Ages, the Roman Catholic Church established an elaborate administrative system that included the control and supervision of a sizable labor force. Ironically, this fine administrative system went largely unnoticed by the ethnic-political society, which developed its system apart from the church.

Later on, the merchant adventurers of England and the Low Countries, who dealt in the shipment of goods in the fifteenth and sixteenth centuries, contributed to the rise of labor-management relations. An Austrian and German group, called the cameralists, emphasized the financial and social aspect of management's responsibility for labor.

More recently, the modern hospital has provided the necessary administrative management techniques for supervision of health care facilities. A number of early writers made contributions in the management field. These include: Frederick W. Taylor, 1911; Henri Fayol, 1916; O. Sheldon, 1923; Russell Robb, 1910; and H. S. Dennison, 1931.

Employer-Employee Sharing of Management

In management there are several trends developing which result in labor sharing with management in the decision-making process. These include the democratic approach, the committee approach, and the employees' representative approach. However, to deal properly with each, it is necessary for the administrator to understand some of the theories concerning management and labor relations. These theories deal with wages, human behavior, social needs, and the labor market.

The *classical wage theorists* emphasize the individual's right to choose his job, with the wages being the prime determinant. The result of this theory, in simple terms, is the equality of the labor market.

Operational labor-management theorists accept the traditional, analytical methods of study of the labor market to advance principles of labor by which one may predict the results of labor-management relations.

The *human behaviorists* emphasize human relations and psychology as the basis of solving worker-management problems.

Finally, *social organizationalists* view the working enterprise as purely a social structure. They emphasize the importance of social relations.

The student of nursing home administration will notice that a portion or all of the theories may be applied to problem-solving. Thus, as the employees and the employer share in management, it may be approached from one or more points of view. The democratic approach may emphasize the majority as opposed to the autocratic concept of the "boss ordering." The committee system has been applied with some success by those who emphasize the social structure of the enterprise. Given these theories and approaches to shared management, it is evident that not all are compatible. Obviously, some administrators may not adapt to sharing the management role, because they are traditional theorists who emphasize analytical methods; others may agree in theory but not in practice. In the nursing home, however, an additional reason for sharing management decision-making with labor is the many professional disciplines that need to be focused on problems of patient care. Thus, no matter what the philosophy of the management or labor, the needs of the patient become more important.

Employee Health Factors

Health is fundamental to work. Good health and good work stand opposed to poor health and poor work. The health of the employee is directly related to his proficiency, dependability, quality of work, attitude, safety, and relationships with fellow employees. Health problems of employees range over the entire list of human needs, none of which should be neglected. Because of the importance of encouraging top performance, the administrator should periodically review his employees' records for evidence of medically related problems which may include: disease, chronic infirmities, disabilities, mental stress, and other special health problems. He should establish a requirement of periodic health examination, including pre-employment examination, and expect the employees to file a physician's report. This requirement should be included in the statement of personnel policies.

The administrator has a responsibility to protect the employee's health with safety measures. This has always been a moral obligation of the management; however, with the passing of the Occupational Safety and Health Act, it is now a legal obligation. A program of education in infection control practices must be coupled with working policies that require the safest working conditions. Proper heat and ventilation, safety equipment and regulations, good lighting, rest breaks, and adequate time for lunch should be provided. Adequate health protection for employees should include a periodic review of the total working program, including job requirements, working conditions, safety, and infection control. There should be a program of education in health and hygiene, provision for first aid and emergency medical attention, and perhaps a liberal sick-leave and sick-pay policy. Health services may include Employer's Liability Insurance, Medical and Health Insurance, periodic health checkups, dental and optical services, counseling, and provision for maternity leave for the working mother.

Drug abuse has become an area of danger in recent years. The fact that the nursing home employee works within an environment that relies heavily on pharmaceuticals, and that the professional nurse—some states permit a medication aide—administers medication, provides opportunity for possible drug abuse, ranging in degree from the confirmed addict to the person who is psychologically dependent on drugs.

The drugs subject to abuse range from the amphetamines, which stimulate the central nervous system, the barbiturates, which are prescribed for sedatives, to narcotics, i.e., opium and its derivatives, morphine, heroin, codeine, meperidine, demerol, and methadone. Marijuana is a narcotic; hallucinogens such as LSD are grouped separately.

The administrator should watch for signs of drug abuse among his employees. Some indicators are: chronic absenteeism or lateness for work, unexplained absences from the work area, lengthy visits to the rest room, visits by strangers or frequent phone calls; physical evidence, such as stupor or drowsiness, personality changes, and poor work habits and judgment.

Employee Safety Factors

Safety should be a way of life in the nursing home. This rule applies not only to the patient but to the employee as well. Nothing maintains morale and the conservation of manpower quite so much as practicing safety. Losses resulting from accidents may be insurmountable; aside from the legal liability, which could be disastrous, the economic effect of the loss of a good worker may decrease the operating margin. Manpower losses will reduce the level of care to the patients, as employees may not be replaced readily, and loss of supplies, equipment, or facilities which result from accidents may lower the standards of care, placing the nursing home below minimum standards established by the licensing agency.

Accidents in the nursing home are classified by the National Fire Protection Association in the order of their occurrence: falls, fires, poisoning, machinery, ingestion of food, a blow by object, medical practice, and electrical shock. An adequate safety program should include education in safety practices, safety rules, safety equipment, etc.

Safety education is provided by posters, bulletins, slogans, records of injuries, talks, demonstrations, or seminars.

The home will make and publish its policy concerning safety. Any rules and regulations related to work habits should be reviewed periodically. Necessary corrective measures should be instituted immediately.

Safety equipment, including guards, fences, locks, clothing, glasses, gloves, etc., must be maintained. Equipment certified as to construction and safety by an underwriters' laboratory should be used.

Compliance with voluntary codes such as the National Electrical Code is a routine safeguard. Regular inspections for safety should be conducted in cooperation with the local fire marshal and local health authorities.

Occupational Safety and Health Act

The nursing home as an employer is regulated by the Williams-Steiger Occupational Safety and Health Act of 1970. The purpose of the act is "to assure so far as possible every working man and woman in the nation safe and healthful working conditions and to preserve our human resources."

The law places the responsibility of compliance on both the employer and the employee. The employer will furnish hazard-free working conditions, while the employee will comply with safety and health standards, rules and regulations. The law is administered by the Secretary of Labor, who not only has power to enforce the act, but also power to set standards for compliance either for all employees or for specific types of work.

The sources of information for rules, regulations, and standards are varied. Much of the original act came from the National Fire Protection and existing Federal Standards, i.e., the Walsh-Healey Act regulating federal contractors. New standards may be recommended by the Secretary of Labor, advisory committees, or others. The act specifies the procedure for changes, new regulations, or revocation of existing rules. Emergency, temporary standards may be established when workers are subjected to excessive dangers. The Secretary of Labor, after a hearing, may grant temporary relief or permanent variance from standards, if an employer is using equally safe practices.

Employees are permitted to file complaints when they believe their job is unsafe. While the charge must be shown the employer, the name of the complainant is not. Investigation of such complaints of violation is required without delay and at reasonable times. Inspectors will be granted full access to facilities, machines, and equipment. The administrator of the nursing home being inspected has a legal right to accompany the inspector. Personnel may be questioned privately.

When a violation is revealed as a result of such an investigation, a citation is issued describing it in detail and fixing a reasonable time for abatement of the hazard. Such notice shall be posted prominently at or near the place of violation. The employer will be notified by certified mail of any penalty. However, the employer may contest a penalty or citation by giving notice to the Labor Department within 15 working days.

Record-keeping of injuries and deaths is a requirement of the law. Such records are required when an occupational injury or illness occurs that requires medical treatment, loss of time, or transfer to another position. In case of death or illness of five or more employees, the Secretary of Labor will be notified. Records of exposure to toxic materials is required. Finally, a summary of accidents and illnesses is to be posted annually by the end of January.

Because many states have been involved in occupational safety and health, the act permits states to develop their own programs. When the individual states can advance programs of occupational safety and health equal to or exceeding federal standards, such states may assume administration. Thus, the nursing home administrator would be accountable to his particular state agency.

Wages

Minimum wages are required under the Fair Labor Standards Act of 1938 as amended in 1966 to include nursing homes. The administrator should understand the interpretation the Secretary of Labor places on what is a "minimum wage." Anything the employer may require of the employee that would reduce his true remuneration below the minimum is prohibited. This includes a requirement that the employee wear a uniform, the cost of which reduces the employee's pay below the minimum wage. Any unfair and unreasonable charge imposed on the employee is forbidden. Piecework, when the total earning per week divided by the number of hours worked results in a rate below that of the minimum wage, or a salary which does not exceed the minimum, is forbidden. In addition, the law sets time and one-half rates for over 40 hours (a later amendment reduced the previous 48-hour requirement for nursing homes) for nursing personnel. Some personnel in the nursing home, i.e., the food service personnel, have another requirement which schedules them to reach the same 40-hour requirement in 1977. The employer is required to record hours daily and weekly to determine overtime. Records will also reflect the basic wage, the hourly rate, weekly total, and overtime pay. The law also includes an equal pay provision.

The administrator should learn how to determine the prevailing wage for the nursing home industry. Techniques in salary classification need to be mastered. Should the administrator overprice, he may expect a poor return on the investment; should he underprice, he may expect poor service to the patients, since he will not be able to secure good workers. There are several means of determining the prevailing wage within a given area, such as make a survey, analyze the costs and profits of the home, or enter into negotiations with the employees, their union, or their representatives.

The administrator will need to develop some method of computing comparative wages. There should be wage differentials between jobs, shifts, and starting salaries. Each job will have a base salary to which may be added incentives, seniority pay, or shift differentials.

A method of increasing wages should be considered. Increases may be based on individual changes and changes in the industry. Of course, increases by law regulating minimum wages have first priority. This is followed by increases for a rise in the cost of living and labor, market pricing, fringe benefits, and prosperity.

One method of rewarding the employee is cost sharing or profit sharing. This may include a partnership agreement for supervisory personnel, excess profits distributed as bonuses, or shares based on merit or skill.

Hours

Again the Fair Labor Standards Act of 1938 will apply to the nursing home in determining the maximum work week for the employee. There is an additional factor: both Medicare and Medicaid contracts limit the length of the day and the work week for most nursing home employees. It should be noted that the law provides for record keeping—daily time, weekly time, and overtime—and defines a work week as any seven consecutive 24-hour periods. If the pay is in any other way, i.e., commission, piecework, meals, monthly salary, etc., the hours still need to be recorded to ensure that the minimum wage is paid, and that overtime requirements are kept. The law provides for enforcement in the event of failure by the employer to pay the statutory minimum and overtime rate. Serious violations of the law may result in civil or criminal action. Records required by law must be made available for inspection by representatives of the U.S. Department of Labor.

The administrator will determine the actual hours worked by excluding such time as may be specifically designated for lunch, portal to portal (travel time), and waiting time, such as the change of shift. A reasonable time for lunch is considered to be at least 30 minutes. Waiting time is considered as five or six minutes, and a coffee break may be considered as work if it is less than 30 minutes. Should the employee change clothes or wash up on the premises, this is considered work. *In other words, if the employee is not completely free of all responsibility, the time is considered as work and shall be paid for as such.*

The administrator will consider the nursing home employee to be working if he is actually on the job, if he is only required to be at his place of duty, if he is getting ready to do his job, if he is learning his job by merely observing, if he is correcting others' work, if he is preparing working materials, if he is receiving medical treatment at the place of work, if he is standing by during a breakdown, if he is required to wait until work is prepared for him, or if he has a travel assignment.

The recording of hours worked and wages paid is the express obligation of the administrator or his assistant. It must be done regularly, that is, at the beginning and ending of each shift, totaled at the end of the week, and the amount of overtime recorded. His pay check will indicate the hourly rate, the number of hours, the gross pay, and all deductions.

The time clock may be used, but it it is not the final legal authority. The employer will ensure that time is recorded accurately. Normally, records are stored for three years at the place of employment or the employer's office.

Fringe Benefits

The modern worker has accumulated many side benefits that are considered as fringe benefits to his employment. Some have come by law, such as Social Security; others have come as a result of the improvement of employer-employee relationship. A listing of fringe benefits may include:

> Pension plans to include both the Old Age, Survivors and Disabled Insurance Act (Social Security), company pension plans, and annuities.

Health services to include health and medical insurance plans, life insurance, accident insurance, sick pay, sick leave, and infirmary, and medical examination.

Financial services such as a credit union, bonuses, incentive pay, savings programs, and deductions for union dues, savings bonds, United Fund, etc.

Food services may include cafeteria service at cost, meals, or a company store and/or discounts.

Educational benefits may include tuition grants, educational programs, and scholarships for employees and their children.

Recreational benefits to include paid vacations, paid holidays, social or recreational clubs.

Nursing home uniforms, uniform laundry service, and special equipment.

There may be a counselor or chaplain available.

Fringe benefits are becoming a major factor in the cost of the employee's services. Side benefits sometimes equal as much as 50 percent of the remuneration for work. This can have a decided effect on the operating cost of the nursing home and should be analyzed for budgetary purposes. Fringe benefits are difficult to estimate because of the variable nature of the service to be offered. It is wise, therefore, for the administrator to establish cost controls. Another aspect of fringe benefits is their influence in the labor market. Job turnover is directly related to the amount of these benefits; personnel planning should take this into consideration. In addition, labor problems, absenteeism, and related personnel needs can be greatly reduced when the administrator has a liberal program of fringe benefits.

Retirement of Employees

The nursing home administrator certainly deals with the problems of retirement, but mostly in regard to patients. However, he should consider also his employees who will face retirement, at which time a number of psychological factors begin to emerge. The nearer the employee is to retirement, the more prevalent these factors become. The first and main concern is uncertainty. Some would call it fear, others anxiety, but it is uncertainty of the future. There is uncertainty about the transition from a working to a nonproductive status; there is uncertainty about the feeling of usefulness; there is uncertainty about finance. Unless the individual has planned well, this always will be a major factor of concern. Overconcern then would give rise to anxiety and worry.

There is no ideal age for retirement, yet certain times have been imposed upon the worker. The companies' setting rigid times of retirement and the payment of benefits by Social Security have imposed the ages of 62, 65, and 69 as traditional ages of retirement. The nursing home should maintain a flexible policy when possible.

A number of elements may affect a decision to retire. The work may become too strenuous for the nurse's aide, for example, or health may be the deciding factor as aging progresses. The administrator should be aware of certain prejudices concerning older people. Society expects the older person to retire to make room for younger people. Society also expects the older person to be nonproductive in retirement, and to accept leisure time as a reward for years of production. However, the administrator should be aware of the Age Discrimination in the Employment Act of 1967, which protects individuals 40 to 65 years of age. The employer may not refuse to hire nor to terminate an employee solely on the basis of age.

The administrator may assist employees in the preparation for retirement in several ways. The best is educational opportunities available. With the enactment of the Older Americans Act, many educational benefits are now available. Services in almost all areas of retirement needs are now being explored and provisions are now being made to bring necessary services to the older American. The administrator could provide counseling and assistance for his employees who are to retire, assist them to make financial preparations or encourage increased leisure activities.

The retiree's financial planning will be his main concern. Social Security is the basic financial base of most retirees, but many continue to work. Others have pension plans or insurance annuities, savings, and accumulated equity or full ownership in their homes. With Medicare and Medicaid, some of the burden of high medical costs is relieved.

Job Security and Equal Opportunity

Job security is related to morale and is basically a psychological factor. However, the assurance of job security to the employees is a result of the total employment policy established and maintained by the administrator. A number of factors the administrator may develop to improve job security should be considered.

Opportunity for advancement is one of the most important benefits that a job can offer. Promotion is another; however, promotion is limited in the organization of the nursing home because of the professional requirements. An aide could advance to the position of charge aide, but will need further education to advance to professional nurse. The rigid division between professional and nonprofessional will be a barrier. In order for the administrator to encourage promotion, he also has to encourage the employee to upgrade his education. Transfer is also important. The opportunity to move to a more acceptable job may be a key consideration.

Recognition for achievement may be the key to job security. Every employee wants due credit for accomplishments. The administrator can plan a seniority or merit program of advancement or recognition; he also should create an atmosphere of respect for the individual employee through friendliness, compliments, and recognition.

Job security is directly related to remuneration. Every attempt should be made to provide a living wage, to make periodic wage increases, to bestow merit incentives or bonuses, fringe benefits, and possibly arrange for profit sharing.

Supervision is also related to job security. When employees respect their supervisor, they feel that authority is used wisely and that they have challenging responsibility. They feel more secure in their work.

A safe and pleasant environment and congenial fellow workers motivate employees to do better work. Finally, equal opportunity is necessary for job security. The employee who feels he is being discriminated against is not happy in his work. In recent years laws have been developed to protect the worker against discrimination for reasons of sex, age, race, color, creed, and national origin. To withhold advancement, promotion, recognition, etc., may be interpreted as discrimination.

The administrator as an employer is forbidden by law to discriminate in employment practices. One of the major laws is the Civil Rights Act of 1964, which is directed to those who receive federal financial assistance. It was amended in 1972 to afford equal opportunity to all persons. While this is usually interpreted to forbid discrimination toward women, it should be remembered that men also have equal rights and may be expected in increasing number to enter professions that have been thought to be exclusively reserved to women, e.g., that of registered nurse.

Specifically, Title VII of the Civil Rights Act as amended protects the rights of all individuals to equality in employment practices. Such practices shall include equal pay for equal jobs and would tend to eliminate differential pay scales for both sexes. Hiring and firing practices will be uniform, and promotional opportunities will not exclude either sex. The administrator will be aware that the positions of administration have historically favored the male employee, but by law such favoritism is forbidden. The administrator should examine his own attitude concerning the law. There are the legal requirements which he can write into his nursing home policy; and then there is the spirit of the law, which should influence his decisions. His attitude concerning employment should rest solely on the ability of the employee to perform the skills needed to meet the nursing home goals and objectives. He will write his personnel policies to reflect this attitude, and train his supervisors to follow his leadership with respect to the spirit of the law.

The administrator will reexamine each stated policy of the nursing home to determine that equal opportunity is in fact written into the published policies. Take, for example, the personnel policy concerning temporary sick leave because of reasons of health, pregnancy, or childbirth. The new law requires reinstatement should the female employee take such leave. Job classifications should be further studied to determine if they tend to discriminate, i.e., placing females in the housekeeping department with the classification of maid, and then hiring males exclusively for janitorial work. The tendency to classify the more strenuous jobs for males and the less strenuous jobs for females could be interpreted as discrimination. The recruiting and selection practices of the administrator will need to be done in keeping with the law. Advertising in the local newspaper for workers of a single sex will not likely be an acceptable practice. Statements made during the interview will be cautious in that promises or declarations of employment practices shall conform to the requirements of the acts. A number of customs and beliefs concerning the "weaker sex" can no longer exist.

Enforcement of the act will be the responsibility of the Equal Employment Opportunity Commission. The nursing home administrator should be aware that his liability under the act is excluded if he has 15 or fewer employees, but that he may still be regulated under Executive Order 11246 concerning employment practices for contractors and subcontractors of government services.

Employees' Family Life

Labor theorists who emphasize the social aspect of the employer-employee relationship stress the fact that the employee is primarily a provider for his family. Of course, the single person will be concerned only with himself. There are numerous trends that affect the provider. The rise of the working class is one: our entire economy is founded upon the production of the worker. At no time in history has the worker found himself quite so important, but, as his prominence rises, so does his obligation. One remarkable area of growth in the labor market has been the growth of service personnel, which includes the nursing home employee. The fluctuation of the economy and recent inflationary trends play a considerable part in the stability of labor relations. Finally, union-management relations affect the stability of the labor market. With rising economic demands on the provider, the increasing cost, and higher standards of living, the provider faces many problems.

The majority of nursing home employees are married. Thus the administrator will need to give some consideration to the spouse. Since most nurses are women, their stability in employment is related to the job opportunity of the husband. His promotion or transfer may mean that the working wife is obliged to resign. Domestic relations between the husband and wife can have some influence on working relationships.

Many employees are parents of small children, and children cause certain problems. The administrator will find his workers affected by such problems as health, delinquency, broken homes, educational needs, child care, etc. The overall family health is another factor. If the provider is ill, the entire family suffers. If a child is ill, the mother is usually required to stay at home. Of course, pregnancy of the working mother will require a leave of absence or termination of employment.

Family recreation is a vital factor in employee-family relationships that affect working habits. With the shorter work week as a trend, and therefore more leisure for the employee, the administrator should consider other types of scheduling duties. Some have found four days on duty with four days off, thus rotating the weekends yet working the employee the equivalent of three and one-half days per week, is desirable. Another schedule may be working five days on duty with three days off, giving each employee the equivalent of four and three-eights days per week and also rotating the weekends. Opportunities in addition to vacations arranged for families to be together make for a favorable influence on employees' performance on the job.

Chapter *21*

Licensing

the Nursing Home Facility

Regulation of the Nursing Home

The administrator seeking to establish and operate a nursing home will need to be familiar with the regulation of nursing homes by government. There are essentially three levels of regulation; local, state, and federal. The local regulation is usually by ordinance within the various counties or municipalities. The individual state regulates by statutes which empower a licensing agency such as the state Department of Public Health to establish minimum standards for regulating such establishments. Normally, the agency is given power to promulgate new regulations in light of advancing knowledge. The federal government in recent years has been establishing minimum standards for participation in such programs as Medicare, Medicaid, and the Veterans Administration nursing care programs. While this does not constitute direct authority nor usurp local and state regulation, there is a definite relationship, the effect being that uniform regulations are being evolved.

The relationship works thus: a state agency, e.g., the state Department of Public Welfare, will contract with the U.S. Department of Health, Education, and Welfare, to share the cost of the state medical assistance program. As a condition of participation in the federal program, the state agency agrees to minimum requirements in standards and services. The state agency then in turn contracts with individual nursing homes to provide services for recipients, making as a condition of the contract the requirements imposed by the federal

262

agency. At this point, there is no obligation on either the state agency or the nursing home, if either the state or the individual nursing home elects not to participate. As to what happens in practice, it may be noted that at the time of this writing no fewer than 48 states have entered into contracts with the federal government. Nursing homes have about the same percentage of participation, with about 60% of their revenue coming from the Medicaid program. It is merely a matter of time until the federal standards become the law of states. In fact, H.R. 1 signed into law October 30, 1972, by President Richard Nixon establishes a nationally uniform system of benefits beginning January 1, 1974, for the needy aged, blind, and disabled.

States and local governments usually maintain their own regulations, updating them only as the need arises. Of course, regulations have a tendency to vary from jurisdiction to jurisdiction. A policy of allowing the higher of two standards to prevail will usually prevent any conflict. However, with the enhanced role of the federal government and even higher standards in its requirements for contracting services, the trend to a uniformity of standards is evident.

There is no common statement of standards that will encompass all state programs in such particulars as the physician's, pharmaceutical, and restorative services. It appears evident that uniformity of regulation will derive from the federal Medicaid and Medicare requirements relating to the skilled nursing home. Uniform standards for intermediate facilities have also been formulated. Public Law 90-248 (Medicaid) Section 234(c) specifically requires nursing homes to be licensed in compliance with state and local laws.

The student should secure copies of local ordinances and state regulations for nursing homes in his particular locale and state. To these may be added the standards for participation in the state medical assistance program and the conditions of participation in the federally funded programs.

Cooperation with Regulatory Agencies

The licensing of the facility is normally prohibitive in nature. First, a person is forbidden to offer care to persons related to himself. Normally, this is qualified by establishing a minimum number, usually four or more persons, to whom care may be offered. An interpretation of what constitutes care is: personal assistance in anything other than room, board, laundry, and recreation. In addition, the prohibition has attached the condition the care must not be offered without licensing.

Thus care may be offered to four or more persons unrelated to the proprietor, if it is regulated by proper licensing. With licensing, certain conditions called regulations or minimum standards must be met.

The second important thing the administrator should learn concerning cooperation with the regulatory agencies is that he is assumed to be the one obeying the law in the operation of his facility. Like the obedient motorist who faithfully stops for the traffic light at the intersection, the administrator is assumed by health inspectors to be in compliance with the requirements imposed by licensing. Thus the inspector makes his survey of the licensed nursing home to ascertain that the interest of the public is being protected, and that the facility is in fact in compliance with regulations. This attitude should reflect the need for the administrator to know the law and initiate corrective actions, and that an inspector is not needed to inform him of his responsibility. Unfortunately, there are many ways that the administrator may not reach this ideal.

A third facet for the administrator to understand is the variance in interpretation of what regulations actually require. In fact, some variance will be noted between inspectors from the authority having jurisdiction. Thus we have regulations applied rather loosely by one jurisdiction and rather strictly by another. The administrator has no defense, except to exceed the minimum requirement wherever possible. He should be just as knowledgeable of the regulation as the inspector, in order to discuss intelligently what the standard actually is.

A fourth thing the administrator should do in his relations with the authorities having jurisdiction is to treat their inspectors with professional courtesy. It is far better to make friends with the inspector than to alienate him, for, in doing so, you make his task more difficult. Being human, he may insist on the letter of the law being obeyed. While strict obedience is the ideal, overly strict regulation will raise an increasing number of problems requiring the administrator to resolve them or lose control of the facility.

Finally, the administrator can expect to be found deficient at some time. When deficiencies are cited, they will require his constant attention until resolved. Normally, deficiencies are cited by the inspector, who will quote the regulation to which compliance is wanting. The administrator will then be given an opportunity to propose a plan of correction, noting the specific time at which the deficiency is corrected. The inspector may disagree as to the amount of time and that the proposed correction is acceptable. In either case, he will cite the facility in writing and note the plan of correction agreed upon. The administrator is then under pressure to comply, since the citation is actually a legal instrument that could lead to grounds for revoking the facility license, withholding state welfare payments, or even criminal charges, if the administrator persists after he has lost his license.

Licensing and Inspection

In order to illustrate the extent of regulations of the nursing home, an analysis of a basic nursing home regulation is given. However, this is not the only requirement imposed on the nursing home administrator. He will note from time to time that this document refers to other documents to which the administrator will also adhere. In addition, certain legal requirements are imposed by reason of related services offered by the nursing home, e.g., the dietary service is also regulated by requirements for food and eating establishments to observe both local ordinances and state health regulations.

The basic document outlined below is *Minimum Standards for Nursing Homes,* Texas State Department of Health, Nursing and Convalescent Homes, Austin, Texas, 78756.

> The purpose of the standards is to promote the public health, safety, and welfare, and provide for the development, establishment, and enforcement of standards (1) for the care of individuals in institutions of the character defined and covered herein; (2) for the establishment, construction, maintenance, and operation of such institution, which, in the light of advancing knowledge, will promote safe and adequate care of individuals in these institutions.

Application for license shall be made to the Texas State Department of Health, Austin, Texas, on the appropriate forms which are provided. License applications shall be accompanied by required documentation and the required fee. Signatures required are that of the representative of the nursing home, the local health officer, and the local fire marshal.

Application shall be made in the name of an individual who shall meet eligibility requirements, i.e., to be a high school graduate, of legal age, of moral character, stable, financially responsible, physically and mentally capable, and having the approval of the city health officer and or the unit director having jurisdiction.

The submission of false information and the use of subterfuge or evasive means are grounds for the denial or revocation of license to operate.

"There shall be a governing body which assumes full legal responsibility for the overall conduct of the facility."

A disclosure of ownership shall be in the form of an affidavit to the state licensing agency. In the case of the corporation, a license is issued in the name of a corporation officer in addition to the full-time administrator. A copy of the articles of incorporation, bylaws, and charter, including the name and address of the individual or agent authorized to receive services, is filed. In addition, a list of all stockholders exercising control over the management is to be filed. The welfare agency specifies that each stockholder shall file an affidavit, if the home has 35 stockholders or fewer, and, if they have over 35, affidavits will be filed by those having 10% or more ownership.

The license is to be displayed prominently, will specify the maximum number of patients, and may not use the term "hospital" in the nursing home name.

Admission and Discharge Policy

The standards require each home to establish its admission and discharge policy to include specific requirements, such as medical attendance, financial agreement, records required, identifying information, etc. The admission policy will specify who may be admitted, the condition under which they may stay, and when discharge may be required.

"Patient" is anyone accepted for care in the institution (nursing home). Nursing care is the situation in which care is offered to four or more persons unrelated to the proprietor. The conditions for patient admission follow.

Identifying information required:
    See Article 4477, Rule 50a, Vernon's *Revised Civil Statutes of Texas*.
Medical attendance required:
    By physician licensed by the State Board of Medical Examiners.
    A quarterly patient examination is recommended.
    A quarterly review of medications and orders is required.
Physical examination required:
    Within 14 days of admission.
    Within 48 hours after admission if the referring physician is not the attending physician.
Written report is required of:
    The physical examination.

The medical history.
The diagnosis.
Physician's orders.
Clothing and personal possessions inventory.
Each visit by the physician, including his progress note.
Medical treatment is to be of a minor nature.

Nursing care is to include food, shelter, and social services.

Maternity patients, alcoholics, drug addicts, children, or persons having or suspected of having mental and/or physical disease endangering other patients shall not be admitted, unless separate facilities are provided. Children shall be completely isolated from all other residents. Patient status refers to the level of care needed and is determined by (1) typing according to welfare standards for medical assistance patients and (2) by the patient's physician for private, paying patients.

Discharge shall be pursuant to a predetermined policy: dismissal by the patient's physician, a relative/guardian's request, the patient's request (the nursing home may require a signed release of responsibility), the health officer's requirement for isolation, because of communicable disease. Provision shall be made to notify the next of kin or responsible person in case of accident, illness, or death.

Staffing and Personnel Policy

The staffing of the nursing home is a matter of discretion on the part of the individual nursing home. However, minimum standards require that certain conditions be met for a minimum staffing of professional workers. All workers shall meet basic mental, physical, and character standards. Duty schedules are limited to the 8-hour day, 48-hour week.

The standards require a full-time administrator who is licensed, of legal age, capable of making mature judgments, and has a two-year associate degree. Generally, he shall be co-licensed on the nursing home license, have authority from the nursing home's governing board to assume full responsibility for the internal operation of the home, shall designate someone to act in his absence, and be physically and mentally capable of carrying out his responsibilities.

An assistant administrator shall meet the same qualification as the administrator, except for the requirement of license and the assignment of responsibility and authority.

A director of nursing shall be employed a minimum of 40 hours per week during the day. The minimum standards recognize either a registered nurse or a licensed vocational nurse who is a graduate of an approved school. Each will be licensed by the appropriate licensing authority in the state of Texas. Normally, the director of nurses helps develop patient-care policies, the orientation of new employees, in-service training, patient-care plans, and she directs the nursing services.

Charge nurses (licensed) are required for the 7:00 A.M. to 3:00 P.M. shift, and the 3:00 P.M. to 11:00 P.M. shift. Non-licensed personnel may staff the 11:00 P.M. to 7:00 A.M. shift. The standards require a ratio of one professional nurse to each 30 patients in a 24 hour period. The state standard for a custodial home is one attendant to each 20 patients. This may be compared to the skilled nursing facility of one professional nurse to each 15 patients.

Additional nursing personnel on duty, awake and dressed, shall be employed in sufficent number to provide a 24-hour nursing service to meet the total needs of the patients.

Nonnursing personnel shall be distinguished from aides and orderlies giving direct patient care. Again, a "sufficient number shall be employed to maintain order, safety, and cleanliness of the home and premises, to keep an adequate supply of clean linens, to assist and supervise the resident in the use of recreational facilities, and to meet the other operational needs of the home."

Certain personnel are not acceptable on nursing home staffs: mentally retarded persons (I.Q. 70 or below), deaf mutes, persons on furlough from state hospitals, persons unable to read and write English, alcoholics, drug addicts, those physically unable to perform their duties (but not necessarily the physically handicapped), and certain persons of disorderly nature. Consumption of alcoholic beverages and acts of moral turpitude are forbidden.

The Facility: Safety, Construction, and Arrangement

The planning for construction, additions, remodeling, or conversion of a nursing home shall conform to the minimum standards for safety and operational requirements (the Life Safety Code has been adopted). Generally, one copy of the preliminary plans has to be approved by the local health officer, the local and state fire marshals, the local building inspector, and the state department of health. Then two copies of the working drawings will be prepared, bearing the seal of a registered engineer, and submitted in like manner for approval. No work may begin until fully approved. New construction, additions, remodeling, or relicensing shall generally meet the requirement of new construction.

Codes, guides, manuals to be used:

> *Planning and Construction Manual,* Texas State Department of Health
>
> *National Building Code*
>
> *National Electrical Code*
>
> *The Life Safety Code* (1967 edition)
>
> *American Standard Safety Code for Elevators, Dumbwaiters, and Escalators*
>
> *National Plumbing Code*
>
> *Heating, Ventilating, and Air Conditioning Guide*
>
> *Illuminating Engineering Society Lighting Handbook*

Conformity to all state and local laws — the more stringent laws shall apply.

Requirements to promote patient safety:

> For fire resistance, resistance to flame spread:
>
>> Carpets, drapes, dividers, etc., to be of fire resistant material in compliance with the law.
>
> Location of the nursing home to be such that service of fire protection unit is not over 5 minutes travel distance.
>
> One-story construction shall have not less than one-hour fire resistive combustible construction.
>
> Two-story construction shall have not less than one-hour fire resistive noncombustible construction.
>
> Three-story construction shall have not less than two-hour fire resistive noncombustible construction.
>
> An approved sprinkler system shall be considered as equal to one-hour fire resistive combustible construction or noncombustible construction.
>
> Exits, corridors, stairways, handrails, doors (bedroom door shall be wide enough to move the patient and his bed), unobstructed hallways (8 feet wide), panic hardware on doors, floors, ramps, stair treads, heating system, an emergency telephone for patient use, and sprinklers in hazardous areas shall meet the minimum standards.
>
> Proper oxygen storage and supervised smoking is required.

Inspections:

Annually by fire department for licensing.

Annually, a gas pressure check on heating systems using natural or petroleum gas at the start of the heating season.

Periodically for maintenance and upkeep.

Periodically by health officer having jurisdiction.

Sewage, water supply, room sizes, ventilation:

Sewage shall be disposed of by system approved by department of health.

Water shall be from an approved system. It is required that patient-use fixture water temperature not exceed 110°F.

Width of bedrooms is to be no less than 10 feet.

Bedrooms shall have exterior exposure equal to no less than 1/10 of their usable floor area. Windows shall have a sill not more than 36″ from the floor and have an operable section at least 36″ wide and 24″ high.

Bedrooms shall open onto an exit, corridor, or living area.

Bedrooms shall have 100 square feet of usable floor space for a one-bed room.

Bedrooms shall have 72 (Medicare, Medicaid require 80) square feet of usable floor space per bed for multiple-bed rooms.

Bedrooms shall not be more than 36″ below outside grade. This would forbid basement bedrooms.

Additional requirements for patient well-being:

Provision shall be made for wheelchair patients such as wide doors, raised lavatories, etc.

One shower or tub may not serve more than 20 patients.

One lavatory or water-closet (commode) may not serve more than 8 patients of one sex.

Doors usually open outward for restrooms. Folding or sliding doors for patient use are not recommended.

Recreation, dining, and day room space shall be provided at not fewer than 10 square feet per patient.

Storage areas shall be maintained in a safe manner.

Cubicle curtains or screens are recommended.

Patient-use laundries shall be supervised.

Furnishings and Equipment

The facility shall be so equipped and furnished as to provide for the total care and safety of the patient. The standards require adequate housekeeping, sanitation, and maintenance to ensure a favorable environment.

Illumination of the facility, either natural or artificial, shall be provided to supply the needs of the patients without eye strain or glare. An emergency electric lighting plant or battery system is recommended for exitways, exit light, and nurses' station. (Required by Medicare, Medicaid.)

The heating system shall maintain a temperature of not less than 72°F at the patient level in all patient-use areas. Cooling shall be provided as necessary.

Arrangement of clean and soiled areas shall be such as to prevent cross-contamination. Sufficient clean and soiled utility areas, linen storage, rest rooms for employees and public, laundry, janitorial use, and working areas shall be provided. Forced-air ventilation is required in patient baths, janitorial area, utility room, and soiled linen room. The janitorial room shall have a service sink and the soiled linen room shall have a flush-type of sink.

The nurses' station shall have a work area with desk, chair, record storage, sufficient lockable enclosed medicine cabinets, medicine preparation area, sink, refrigerator, and other storage.

The patient bedroom shall not exceed a four-bed ward (Medicaid has required that no more than 50% of the bed capacity shall be in wards). It should be arranged for comfort and privacy, have a bed with moisture-proof mattress at least 36″ wide, and not closer than 36″ to another bed. There shall be a suitable chair, table or dresser, and clothes storage (closet or wardrobe). A patient-call device shall be provided; the electrical type is recommended (required by Medicare, Medicaid). Each bed shall have a reading light; fire-retardant cubicle curtains and draperies are provided.

Bathrooms shall have safety grab bars capable of supporting 200 pounds dead weight, provision for separate towel racks (or paper towel containers) and separate soap and toothbrush holders. Showers and tubs shall have slip-proof bottoms.

Community living areas shall be appropriately equipped for the convenience and recreation of the patients and their guests.

An isolation and examination room is recommended (it is required for skilled facilities).

Patient Care, Rehabilitation, and Ancillary Services

The patient-care plan, to be developed under the supervision of the director of nurses, shall be comprehensive and include: medical attendance, rehabilitation, dietary care, social adjustments, and ancillary services.

Medical attendance shall be arranged by the person placing a patient in the nursing home. Only a duly licensed physician shall give orders for medical treatment and medication. The patient-care plan will be in accordance with physician's orders.

The patient-care plan will also cover rehabilitation of the patient and related restorative services. Therapy will be prescribed by the physician, and his advice shall be sought for the total plan.

Dietary care requirements shall include special or modified diets, assistance in eating, special assistance owing to physical and/or social needs, and consideration for any dietary restrictions because of religious belief.

Social adjustments, social needs, recreation, and occupational therapy shall be a part of the patient-care plan. "It is recommended that the nursing home provide opportunities for meaningful activities and social relationships. These may include holiday celebrations, parties, indoor or outdoor games, or personal hobbies. Educational or recreational sessions, sponsored by groups within the community, should be encouraged and planned for with such community groups or agencies. Church groups should be encouraged to provide means for church attendance of ambulatory patients." The patient-care plan shall reflect the ability and need of the patient to participate.

Ancillary services such as physical therapy, occupational therapy, speech therapy, beauty and barber services, laundry, etc., shall be included in the patient-care plan.

The patient-care plan shall reflect the preparation for emergency medical care such as an alternate physician, specified hospital in case of transfer, ambulance service preferred, and PRN orders for known physical needs, e.g., oxygen.

Dietary Requirements

Supervision of the dietary department shall be by a person designated by the administrator. If such person is not a professional dietitian, a consulting nutritionist shall be employed for a minimum of four hours per month. Sufficient other personnel shall be employed to meet the dietary needs of the patients. Food service employees shall be trained by selected, in-service educational programs.

Food service requirements:
   Three meals per day.
   No more than 14 hours between evening meal and breakfast.
   Menus planned at least one week in advance.

Food to meet the nutritional needs of the patients.

Sufficient variety of foods.

Different menus for days of the week.

Menus adjusted according to the seasons.

Substitutions shall be recorded.

Menus shall be kept on record for 30 days.

Supplies of staple food for a minimum of one week's need.

Supplies of perishable food for a minimum of two days' need.

Food preferences of the patients shall be considered.

Food must be ground or chopped to meet patient needs.

Food service equipment:

Sufficient equipment shall be available.

Procedures established to ensure maintaining food at proper temperature prior to and during serving.

Sufficient to meet the needs of refrigeration, storage, preparation, and serving of food.

Therapeutic diets:

Modified diets shall be prepared and served as prescribed by a patient's attending physician.

A current diet manual shall be available to guide preparation.

Consulting nutritionist shall recommend food exchanges.

Equipment for dish and utensil cleaning and refuse storage and removal.

Separate areas for clean operations and soiled clean-up shall be established.

Sanitary conditions shall comply:

With local health and food handling codes.

With effective procedures for cleaning and sanitizing.

Dishwashing procedures and techniques:

Shall comply with state and local health laws.

Waste shall be kept in leak-proof nonabsorbent containers with close-fitting covers.

Records Required in the Nursing Home

The standards specify a certain number of records that shall be kept and, when outdated, stored for documentation. These records shall not be destroyed until the statute of limitations expires. In the case of admission and death records, they are to be kept permanently. When a home is closing or ownership is being transferred, the licensee shall apply to the state department of health for instructions as to the disposition of them. All records are to be kept confidential.

Identification information, as outlined in Section VII, Paragraph C of the standards shall be secured at the time of admission. A medication and treatment record, including all medication, treatments, and special procedures performed for the safety and well-being of the patient, shall be kept on a daily basis. Daily nurses' notes containing observations shall be maintained. Physicians' progress notes of each visit or consultation shall be kept. Laboratory and x-ray reports shall be kept on file.

Incident reports shall be kept of (1) any injury, (2) every adverse incident, and (3) any allegation of mistreatment. One copy shall be placed with patient records; one copy shall be filed in the administrator's office. The report shall name persons, witnesses, date, time, extent of incident, circumstances, action, and final disposition. The report shall be completed under the direction of the charge nurse at the time of the incident.

A personal possessions and clothing list shall be kept of all valuables at the time of admission, corrected with additions and deletions. Two copies are to be made, one copy for the patient and/or representative and one copy to be kept with the patient's records.

Financial records shall be maintained of all transactions with the patient or in his behalf. This shall be for his petty cash, if it is managed by the home, and for his general account. A statement of policies governing the operation of the home shall be made available for distribution.

Medical Attendance, Drugs, Narcotics, Isolation, and Humane Treatment

Medical attendance, including emergency medical care, shall be under the supervision of a local physician designated by the patient or his guardian. The home shall have one or more physicians to be called in emergency (when the designated physician for a patient is not available). Each patient shall have unlimited right to choose and change the physician, dentist, or pharmacist. When medical attention needed by the patient exceeds the limit of services offered within the home, the physician may transfer the patient to a hospital. In case of serious accident, acute illness or death, the next of kin or person responsible shall be notified by the charge nurse on duty.

Isolation shall be provided for a person having or suspected of having a communicable disease. His name shall be immediately reported to the health officer having jurisdiction. Such a person may be required to move to a hospital supplying adequate isolation.

Procedures for proper medication administration:

  Medications are given on written orders of a physician.

  Medications are prescribed to an individual patient.

  Medications are labeled on the container.

  Medications are stored in the original container.

  Transferring between containers is forbidden.

Proper storage of medications:

  In a locked cabinet.

  Under refrigeration when needed.

  Controlled drugs are to be kept in a separately locked, securely fastened cabinet within the medicine cabinet (also locked).

  Poisions and "External Use Only" medications are stored separately.

  Discontinued medications are stored separately and disposed of in accordance with the state pharmacy law.

Release of medications:

  To individual patients on discharge.

  On written orders of the physician.

Medication orders:

  To be in writing by the physician.

  Oral orders may be taken only by a licensed nurse.

  Oral orders must be reduced to writing immediately, signed by the nurse receiving the order, and countersigned by the physician within 72 hours (Medicare, Medicaid require 48 hours).

  Reorders should be made at least 24 hours prior to administering the last dose in a container.

  Review of medication orders shall be at least quarterly (Medicare, Medicaid require a monthly review in a skilled facility).

Appropriate stop-orders for medications:

  All medication orders which do not specifically indicate the number of doses to be administered are automatically stopped after a given period.

  Stop-orders are specified in section IX, paragraph E, of the standards.

  The manufacturer's control number indicates an expiration date.

Administration of medications shall be properly done so as to ascertain that the medicine is in fact taken by the patient. Each dose administered shall be properly recorded. Medications prescribed for one patient are not to be administered to any other patient. Self-administration of medications is not permitted, except for emergency drugs or on special order of the patient's physician. Medication errors and drug reactions are reported immediately to the patient's physician and the issuing pharmacist, and an incident report is made.

Narcotics, hypnotics, amphetamines, and other controlled drugs are to be accounted for separately. A count should be made at the change of each shift. A separate record will be kept on each controlled drug to contain: name of patient, date, time, dose, name of drug, physician, signature of nurse, and balance in inventory. All "class A" narcotics can be dispensed only after receiving a signed prescription.

The standards suggest an emergency equipment tray, listing specific items to be included as well as suggested sterile supplies. An emergency drug supply of legend drugs may be left in the home by a licensed practitioner, in a locked box with his name on it. "It is the privilege of the practitioner to ask the appropriate individual to administer a dose from his medication container to his patient." The standards suggest which medications may be left for such an emergency.

If the facility has a pharmacy, a licensed pharamacist in good standing and licensed to practice his profession under the laws of the state shall be employed to administer the pharmacy. The pharmacy is to operate in compliance with pharmacy laws and regulations. If the facility does not have such a pharmacy, it is recommended that a consultant pharmacist be employed.

Humane treatment required:

Restrictive rules shall be kept to a minimum.

Patients shall be allowed the right of privacy, self-determination, and personal dignity.

Patients shall be allowed to function as adults.

Abuse or punishment of patients is forbidden. This includes injury, physical suffering, or mental anguish.

Patients shall have unlimited freedom to move. The home is privileged to secure a signed release from the patient or his guardian/relative.

Patients shall manage their own money. If a patient cannot, a legal guardian shall be secured. This may not be the licensee or an employee.

Patients shall have the right to participate in religious services as they choose, or to abstain.

Patients shall have freedom of communication. A patient may send and receive unopened mail. Only the physician or the patient's representative may make exceptions to this freedom.

Patients shall have the right to receive visitors, frequently, and at reasonable hours. Visiting hours shall be conspicuously posted.

Patients shall have freedom of choice of clothing.

Beautician and barber services shall be available.

Opportunities for meaningful and social relationships shall be afforded by the home.

Chapter 22

Medicaid: Title XIX

Assistance Programs in the Nursing Home

There are several types of assistance programs available for the patient in the nursing home. The patient may have purchased a plan from his insurance company. He may be eligible for the Veteran Administration program for veterans of the armed services. By reason of age (that is, the patient is 65 years of age or older), the patient may be eligible for Medicare benefits in a skilled nursing facility. Finally, he may be eligible for Medicaid because of financial need. All these are third parties to the agreement the nursing home may make with the patient for admission.

The Veterans Administration program is a limited (six months) program available to veterans only. Normally, The Veterans Administration contracts with skilled nursing homes to admit veterans in need of skilled nursing care. The total cost is paid by the Veterans Administration for all care, pharmaceuticals, and services.

The individual having a health care insurance policy with nursing home benefits will need to refer to his individual policy to determine eligibility. A number of types of policies include some benefits.

Because Medicare has been discussed, Medicaid assistance will be taken up in this chapter. It should be pointed out that Medicaid was established as a part of Public Law 89-97 and Public Law 90-248. It is known as Title XIX, although intermediate care facilities are regulated under additional legislation. Medicaid is an assistance program administered by the individual states, but matching funds are contributed by federal financing when a contract between the state department of public welfare and the Department of Health, Education, and Welfare is in effect. The states agree to meet certain basic requirements (licensure of nursing home administrators is a requirement) in order to receive funds. Each state, however, can administer its own unique program. Because of the variations among states, the program as administered in the state of Texas is described.

Eligibility for nursing home benefits falls into four categories for all ages except for one, old age assistance, which is limited to those 65 years of age and over. The other categories are aid to the totally disabled, aid to the blind, and aid to dependent children and/or their parents.

Eligibility is established as to financial need, known as being indigent, upon request to the Texas State Department of Public Welfare. Usually, an investigation is made (normally within 30 days) to determine need. The present maximum worth allowable is set at $1800 per person. A person having a net worth less than this figure (excluding a homestead in Texas) and insufficient income to meet a basic standard of living may be found eligible.

With the beginning of Supplemental Security Income, the Social Security program of assistance which began in 1974, eligibility may already have been established. If the individual's monthly income is above the figure established for eligibility for Supplemental Security Income (1974: $142 per month), yet below a maximum figure established by the welfare agency (1974: $363 per month), the individual may establish need for medical assistance.

For a medically indigent person, his need is for nursing care, medication, and personal needs. Normally, eligibility is a dual process. The individual first establishes that he is indigent, after which he is placed on the assistance rolls; then his need for nursing care is determined.

A patient in need of nursing care is graded (referred to as typing) to determine his need for a particular level of care. This is known as medical review. The patient's physician completes a form, the director of nurses completes a form, and the welfare caseworker makes his recommendations for alternate care provisions that may be made. This information is forwarded to the state headquarters and its medical assistance unit, where a medical review is made to determine the appropriate level of care. The patient may be determined to need Skilled IV nursing care, Intermediate Care Facility III nursing care, or Intermediate Care Facility II custodial care. It is expected that the individual will then be placed in a facility contracting for services matching the type of care he is determined to need.

Typing is not permanent but must be done every six months for intermediate patients or every three months for the skilled patient. A significant change in the condition of the patient may be grounds for a new determination. In addition, medical assistance unit teams composed of a physician, registered nurse, social worker, and other appropriate consultants make at least one on-site review of each facility and every assistance patient in any given calendar year. Retyping may be instantly accomplished by the review team.

Contracting to Provide Nursing Services

The procedure for the facility to use in contracting with the State Department of Public Welfare (or other appropriate state agency which may be designated in a particular state) is given in the "Standards for Participation," which indicates the services to be furnished by the facility. In requesting the booklets giving these standards, the administrator should indicate the level of care he expects to offer; Skilled, ICF III, or ICF II. The actual agreement is in the form of a signed and notarized contract between the legal representative of the nursing home and the State Department of Public Welfare. The nursing home agrees to remain "in compliance" with the standards at all time. Actually, the standards have been written to compare favorably with the state health department's "Minimum Standards," which we reviewed in the last chapter. It is good practice to learn the basic licensing agencies' standards and then to learn where the welfare standards vary from it.

The nursing home will agree to the right of inspection to ensure continuing compliance with the standards. Such inspection is to be made by authorized representatives of the Texas State Department of Health (the nursing home licensing agency), the Texas State Department of Public Welfare (the contractual agency), and the Department of Health, Education, and Welfare (the federal agency participating by contract with the state contractual agency). Inspection may be made at all times.

The welfare agency may reject the contract of participation for a facility being out of compliance with the "Standards for Participation." The conditions for rejection include evidence of abuse to patients, their neglect, or practices not in the best interest of the recipients. They may, upon receipt of documentation of alleged deficiencies discovered by either their inspectors or those of the licensing agency, withhold payments for service after the expiration date agreed by the administrator to have corrections made. The payments, called "Vendor Payment," amount to about 50% of the revenue of the average Texas nursing home. An administrator will note the seriousness of his seeking to stay in compliance.

To be in full compliance is to be in obedience to not only the welfare standards, but also those of the licensing agency and those of the local municipality. All of the following personnel regulated by state licensing boards will hold current licenses or registry: administrator, registered nurse, licensed vocational nurse, physician, pharmacist, physical therapist, occupational therapist, speech therapist, dietitian, dentist, inhalation therapist, and any other paramedical personnel. Nurses aides and orderlies are not licensed at this time. However, certain unlicensed personnel are now being required to have minimum educational experience. Recently the activities director was required to have training or experience, and the food service manager was required to have training of at least a 90-hour course, such as one accredited by the American Dietetic Association.

On January 12, 1974, the Secretary of Health, Education, and Welfare published in the *Federal Register* its official regulations for "Skilled Nursing Facilities" (the full text appears in Chapter Four) and "Intermediate Care Facilities." The length of a provider agreement was limited to one year. The regulations specify that, when a facility is out of compliance and a plan of correction is made, the contract may continue but not to exceed one year (the plan of correction may be for a shorter period). When a facility's deficiencies are not corrected within the time set by the plan of correction, only one extension may be made but not to exceed two additional months. The facility will then be given notice that his contract will not be renewed; the notice must be at least 30 days. Should the provider choose not to renew his contract, he must give the state agency 15 days' notice; however, the state agency may extend the closing date up to 6 months.

Civil Rights Compliance

Compliance with the Civil Rights Act of 1964, section 601, title VI, is a requirement for the facility to receive federal money such as payments as a provider of services under Medicare, Medicaid, Veterans Administration, and CHAMPUS (Civilian Health and Medical Program of the Uniformed Services).

This section stipulates that:

> No person in the United States shall, on the ground of race, color, or national origin, be excluded from participation in, be denied the benefits of, or be subjected to discrimination under any program or activity receiving Federal financial assistance.

Enforcement of the provisions of the act as they may relate to nursing homes is normally performed by appropriate state agencies that receive federal funds, e.g., the state department of public welfare, which in turn are disbursed to providers of medical assistance recipients. However, general oversight of civil rights compliance is given to the Department of Health, Education, and Welfare.

The normal experience confronting the administrator is an inspection of a new facility, an investigation into a complaint, or a periodic review appropriately entitled, "Nursing Home Civil Right Compliance Review." The actual review consists of filling out the review form by answering specifically a number of questions concerning the practices and policies of the nursing home. The administrator will be expected to document his answers to the review questions. Also, the inspector will make a visual inspection of the facility.

Specifically, the questionnaire will ask for the identity of the chief administrative officer and the type of governing board with the names of officers. In the case of the nonprofit corporation, a direct question is asked concerning membership restrictions and requirements.

The administrator will be asked to determine the percentage of occupancy given over to minority groups, which usually are Negro, American Indian, Oriental, or Spanish, but they may be of any other nationality depending on the area served by the nursing home.

The review will determine if a policy of nondiscrimination is written, practiced, and disseminated to all within the scope of the nursing home, including referral groups, minority groups, employees or prospective employees, and all patients or prospective patients. The administrator will be asked to document his efforts to inform properly all concerned by properly posting a written nondiscrimination policy, including it in publications for the staff, employees, patients, and the general public, and showing the basis for selection of patients from the waiting list.

The admission policy of the home will be evaluated to show who was accepted, where they were placed within the home, and the services they received without regard to discrimination. The staff will be reviewed as to ethnic background, whether discrimination exists in hiring practices, and whether favoritism is given in making job assignments. Even the training programs and volunteers of the nursing home may be surveyed.

As is the accepted practice of inspections made by regulatory agencies, compliance, in this case with Civil Rights Act, is the primary aim. Thus, if deficiencies are indicated by an appropriate inspector, these are discussed with the representatives of the nursing home and a plan for correction, including the time required, is indicated in the report. The administrator or other representative of the nursing home may be required to document such compliance. Noncompliance could result in federal funds being withheld under provision of the provider contract between the nursing home and any agency disbursing federal funds.

Intermediate Care Facilities

Uniform standards for intermediate care facilities participating in the Medicaid program were approved January 10, 1974, by Caspar W. Weinberger, Secretary of the Department of Health, Education, and Welfare. Unlike the skilled nursing facility regulation also published in the *Federal Register* the intermediate regulations are more general in terminology, which will allow state agencies more flexibility in instituting them.

We have published a portion of those regulations in the following pages. The student will note the reference to "institutions for the mentally retarded," in the ICF regulations. This is because there follows section 249.13 dealing with such institutions which will also function under the intermediate regulations. The agency responsible for the medical assistance program in each state will write its own specific regulations based on these requirements.

§ 249.12 **Standards for intermediate care facilities.***

(a) The standards for an intermediate care facility (as defined in § 249.10 (b) (15) of this part) which are specified by the Secretary pursuant to section 1905 (c) and (d) of the Social Security Act and are applicable to all intermediate care facilities are as follows. The facility:

(1) Maintains methods of administrative management which assure that:

(i) There are on duty during all hours of each day staff sufficient in numbers and qualifications to carry out the policies, responsibilities, and programs of the facility. The numbers and categories of personnel are determined by the number of res-idents and their particular needs in accordance with guidelines issued by the Social and Rehabilitation Service;

(ii) There are written policies and procedures available to staff, residents and the public which:

(A) Govern all areas of service provided by the facility:

(1) Admission, transfer, and discharge of residents policies shall assure that:

(i) Only those persons are accepted whose needs can be met by the facility directly or in cooperation with community resources or other providers of care with which it is affiliated or has contracts;

(ii) As changes occur in their physical or mental condition, necessitating service or care which cannot be adequately provided

*Reprinted from the *Federal Register* Vol. 39, No. 12, Part II (Thursday, January 17, 1974), pp. 2223–2225. The sponsor of these standards is the Department of Health, Education, and Welfare: Social and Rehabilitation Service and Medical Assistance Program.

by the facility, residents are transferred promptly to hospitals, skilled nursing facilities, or other appropriate facilities; and

(*iii*) Except in the case of an emergency, the resident, his next of kin, attending physician, and the responsible agency, if any, are consulted in advance of the transfer or discharge of any resident, and casework services or other means are utilized to assure that adequate arrangements exist for meeting his needs through other resources; and

(2) In the case of institution's for the mentally retarded or persons with related conditions, policies define the uses of physical restraints, the staff members who must authorize their use, and a mechanism for monitoring and controlling their use;

(B) Set forth the rights of residents and prohibits their mistreatment or abuse;

(C) Provide for the registration and disposition of complaints without threat of discharge or other reprisal against any employee or resident;

(iii) A written account, available to residents and their families, is maintained on a current basis for each resident with written receipts for all personal possessions and funds received by or deposited with the facility and for all disbursements made to or on behalf of the resident;

(iv) The facility has a written and regularly rehearsed plan for staff and residents to be followed in case of fire, explosion or other emergency;

(v) There are written procedures for personnel to follow in an emergency, including care of the resident, notification of the attending physician and other persons responsible for the resident, arrangements for transportation, for hospitalization, or other appropriate services;

(iv) There is an orientation program for all new employees that includes review of all facility policies. An inservice education program is planned and conducted for the development and improvement of skills of all the facility's personnel. Records are maintained which indicate the content of, and participation in, all such orientation and staff development programs;

(vii) The facility is in conformity with Federal, State, and local laws, codes, and regulations pertaining to health and safety, including procurement, dispensing, ad-

ministration, safeguarding and disposal of medications and controlled substances; building, construction, maintenance and equipment standards; sanitation; communicable and reportable diseases; and post-mortem procedures.

(2) Has in effect a transfer agreement with one or more hospitals sufficiently close to the facility to make feasible the transfer between them of residents and their records, which provide the basis for effective working arrangements under which inpatient hospital care or other hospital services are available promptly to the facility's residents when needed. Any facility which does not have such an agreement in effect but which is found by the survey agency to have attempted in good faith to enter into such an agreement with a hospital shall be considered to have such an agreement in effect if and for so long as the survey agency finds that to do so is in the public interest and essential to assuring intermediate care facility services for eligible persons in the community.

(3) Maintains effective arrangements

(i) For required institutional services through a written agreement with an outside resource in those instances where the facility does not employ a qualified professional person to render a required service. The responsibilities, functions, and objectives and the terms of agreement with each such resource are delineated in writing and signed by the administrator or authorized representative and the resource;

(ii) Through which medical and remedial services required by the resident but not regularly provided within the facility can be obtained promptly when needed.

(4) Maintains an organized resident record system which assures that:

(i) There is available to professional and other staff directly involved with the resident and to appropriate representatives of the State agency a record for each resident which includes as a minimum:

(A) Identification information and admission data including past resident medical and social history;

(B) Copies of initial and periodic examinations, evaluations, and progress notes including all plans of care and any modifications thereto, and discharge summaries;

(C) An overall plan of care setting forth goals to be accomplished, prescribing an integrated program of individually designed activities, therapies, and treatments necessary to achieve such goals, and indicating which professional service or individual is responsible for each element of care or service prescribed in the plan;

(D) Entries describing treatments and services rendered and medications administered;

(E) All symptoms and other indications of illness or injury including the date, time, and action taken regarding each; and

(F) In the case of institutions for the mentally retarded or persons with related conditions, the resident's legal status, developmental history, a copy of the post-institutionalization plan of care and a signed order for any physical restraints including justification and duration of application;

(ii) Records are adequately safeguarded against destruction, loss, or unauthorized use; and

(iii) Records are retained for a minimum of 3 years following a resident's discharge.

(5) Meets such provisions of the Life Safety Code of the National Fire Protection Association (21st Edition, 1967) as are applicable to institutional occupancies; except that:

(i) For facilities of 15 beds or less, the State survey agency may apply the Lodging or Rooming Houses section of the residential occupancy requirements of the Code for institutions for the mentally retarded or persons with related conditions and intermediate care facilities primarily engaged in the treatment of alcoholism and drug abuse, all of whose residents are currently certified by a physician or in the case of an institution for the mentally retarded or persons with related conditions by a physician or psychologist as defied in paragraph (c) (3) (i) of this section, as:

(A) Ambulatory;

(B) Engaged in active programs for rehabilitation which are designed to and can reasonably be expected to lead to independent living, or in the case of an institution for the mentally retarded or persons with related conditions, receiving active treatment; and

(C) Capable of following directions and taking appropriate action for self-preservation under emergency conditions;

(ii) In accordance with criteria issued by the Secretary, the State survey agency may waive the application to any such facility of specific provisions of such Code, for such periods as it deems appropriate, which provisions if rigidly applied would result in unreasonable hardship upon a facility, but only if such waiver will not adversely affect the health and safety of the residents; and

(iii) The Life Safety Code shall not apply in any State if the Secretary makes a finding that in such State there is in effect a fire and safety code, imposed by State law, which adequately protects residents in intermediate care facilities.

Where waivers permit the participation of an existing facility of two or more stories which is not of at least 2-hour fire resistive construction, blind, nonambulatory or physically handicapped residents are not housed above the street level floor unless the facility is of 1-hour protected noncombustible construction (as defined in National Fire Protection Association Standard #220), fully sprinklered 1-hour protected ordinary construction or fully sprinklered 1-hour protected wood frame construction.

(6) Maintains conditions relating to environment and sanitation as set forth below:

(i) Resident living areas are designed and equipped for the comfort and privacy of the resident. Each room is equipped with or conveniently located near adequate toilet and bathing facilities appropriate in number, size, and design to meet the needs of residents. Each room is at or above grade level and each resident room contains a suitable bed, closet space which provides security and privacy for clothing and personal belongings, and other appropriate furniture;

(A) Resident bedrooms have no more than 4 beds. Single resident rooms measure at least 100 square feet, and multi-resident rooms provide a minimum of 80 square feet per bed. The survey agency may waive in existing buildings, for such periods as deemed appropriate, provisions which, if rigidly enforced, would result in unreasonable hardship upon the facility but only if such waiver is in accordance with the particular needs of the residents and will not adversely affect their health and safety. Each room is equipped with a resident call system; or

(B) In the case of institutions for the mentally retarded or persons with related conditions, the number of residents in multi-resident bedrooms does not exceed 12 persons. Single resident rooms measure 100 square feet, and multi-resident rooms provide a minimum of 80 square feet per bed. The survey agency may waive in existing buildings, for such periods as deemed appropriate, provisions which, if rigidly enforced, would result in unreasonable hardship upon the insitution but only if such waiver is in accordance with the particular needs of the residents and will not adversely affect their health and safety; and

(ii) The facility has available at all times a quantity of linen essential for proper care and comfort of residents. Each bed is equipped with clean linen;

(iii) An adequate supply of hot water for resident use is available at all times. Temperature of hot water at plumbing fixtures used by residents is automatically regulated by control valves;

(iv) Except in the case of an institution for the mentally retarded or persons with related conditions, corridors used by residents are equipped with firmly secured handrails;

(v) Provision is made for isolating residents with infectious diseases;

(vi) Areas utilized to provide therapy services are of sufficient size and appropriate design to accommodate necessary equipment, conduct examinations, and provide treatment;

(vii) The facility provides one or more areas for resident dining, diversional, and social activities; and areas used for corridor traffic shall not be considered as areas for dining, diversional or social activities;

(viii) If a multipurpose room is used for dining and diversional and social activities, there is sufficient space to accommodate all activities and prevent their interference with each other;

(ix) The facility is accessible to and functional for residents, personnel, and the public. All necessary accommodations are made to meet the needs of persons with semi-ambulatory disabilities, sight and hearing disabilities, disabilities of coordination, as well as other disabilities in accordance with the American National Standards Institute (ANSI) Standard No. A117.1 (1961) American Standard Specifications for Making Buildings and Facilities Accessible to, and Usable by, the Physically Handicapped. The survey agency may waive in existing buildings, for such periods as deemed appropriate, specific provisions of ANSI Standard No. A117.1 (1961) which, if rigidly enforced, would result in unreasonable hardship upon the facility, but only if such waiver will not adversely affect the health and safety of residents. For purposes of ANSI Standard No. A117.1 (1961), "existing buildings" are defined as those facilities or parts thereof whose construction plans are approved and stamped by the appropriate State agency responsible therefor before the date these regulations become effective.

(7) Provides or arranges menus and meal service so that:

(i) At least three meals or their equivalent are served daily, at regular times with not more than 14 hours between a substantial evening meal and breakfast;

(ii) A designated staff member suited by training or experience in food management or nutrition is responsible for planning and supervision of menus and meal service;

(iii) If the facility accepts or retains individuals in need of medically prescribed special diets, the menus for such diets are planned by a professionally qualified dietitian, or are reviewed and approved by the attending physician, and the facility provides supervision of the preparation and serving of the meals and their acceptance by the resident;

(iv) Menus are planned and followed to meet nutritional needs of residents, in accordance with physicians' orders and to the extent medically possible, in accordance with the recommended dietary allowances of the Food and Nutrition Board of the National Research Council, National Academy of Sciences;

(v) Records of menus as actually served are retained for 30 days;

(vi) All food is procured, stored, prepared, distributed, and served under sanitary conditions; and

(vii) Individuals needing special equipment, implements, or utensils to assist them when eating have such items provided.

(8) Implements methods and procedures relating to drugs and biologicals which assure that:

(i) If the facility does not employ a licensed pharmacist, it has formal arrangements with a licensed pharmacist to provide consultation on methods and procedures for ordering, storage, administration and disposal and recordkeeping of drugs and biologicals;

(ii) Medications administered to a resident are ordered either in writing or orally by the resident's attending or staff physician. Physician's oral orders for prescription drugs are given only to a licensed nurse, pharmacist, or physician. All oral orders for medication are immediately recorded and signed by the person receiving them and are countersigned by the attending physician in a manner consistent with good medical practice;

(iii) Medications not specifically limited as to time or number of doses when ordered are controlled by automatic stop orders or other methods in accordance with written policies and the attending physician is notified;

(iv) Self-administration of medication is allowed only with permission of the resident's attending physician;

(v) A registered nurse reviews monthly each resident's medications and notifies the physician when changes are appropriate. Medications are reviewed quarterly by the attending or staff physician; and

(vi) All personnel administering medications must have completed a State-approved training program in medication administration.

(9) Provides health services which assure that each resident receives treatments, medications, diet, and other health services as prescribed and planned, all hours of each day, in accordance with the following:

(i) Immediate supervision of the facility's health services on all days of each week is by a registered nurse or licensed practical (or vocational) nurse employed full-time on the day shift in the intermediate care facility and who is currently licensed to practice in the State: *Provided*, That:

(A) In the case of facilities where a licensed practical (or vocational) nurse serves as the supervisor of health services, consultation is provided by a registered nurse, through formal contract, at regular intervals, but not less than 4 hours weekly;

(B) By January 1975, licensed practical (or vocational) nurses serving as health services supervisors have training that includes either graduation from a State approved school of practical nursing or education and other training that is considered by the State authority responsible for licensing of practical nurses to provide a background that is equivalent to graduation from a State approved school of practical nursing, or have successfully completed the Public Health Service examination for waivered licensed practical (vocational) nurses; and

(C) Other categories of licensed personnel with special training in the care of residents may serve as charge nurse: *Provided*, That such person is licensed by the State in such category following completion of a course of training which includes at least the number of classroom and practice hours in all of the nursing subjects included in the program of a State approved school of practical (or vocational) nursing as evidenced by a report to the single State agency by the agency or agencies of the State responsible for the licensure of such personnel comparing the courses in the respective curricula; and

(ii) Responsible staff members are on duty and awake at all times to assure prompt, appropriate action in cases of injury, illness, fire or other emergencies;

(iii) In the case of an institution for the mentally retarded or persons with related conditions, with less than 15 beds, which has only residents certified by a physician as not in need of professional nursing services, paragraph (a) (9) (i) and (ii) of this section may be met if the institution arranges through formal contract for the services of a registered nurse or public health nurse to visit as required for the care of minor illnesses, injuries, or emergencies, and consultation on the health aspects of the individual plan of care; and if a responsible staff member is on duty at all times who is immediately accessible, to whom residents can report injuries, symptoms of illness, and emergencies;

(iv) A written health care plan is developed and implemented by appropriate staff for each resident in accordance with instructions of the attending or staff physician. The plan is reviewed and revised as needed, but not less often than quarterly;

(v) Nursing services are provided in accordance with the needs of the residents and, in the case of a facility other than an institution for the mentally retarded or persons with related conditions, restorative nursing care is provided to each resident to achieve and maintain the highest possible degree of function, self-care and independence.

(b) In addition, for intermediate care facilities other than institutions for the mentally retarded or persons with related conditions, the following standards specified pursuant to section 1905(c) of the Social Security Act shall apply.

(1) The facility is administered by a person licensed in the State as a nursing home administrator or, in the case of a hospital qualifying as an intermediate care facility, by the hospital administrator, with the necessary authority and responsibility for management of the facility and implementation of administrative policies.

(2) The administrator or an individual on the professional staff of the facility is designated as resident services director and is assigned responsibility for the coordination and monitoring of the residents' overall plans of care.

(3) The facility provides, according to the needs of each resident, specialized and supportive rehabilitative services either directly or through arrangements with qualified outside resources, which are designed to preserve and improve abilities for independent function, prevent insofar as possible progressive disabilities, and restore maximum function, and which are:

(i) Provided under a written plan of care, developed in consultation with the attending physician and if necessary, an appropriate therapist. The plan is based on the attending physician's orders and an assessment of the resident's needs. The resident's progress is reviewed regularly, and the plan is altered or revised as necessary;

(ii) Provided in accordance with accepted professional practices by qualified therapists or by qualified assistants as defined in 20 CFR 405.1101(m), (n), (q), (r), and (t) or other supportive personnel under appropriate supervision.

(4) The facility provides or arranges for social services as needed by the resident, designed to promote preservation of the resident's physical and mental health.

(i) A designated staff member suited by training or experience is responsible for arranging for social services and for the integration of social services with other elements of the plan of care.

(ii) A plan for such care is recorded in the resident's record and is periodically evaluated in conjunction with the resident's total plan of care.

(5) The facility provides an activities program designed to encourage restoration to self-care and maintenance of normal activity which assures that:

(i) A staff member qualified by experience or training in directing group activity is responsible for the direction and supervision of the activities program;

(ii) A plan for independent and group activities is developed for each resident in accordance with his needs and interests;

(iii) The plan is incorporated in his overall plan of care and is reviewed with the resident's participation at least quarterly and altered as needed;

(iv) Adequate recreation areas are provided with sufficient equipment and materials available to support independent and group activities; and

(6) The facility maintains policies and procedures to assure that each resident's health care is under the continuing supervision of a physician who sees the resident as needed and in no case less often than every 60 days, unless justified otherwise and documented by the attending physician.

Chapter 23

Counseling

and Patient Psychology

Some Principles of Counseling

The nursing home administrator will soon discover that problem-solving will occupy a large portion of his time. He will have discussions with the patients, with the employees, with other professionals, and with the guardian/relatives of the patients. Of course, not all his dealings with these will be with the aim of problem-solving. However, he will find that a knowledge of counseling will greatly enhance his ability to keep good relationships with them. Counseling in its truest sense is a skill of the social worker, the psychologist or psychiatrist, or the minister and the administrator will not engage in it if such professional services are available, and if, by doing so, he would infringe upon their professional disciplines. It should also be noted that some states license the professional counselor. However, the administrator may, in the normal course of his business, discuss the problems of employment, patient care, and personnel relationships.

There are three basic approaches to counseling. In *directive counseling* the counselor tries to lead a person to a predetermined action. He may advise or persuade. Ultimately, he is trying to lead a counselee to make a decision to do what he, the counselor, feels is the best action. In *nondirective counseling* the counselor guides the counselee to discover the best action for himself. Mostly, the counselor listens for insight, uses questions, and interprets the statements of the counselee. *Cooperative counseling* is the use of several methods, including those above, plus the several types of therapy. An example would be the administrator, the staff, and the patients joining together to deal with hostility in a particular patient. It could be termed interdisciplinary cooperation.

Psychiatry is an advanced method of counseling practiced by the professional psychiatrist in the treatment of a mentally defective, or injured personality. Only a psychiatrist should deal with such cases. It is necessary, however, for the counselor to know the difference between simple problem-solving and mental defect.

The counselor must be able to understand the nature of people, to love people, to have the ability to listen, to keep confidences, and to be skilled in the techniques of counseling. Among the several techniques available to him, listening is perhaps the best. Listening involves the counselor sublimating his desire to dominate the conversation. The most difficult thing will be for him not to make comparisons with his own experience or to try to advise on the basis of his own problems. By listening carefully, he will discover that each individual's problems are unique to that individual and usually cannot be solved as another has solved his problems. Not becoming emotionally involved in the problems of the counselee is another technique to be mastered. An honest search for causes and solutions will best aid the counselee. The counselor may use his faith in the individual, in society, in God, to successfully guide a counselee in the solution of a problem.

Counseling with a View to Admission

The most important counseling session is counseling with a view to admission. There are many areas to be covered, including finances, eligibility, alternative care, policies, and psychological problems of placement. In essence, the administrator is guiding the family to find the best solution, even an early discharge, to the need of nursing care for a particular patient. There may be related problems to be dealt with during the interview.

First in importance is the establishment of a friendly relationship between the patient, the relative/guardian, and the administrator. Often the relative will feel guilty in making the placement, or the patient will show remorse for having to leave home, spouse, or friends. The second point is determining the eligibility of the patient. Does the patient need the type of nursing care furnished by the home? Does the home offer the type of care needed by the patient? If an alternate service, i.e., a homemaker's service, foster care, day care, meals-on-wheels, or another level of care would be more suitable, the administrator should counsel its acceptance.

It is sometimes necessary to refer the patient to another agency. The counsel of the social worker or welfare caseworker should be sought in making such referrals.

The administrator will review carefully with the prospective patient the policies of the home. Each point will be discussed. He will also place a written copy of these policies in the hands of the patient and/or the responsible person. This is an important part of the interview, as he will wish to guide the prospective resident to a full acceptance of living within the nursing home.

Finances often determine whether a person will be placed or not. Does the patient understand the exact terms? Does he understand extra charges, the refund policy, the reservation policy, and the payment schedule? If the patient is expecting Medicaid or Medicare assistance, these arrangements must be clarified. Often, the administrator will be using directive counseling, since basically he is telling the patient the conditions of admission. He may also be convincing the patient that a solution to his need for care can be found.

Counseling for admission also includes preparing the staff for the patient's arrival. The staff will want to know the type of patient to expect, whether he is bedridden or ambulatory, whether hostile or confused, and what special problems may exist. Thus the admission of a patient may spawn many related problems, giving the administrator need for continual discussion with and guidance of his staff.

Counseling Patient-Family Related Problems

Counseling in patient-family related problems should be done by a skilled social worker; however, the administrator will usually be called upon first, since he is ultimately responsible for the operation of the home and is closer to the problem. There are some things for the administrator to remember. His involvement in patient-related problems should concern primarily the patient's placement and care from the administrative viewpoint, because it is necessary to inform the family of problems of patient care and enlist their involvement with it, and because other patients may be involved in such problems, counseling may be necessary.

The administrator is primarily concerned with the adaptive behavior of the patient, how he utilizes his past experience to adjust to the reality of living in a nursing home.

One problem area concerns placement. Prejudices concerning the nursing, such as the "tales" they have heard, or preconceived notions about institutional living may add to the apprehensions a family may have. The "poor farm" stigma of welfare assistance may add to the burden, thus giving rise to the need for family counseling. Another serious area is the breaking up of the home and the separation of the spouses. Leaving one's home and disposing of possessions is extremely difficult for the patient and his family. While the administrator will not assume any direct responsibility for these, he will nevertheless be dealing with the individual patient who develops anxiety because of such problems. His sympathy, kindness, and concern may be voiced as friendly counsel.

Perhaps the greatest need for counseling will arise when the administrator and his staff prepare the patient for his acceptance of the nursing home as a place of residence. The loss of independence and privacy that may result from routine nursing care, the problems of community living, the change of routines, the medication regimen, new leisure activities, and the loneliness some patients experience must be dealt with. The administrator cannot take a passive attitude nor can his staff ignore the patient's emotional needs. Certainly, the practice of employees giving "advice" is not what the patient needs. He needs to be led to discover new activities, new interests, new friends, and new appreciation for his life in the nursing home.

Some problems are imagined by the patient. When the administrator is certain this is the case, he should seek the services of a social worker. Problems that are psychotic in nature must be dealt with by the psychiatrist.

The nursing home staff will encounter a variety of problems, emotions, and characteristics of nursing home patients. Following is a list of words with brief comments or definitions that may prove helpful.

Anxiety: Apprehension or excessive worry; usually is a result of chronic illness.

Attitude: Mood, mental state, or feelings.

Behavior: Conduct of individuals. May be physical or psychological; may be interpersonal, interprofessional, or interdisciplinary.

Conflict: Controversy or disagreement with or between patients. The staff or a social worker may counsel or discuss the problem with the patients involved.

Criticism: Opinion or judgment. Some elderly persons become critical in personality.

Daydreaming: The musing or fantasy of the elderly who have difficulty projecting themselves into the future. It is easier to reminisce about the past.

Death, approach of: The staff should provide privacy and helpfulness to the family. Use cautionary speech, as the patient is usually aware of approaching death. Even the apparent semiconscious patient may be aware of those around him.

Dependency: Being unable to live without the aid and assistance of another person, a tendency of the aged owing to physical, social, and psychological needs.

Depression: A state of emotional dejection or despair. Depression may overcome a person very quickly.

Discipline: Self-control.

Ego: The inner self that controls behavior by making one aware of internal and external stimuli, integrating knowledge, and affecting actions. It functions when the elderly person has hope and is relatively free of disease.

Emotions: Strong inner feelings such as love, fear, sorrow, etc., which characterize all age groups.

Fear: Anxiety or deep emotion over an external or environmental threat to one's safety. It may be real or imaginary.

Food phobia: Fears and apprehensions of eating certain foods because of imaginary or cultural reasons.

Freedom of choice: Permitting the patient his preferences in keeping with human dignity and the licensing agency's requirement.

Grief: Sorrow or mental anguish, such as sorrow over the death or a close family member.

Hostility: Deep anger and threatening harm or injury to another.

Illness, imagined: Pseudoesthesia or false sensation of illness, i.e., hypochondria.

Incompatibility: Inability to co-exist harmoniously, such as roommates not being able to get along socially.

Independent living: Self-reliance, self-sustaining, autonomous living.

Indigence: Being without means of financial support.

Interdisciplinary cooperation: Both the staff and the patients sharing in the responsibility of correcting attitudes and behavior.

Interpersonal relationships: Social interaction on a personal level, as between roommates.

Isolation, social: Self-imposed social restrictions for environmental or psychological reasons. A recluse. Causes: smaller family units, urbanization, difficulties in socialization, or institutional living.

Leisure: Time free of obligation for relative nonproductivity, usually social and recreational, which society expects of the elderly. Leisure time does not provide status, self-esteem, or productivity (financial return).

Loneliness: Result of social isolation caused by physical handicaps, psychological reasons, loss of companions, environmental barriers, and neglect by family and friends.

Loss of possessions: Traumatic experience often attended by psychological, social, and physical considerations.

Melancholy: Deep state of sadness.

Memory defect: Forgetfulness. Memory in the elderly tends to be stronger for remote experience.

Personal dignity: Sense of honor, self-worth, or self-esteem. Pride in one's self.

Privacy: Right of a patient to maintain seclusion for personal reasons.

Productivity: Problems arise in the elderly because of the lack of productivity.

Reality: Pertaining to that which is true or real, i.e., illness, economic problems, separation, daily living habits.

Recognition: To acknowledge the worth or status of the individual; a social satisfaction.

Reconciliation: To bring together; to reunite hostile parties. To reestablish friendship.

Regression: To return to a former state, i.e., to the characteristics of one's childhood behavior.

Security: Feeling or state of being safe from harm.

Separation: In the nursing home, it means loss of companions, i.e., the husband or wife, separation from family, and ultimately death. It is because of the severity of separation and loss of status and its psychological effect that the nursing home provides activities, social services, and counseling.

Social involvement: Companionship, i.e., male and female. Considerations: continuing activity, complexity, usefulness.

Status: A personal feeling of social acceptance. The elderly tend to lose status as they are less active and less productive in society.

Stress: Strain or pressure. Tension. Distress or disruption of emotional stability.

Suffering: To experience or endure pain or mental anguish. Psychiatrists believe a person suffers because of illness, economic reasons, separation, culture, and internal conflicts.

Theft: Loss of possessions. An interpersonal relationship.

Touch: Tactile sense. The elderly are usually deprived of the natural sense.

Trauma: An emotional shock or experience which may be extended over a period of time, such as fear of the loss of the ability to live independently, worry over inadequate finances, anxiety over separation. However, it may be sudden, such as illness, injury, or accident.

Withdrawal: Self-imposed isolation.

Suicide among the elderly has increased at an alarming rate in recent times with the age group 65 and over having the largest rate of incidence among the male population. Suicide usually results from severe depression or melancholia. Obviously, the nursing approach is one of watchfulness, caution, and encouragement of the patient to enter into activities that elevate him to better self-esteem. However, competitiveness with resultant irritation, stress, pressure, and frustration will only increase the danger.

The administrator will survey his nursing home for contributing causes of the patient's becoming overly depressed. Some probable causes are strict visiting rules, hostility between roommates, an unsympathetic nursing staff, the absence of activities, rigid and inflexible scheduling of patient care, and factors which deny the patient self-respect and dignity. Certain conditions should be corrected, such as allowing patients to have items and instruments that may be dangerous, leaving the medicine room unlocked and unattended, leaving janitorial supplies unattended and not stored under lock, or ignoring the suicidal remarks of a patient.

The Social Worker in the Nursing Home

The social worker is a professional worker skilled in dealing with the social-medical aspects of patient care. Because of the complementary nature of medical and social psychology of patient care, such a worker will be invaluable in dealing with behavioral problems of the aging.

The social worker may make the initial social evaluation at the admission of the patient. His findings will be used by the supervising nurse and the physician in developing the patient-care plan. A particular interest to the social worker will be the emotional stability of the patient, his relationships with his family, his ability to socialize, his ability to adjust to his new surroundings, and related problems of living. He could assist the patient in several areas: counseling concerning financial problems, interfamily relationship, personal motivation, referrals, attitudes toward health care, etc.

The social worker should be familiar with community resources, i.e., social services, legal aid, etc. He may assist in making referrals for care such as meals-on-wheels, visiting nurse, homemakers service, etc., when these will allow him the independence of living at home. The social worker may deal with specific problems, i.e., hostility, criticism, isolation, etc.

ALTERNATIVES TO NURSING CARE:

Day care: Institutional care during the day only. This may allow a working member to continue working during which time a family member could receive care.

Foster care: The aged person living with another family. Considerations: living with relatives; violation of nursing care licensing acts; safety; adequacy of care.

Homemaking service: A housekeeper who will maintain the household during times of confinement. This may be accomplished by a relative, an employee, or an organized Homemaker Service.

Living in congregate settings: The grouping of elderly persons into congregate residential facilities, e.g., senior citizens' village, apartments, duplex, or subdivision. Considerations: health care, shopping, transportation, fire protection, recreation, social services, and dietary services.

Meal services: Cafeteria, community meal service, meals-on-wheels. Considerations: Hot meals, nutritionally balanced, regularity, reasonable prices, social relationships.

Phone calling service: Organized effort to telephone regularly the shut-ins. Purpose: discovery of need for assistance; social contact.

Social service agency: Organization providing professional social counseling and guidance.

Visiting nurse: Home Health Agency. The physician prescribes treatments and medication requiring the services of a professional nurse who makes house calls to provide this care.

Visitors service: Organized effort to make periodic calls on the shut-ins. Considerations: isolation; safety; security; social interaction.

AGENCIES AND PROGRAMS FOR THE ELDERLY

Area Office on Aging: The Older Americans Act has provided funding for organized efforts by local communities to study, identify, and develop programs to benefit the elderly.

Consumer protection: Consumer Credit Commission, Chamber of Commerce, Better Business Bureau.

Employment and Volunteer Opportunities: Volunteer Employment, Foster Grandparents, Retired Senior Volunteer Program (RSVP), Volunteers in Service to America (VISTA), Service Corps of Retired Executives (SCORE).

Housing: Assistance in buying a house. Contact the local office of the Department of Housing and Urban Development or FHA.

Nutrition: Assistance is available through the county extension office, local Area Office on Aging, or senior citizens nutritional projects.

Legal Aid Society: Provides free legal assistance.

Medicare: Hospital Insurance, Supplementary Medical Insurance, Home Health Care, Skilled Nursing Facility benefits.

Medicaid: Old Age Assistance, Aid to the Blind, Aid to the Permanently and Totally Disabled. Benefits include: in-patient hospital services, out-patient hospital services, medical assistance in the nursing home, laboratory and x-ray services, radiation therapy, physician's services, ambulance services.

Railroad Employee Benefits: Supplemental benefits, disability benefits, survivors' benefits.

Social Security Benefits: Retirement insurance, dependents, and the beneficiary's retirement income, survivors' benefits, disability insurance, supplemental security income.

Taxation: Certain exemptions are available: second deduction for those 65 and above on their federal income taxes; higher exemption for homesteads for those 65 and above; retirement credits.

Recreational opportunities: Most municipalities are sponsoring clubs, activities, and services for the elderly.

Veterans Administration: Compensation for disability, pensions, hospitalization, nursing home care, domiciliary care, insurance, dependency and indemnity compensation, nonservice connected death pension.

Voting privileges: Voting absentee in person, voting absentee by mail.

Psychological Problems of Aging

There are several cardinal principles to remember in dealing with the patient suffering psychological problems. The first we have mentioned: the nonprofessional should not deal with such problem-solving. Also, the licensing agency will not permit the nursing home to keep patients whose behavior is detrimental to themselves and others. The nursing staff, therefore, should know the signs and symptoms of mental illness. While it is difficult for the lay person to recognize them, it is nevertheless well for the administrator and his staff to study psychological difficulties. Among the elderly, what some may think is mental illness may not be this at all, but only a simple neurosis.

The administrator should look at the milder abnormal emotional conditions of the aged and recognize them for what they are, temporary periods of emotional upset. The state may be one in which the patient is "out of character" because of an outburst to relieve his feelings. No pattern or consistent repetition is noticeable. It may be a simple neurosis, which is a minor disorder of the personality. In some cases, the elderly suffer from undue nervousness; in others, anxiety or depression may set in. Anxiety is a state of fear, and fear focuses on the external. Depression is deep remorse, rejection, or melancholy, which focuses on the internal or psychological.

Emotional states give rise to behavior problems, and thus the patient may be characterized as having a mental illness which he probably does not have. All emotions center around states of the mind or within one's belief. Attitudes are the feelings and thoughts a patient may have about himself, the administrator, the staff, or the nursing home. Emotions may be identified as love, hate, fear, suspiciousness, grief, joy, etc., all of which are common to all ages. However, emotions may also be identified by such neuroses as anxiety, hysteria, apprehension, impulsiveness, fatigue, or obsession. The administrator should learn personality defects for what they are, a part of the human experience, common to all ages, and not changing merely because of age, but because of chronic illness and body deterioration.

Closely related to these problems is that of senility caused by arteriosclerosis or cerebrosclerosis. Its characteristics are loss of memory, faulty judgment, inability to reason, loss of the sense of time, and "living in the past." The stroke patient may exhibit some of these mental defects; however, this is caused by a lesion or injury in the brain. The severity of the injury will determine the type of defect; e.g., aphasia, the inability to form words because of injury to the speech control in the brain, or paralysis to a portion of the body.

The administrator should be aware that some symptoms of a simple neurotic condition may be also those of a major psychotic state. The ability of the administrator to tell the difference will be improved by study and observation. This, however, could give rise to a dangerous practice, that of characterizing patients on the basis of nonprofessional diagnosis. Such practice is considered legally libelous and should not be permitted to anyone on the nursing staff. *The administrator should recognize the characteristics of mental illness only enough to realize that professional help is needed. Even then, the judgment will be left to the attending physician.*

Symptoms of Mental Illness

Some psychoses may result from organic disease such as arteriosclerosis, epilepsy, brain tumor, stroke, and encephalitis. A toxicity to medications may produce a psychosis. The patient experiencing high temperature, a reaction to drugs, or an accumulation of toxins from disease may have psychotic symptoms. These are usually characterized by sudden onset and sudden termination. Alcoholism may produce delirium tremors.

The symptoms accompanying mental illness can be illusive or predominant, can be deceiving, and can initiate several types of illness. The nurse or administrator will not attempt to diagnose, merely to recognize the symptoms and report them to the physician objectively. Normally, the doctor can warn the nursing staff to be aware of possible toxic conditions or organic psychoses. He can advise as to the symptoms.

Toxic psychoses may be accompanied by confusion, hallucinations, and fear. Alcoholism usually requires large doses of sedatives and may be accompanied by tremor and hallucination. Schizophrenia has many symptoms, but the more recognizable ones are the tendency to withdraw, dullness, delusions of persecution, dual personality, excitableness, and hallucinations.

The manic-depressive psychosis is usually identified by erratic elation and depression cycles. The paranoid condition is characterized by delusions of grandeur and persecution. The psychoneuroses are simply advanced states of the simple neurosis, i.e., anxiety, hysteria, or certain obsessions. Sometimes noticeable in the elderly are the obsession for medicine, called hypochondria, and an extreme state of apprehension.

Because the administrator should be reminded that he is charged with caring for adults who are individuals with all the rights and privileges of any person, the following example is included as copied from the personnel policy of the Cedar Crest Nursing Home, Waco, Texas:

OUR PATIENTS' BILL OF RIGHTS

All patients will be treated as adult individuals.

Patients will not be subjected to punishment, ridicule, criticism, or unethical treatment.

Each patient has the right to worship as he chooses or not to participate in religious activities.

Each patient shall have the right to send and receive uncensored mail without undue delay.

Patients may receive visitors at times suggested by our visiting hours and at any other time with the approval of the nursing supervisor or the physician.

Patients (if able) are allowed to select their own clothing.

Patients' possessions remain their own property, including the most trivial or the most valuable.

Patients are paying guests and may expect full services without further tipping or promise of valuables. Staff members are not allowed to accept money or valuables from patients.

The patient's inventory will reflect his property and will be updated with additions; items outdated or discarded shall be deleted.

Possessions will be marked with the patient's name.

Patients will not be subjected to unsanitary conditions. Contaminated materials shall be disposed of in appropriate containers. Accidental filth will be promptly removed.

Patients will be protected from hazards that may cause injury. Loose objects on the floors, wet or slick places, and hazardous conditions will be corrected immediately.

Patients will be protected from undue solicitation.

Complaints shall be considered valid and are to be reported. Corrective measures shall be taken if at all possible.

Patients will recognize our limitations when we show them our concern, kindness, and consideration for the limitations that age and time has imposed upon them.

Chapter *24*

Recreation and

Religious Activities

The Role and Importance of Recreation

Recreation can meet several needs of the elderly. For example, it can fill in leisure time, it can serve as psychological therapy, it may substitute for cultural concepts, and it can assist in health care. Like all activities, recreation is voluntary for the patients. The best use of recreation is to benefit the health of the patient. As a result of exercise, the patient will rest and relax better. Stimulating recreation will help prejudice a person's mental attitude toward health needs. A whole series of physical difficulties are improved with exercise, such as obesity, poor muscle tone, bad posture, breathing problems, faulty elimination, abnormal blood pressure, poor circulation, and problems with diet.

Recreation may serve as an aid to psychotherapy or to socialization among the patients. There is much need for the patient to keep a healthy, wholesome, and cheerful outlook on life. He needs to continue to have fun, to laugh, to belong to the group, to win, and to succeed. Games bring people together, the sexes find companionship, and the socialization need is fulfilled.

Recreation can fill leisure time. The time of retirement may mean empty hours unless some assistance is given to make them beneficial. Retirement changes the entire regimen of the average person. Without normal responsibilities, with the withdrawal from productive life, and because of the physical limitations that may be experienced by the elderly, unoccupied time will be more in abundance. Consequently,

302

boredom and melancholy will increase, and monotony will prevail. Recreation can revive the spirit and attitude of the nursing home patient. When time is occupied with activities that bring pleasure, the patient can find social identification. It is the belief of social workers that a person needs to continue to have experiences and interaction for the purpose of self-identification.

A Planned Recreational Program

The recreational program should be started with a survey of the patients to discover their preferences and their limitations. Participation in any recreational program will be voluntary and within the ability of the individual.

The social activities director should seek expert advice and assistance. The administrator may assign a person to be responsible for the recreational program. Assistance by the National Recreation Association, the Area Office on Aging, the local library, and the American Red Cross are but a few of the resources available. In 1965 Congress established the Older Americans Act. OAA is the federal focal point for activities on behalf of aging. Title III is for community planning and services, Title IV is for research and demonstration, Title V is for training, and Title VI is for special programs.

Equipment for the recreational program should be assembled in one place and storage provided for it. Projectors, tape recorders, stereo players, and mechanical equipment should be included. Outdoor equipment also may be provided. Indoor games will serve as a basis for the program; arts and crafts may be considered. A library will supplement the program. Some suggested activities for groups are:

Group games	Variety shows	Plays and pageants
Birthday parties	Arts and crafts	Sewing groups
Singing	Movies	Religious programs
Picnics	Trips	Library time
Choir	Celebrations	Orchestra

Some suggested activities for individual patients are:

Games	Hobbies	Artwork
Shopping	Needlework	Letter writing
Walking	Hair grooming	Mending
Reading	Music listening	Conversation
Puzzles	Gardening	Crafts

Scheduling activities should not be too difficult. A calendar of activities should be kept in order that all recreational activities may be coordinated with the daily program. It should be updated daily and referred to when making other new schedules. Consideration for the supervisory personnel, the daily schedule of the patients, the season of the year, and the physical limitations of the patients will determine priorities for activities.

The place for recreation should be considered in the arrangement of the nursing home. Certain designated areas should be set aside for it. In the scheduling of activities, the reservation of certain space and equipment should be requested.

SOCIAL ACTIVITIES DIRECTOR'S JOB DESCRIPTION

The social activities director will assume responsibility for those social activities that are for the personal enjoyment and benefit of the individual patient. He or she will coordinate a calendar of activities with other patients' activities. It is his or her responsibility to arrange, schedule, and supervise these activities. Work will be at a minimum of 20 hours per week.

The social activities director will be trained in recreational skills or have a minimum of two years experience in a nursing home activities program.

It is suggested that the director meet regularly with the local activities directors' association and to attend in-service training seminars and courses.

Periodically, the director will conduct a survey of patients' preferences and adjust scheduled activities to conform with survey results. New patients are to be surveyed immediately after admission.

The activities director will be responsible for the nursing home recreational equipment, its care, storage, and maintenance. Equipment will be checked out to patients, recreational facilities scheduled, and a budget recommended.

The calendar of patient activities will be publicized.

Recreational and social activities will be coordinated with nursing schedule. All patient activities will be voluntary.

Reports on patient participation will be kept and recorded in the patients' clinical charts. A plan is prepared for each resident, reviewed quarterly, and updated as needed.

The director will assume responsibility for supervision of the volunteers program. Supervision will include:

The selection of volunteers from those recruited.
An orientation and training session.
The placement of volunteers in assigned positions.
Supervision of volunteers and attendance records.
Evaluation and discipline, in cooperation with the administrator.
Annual recognition of services rendered by volunteers. The social activities director will be a paid employee and will abide by all personnel policies of the nursing home.

SOCIAL ACTIVITIES POLICY

Social rehabilitation services for the nursing home have been designed to include the services of a social activity director, a volunteer program, and a staff member designated to handle social needs of patients. In addition, the entire staff work together to assist the patient in adjustment to the nursing home, to involve the family in patient care, to involve the patients in intrapersonal, social, and community activities.

Recreational activities are arranged for and scheduled in order to make the resident enjoy and benefit from his stay at the nursing home.

Volunteer Workers and Their Supervision

The selection of volunteers will ensure that each is socially acceptable, in reasonably good health, both mentally and physically, free from communicable disease, and is motivated by love. Volunteers should be aware of the type of patients with whom they are to work. An application for volunteer service may be provided. Parents' permission for volunteers under 18 years of age should be secured.

An orientation and training session should be provided for the volunteer that will cover such subjects as the qualifications of the volunteer, patient relations, a survey of the nursing home, emotional problems of the aging, a review of the volunteer program of the nursing home including job descriptions of each type of volunteer service, the resouces available, and a tour of the institution.

The placement of the volunteer should fit both his qualifications and desire to serve in the assigned position. He should be trained first and then later given his assignment, accompanied by a job description. He should be made aware of the limitations of his responsibility, his relation to the staff, and the supervision he may expect.

An evaluation and recognition plan should be provided. This should include not only the counting of hours contributed, but the actual work being done. A recognition service may be scheduled annually.

Development of the volunteer policy should be accomplished by the administrator. This policy will outline:

Qualifications expected of the volunteers.
Supervision of volunteers.
Training activities.
Scheduling of activities including requests for the use of facilities needed: living room, dining room, recreation room, game room, lawn facilities, piano, projector, etc.
Restriction on refreshments, e.g., for diabetics.
Restrictions on types of activities.
Restrictions on activities of volunteers.
Recognition program.

The resident's council is a variation on the use of volunteer workers. In the council, the patients themselves voluntarily join together for self-discipline and active promotion of recreational activities. There are several outcomes related to the council: planning activities, evaluation of the food service, evaluation of housekeeping, self-discipline, continuing activity, organization, and complexity. The council may be organized in two ways: as an advisory committee appointed by the administrator, or a group elected by the patients.

The Importance of Religion to the Aging

America lives under a religious heritage. Many of our older Americans and their ancestors contributed greatly to this heritage. We may trace religion to the founding fathers of Plymouth Bay. through the colonization of the original thirteen states, as a cause of the Revolution for Independence, as a part of the Bill of Rights, as a phrase included in the pledge to the flag, in the expansion of the nation, and now as an integral part of American society.

Americans have founded their belief on the authority of the Bible, the apostolic fathers, in religious tradition, and through spiritual revelation.

The nursing home administrator will discover a very positive correlation between patient attitudes and religious conviction. This type of patient will hope in the face of death, will find joy and happiness in the midst of suffering, will have high morale and a sense of victory over discouragement.

Religious conviction has a relationship to the physical needs of the patients. The deeply religious person may be more tolerant of the handicaps of himself and others. There may be less awareness of handicaps and more interest in other things. Some believe in divine healing and use religious practitioners. The administrator will recognize and cooperate with this practice when it is a matter of faith by the patient.

Religious conviction may be related to psychoses. Beliefs may reduce fear and anxiety. However, religious belief could increase guilt-related complexes when the patient is undergoing periods of doubt. In the mental patient, religious belief will tend to be exaggerated.

Religious conviction is definitely related to social adjustment and to the social needs of the patient. Joining with those of one's own faith will help to fill the need for companionship. It would help to make one more considerate of others in the room with several occupants and should increase harmony among roommates. Religious belief engenders a sense of sharing that is helpful in institutional living.

Religious conviction is related to ethics and will contribute to the sense of fairness in dealing with the patients. That which is just and right is established through the religious conviction of both patients and the nursing home staff.

A place of prayer and worship in the nursing home is the right of the patient, and opportunities for both should be provided by the administrator.

Planning Religious Activities

The nursing home should provide for many types of religious observances. The administrator must allow the scheduling of regular worship services and rites, seasonal religious observances and programs, classes in religious education, and individual religious observances. He has to be prepared to make dietary substitutions when this is a part of the patient's beliefs.

The administrator will exercise supervision over the religious activities, not to restrict such activities or to impose religious beliefs on the patients but to ensure this does not result with the use of volunteer leadership. The selection of the religious leadership will be a matter of careful concern. Normally, the administrator may consult the local ministerial association for counsel, advice, and assistance. Realistic goals and schedules should be set. The leadership should have a period of orientation to acquaint themselves with the physical, social, and emotional needs of the patients. Religious freedom will be discussed and ensured. It is best that a nurse's aide be present at each gathering to deal with the physical needs of the patients.

Religious activities need to be scheduled along with all other patient activities. Each event should be correlated with the total program and entered on the calendar of activities. Full consideration to all faiths should be given. Attendance at religious activities is always to be voluntary to ensure religious freedom. Restriction against attendance is for medical reasons only.

The site of religious activities in the nursing home need not be elaborate. While a chapel is nice and would serve as a focal point of activity, the living room or any other assembly room is adequate.

There are many different types of religious activities for which the nursing home administrator should make some provision to meet the needs of the patients. These may include sabbath day worship services and for all faiths represented in the nursing home special holy day observances. Some provision for prayer either at meals, individually, or as a group activity may be inaugurated.

Minister-Patient Relationships

The minister is the spiritual guide to the patient. He is the link to the patient's church. There is an attachment the patient develops between himself and his minister that helps in overcoming the difficulties of old age. It may inspire peace and comfort in the face of physical handicaps. Often the minister is the only other person permitted when a critical illness develops. The minister's title will vary with the faith, such as Rabbi, Father, Reverend, Sister, Reverend Mother, Brother, etc.

The minister is skilled in counseling, since much of his training and the practice of his efforts to help others will be directed in this manner. He may be able to give an objective view of the patient's need and to recognize symptoms of anxiety, fear, depression, and melancholy. He may be the only person that the patient will need in the endeavor to overcome his difficulties. While not a psychiatrist, he may be prepared, nevertheless, to deal with mild psychoneurotics; he is an important link in the healing team. Many ministers are given advanced training in pastoral counseling of the sick and infirm.

There are many relationships between the patient and his minister. Certainly, he will be a regular visitor and perhaps a prayer partner. Prayer holds a vital place in the spiritual life of the individual. The minister who says prayer at the visit will find great response and even change in the attitude of the patient. Each faith will hold to a number of individual practices that strengthen the individual's faith. The minister may be a regular visiting speaker at services or conduct Bible classes. His name should be recorded on the patient's records in case of need in patient-family problems and other problems related to the patient's well-being. He may break the news to the patient of a tragedy in the family or he may be the comforter to the family when the patient faces death. Some ministers will expect to be called to the death bed to administer last rites. Certainly, the minister will be called upon to conduct the funeral.

The administrator of the home will remember that in the interest of religious freedom the patient may refuse a minister's visit and that religious cranks may be denied visiting privileges when it is detrimental to the health and well-being of the patient. The administrator should know the various ministers and enlist their cooperation in the care of the patients.

For Further Study

Selected Readings in Personal and Auxiliary Relationships in the Nursing Home

Colman, Luciene E., JR., *Understanding Adults*. Nashville: Convention Press, 1969.

Current Literature on Aging (quarterly). National Council on the Aging, 1828 L Street, N.W., Washington, D.C.

Heckman, I. L., and Huneryager, S. G., *Human Relations in Management*. Cincinnati: South-Western Publishing Co., 1967.

Laird, Donald A., and Laird, Eleanor, *Practical Business Psychology*. New York: Gregg Publishing Division of McGraw-Hill, Inc.,1961.

Laird, Donald A., and Laird, Eleanor, *Psychology, Human Relations and Motivation*. New York: Gregg Publishing Division of McGraw-Hill, Inc., 1967.

Routh, Thomas A., *Choosing a Nursing Home*. Springfield, Ill.: Charles C. Thomas, 1970.

Shrope, Wayne Austin, *Speaking and Listening*. New York: Harcourt, Brace, and World, Inc., 1970.

Williams, James D., *Guiding Adults*. Nashville: Convention Press, 1969.

PART FOUR

Financial Management of the Nursing Home

The administrator will establish good financial management. He will establish a sound accounting system, using either cash accounting or accrual accounting, adequate alpha-numerical control of accounts, a system of depreciation to allocate costs, control of accounts receivable and flow of cash, proper billing procedures, adequate credit investigation, procedure for handling cash, depositing and reconciling of bank statement, proper payroll accounting, and the proper classification of accounts.

The administrator must make adequate use of financial statements and the basic accounting equation or balance sheet, and know how to compare and analyze the periodic financial statement.

The administrator will develop proper cost accounting and determine reasonable costs, cost per unit, cost per patient-day. He may use ratio of cost to charges, average daily cost, percentages of charges, and allocation of costs to departments.

The administrator will make a formal statement of charges and refund policy.

The administrator may use interim reimbursement from Medicare and should be ready to document cost by an annual audit.

He will control purchases and inventory, using a purchase order system, perpetual inventory, or periodic inventory.

He will adopt good budgeting practices to forecast future expenditures and anticipated income.

The administrator will use his financial ability constantly to improve the working conditions of the employees through better payroll practices.

The administrator will be aware of his professional position, his obligation to serve the aging, and his relation to the health care community. He should have a high-minded philosophy, a good sense of ethics, good financial business practices, and keep himself morally beyond reproach. He shall engage in comprehensive health care planning with his community, his government, and his peers. He should seek to discover and develop new horizons in nursing home administration.

Chapter 25

General Principles
of Accounting

Fundamentals of the Accounting Process

Accounting is developed according to a fundamental equation which may be stated in three different ways. In its simplest terms it is given as:

Assets equal equity.

However, because the term equity implies that one does not own an asset completely, the formula may be modified thus:

Assets equal equity plus liabilities.

The businessman usually desires to know how much his proprietorship (or capital) is worth, so we may transpose the formula to read:

Assets less liabilities equal net worth.

This now becomes the fundamental equation that concerns the balance sheet of any business at a particular time.

Assets may be anything that is owned. In order that something may be an asset, it must have value. Value is an illusive term, subject to many modifications, such as demand, age, exchange value, depreciation, cost, etc. Some assets we classify as fixed assets, because they

313

are durable or of a permanent nature, e.g., real estate or fixtures. Other assets are classified as current assets because they are of a short-term nature and are readily convertible, e.g., goods to be sold, accounts receivable, notes due, cash, etc. Some assets have an intangible value, for example, goodwill, copyrights, etc.

Liabilities are debts and obligations. It may be an obligation of service to be rendered. Liabilities, like assets, are classified as to current and long-term obligations. Typically, the mortgage on the nursing home property is a long-term obligation. If an obligation is due within one year, including the note payments of long-term obligations, it is usually classified as current. Examples include payments, accounts payable, wages due, taxes, etc.

The basic terminology of finance and accounting includes the major terms used in this text. However, the administrator should be able to identify and use several of those that pertain directly to his business.

Transaction Recording

Since time began and records have been kept, man has been recording his business transactions. Now, modern man has devised ways of making the record more meaningful than the recording of the item, the date, and the amount. He uses the philosophy that every transaction either credits or debits his assets, his liabilities, or his proprietorship. In other words, the businessman wishes to know how transactions affect his business.

These effects are shown on the balance sheet, which we commonly call a statement of capital or net worth. What the businessman wishes to know is the change that may result, i.e., an increase or decrease in net worth when a transaction is recorded. Some confusion results when we adopt the terms credit and debit to classify the effect of a transaction, since they may, but do not necessarily, mean decrease or increase.

The use of the "T" system of recording is a method to show the balance of accounts at each transaction. On the left side of the "T" debits are recorded and on the right side, credits. Using this method, we note that debits indicate increases in assets, and decreases in liabilities and proprietorship. Credits indicate decreases in assets, and increases in liability and proprietorship. Note:

Assets	Liabilities	Net worth
Debit, Credit	Debit, Credit	Debit, Credit
Increase, Decrease	Decrease, Increase	Decrease, Increase

The accountant should adopt a simple yet efficient method of recording a transaction. The adoption of the debit and credit system means he records each account to show the increase and decrease. Transactions may be, as we have said, those which affect either the assets, the liabilities, or the proprietorship. Asset transactions to be recorded include cash receipts, accounts receivable, prepaid accounts, equipment and fixtures, and real estate.

Transactions that affect liability accounts are: accounts payable, notes, wages, taxes, short-term payables, mortgages, long-term payables, and operational expenses. Proprietorship transactions naturally are affected by all the above, and may include the withdrawals of the owner, distribution of profits, etc.

The Business Statement

Normally, the business statement, sometimes called profit-loss statement, is for a specified period, e.g., January 1 to 31, with the statement prepared on a cash basis or an accrual basis. Cash accounting involves only the cash received or disbursed during the accounting period as the basis of the financial statement. Accrual accounting is when all transactions made during the accounting period are recorded in the financial statement. Thus, in accrual accounting, any cash or earned income, and any expense or liability will be accounted for in the period in which they are incurred, whether or not cash was received or disbursed at the time of transaction. The administrator will decide whether he is to use either accrual accounting or cash accounting and establishing his accounting system accordingly, Internal Revenue Service will expect one, and only one, system be used, and that it not be changed without advising them. A typical nursing home profit and loss statement will contain at least the following items with additional ones to fit the need of the individual home. We are using a departmental allocation of costs.

Income or revenue:
    Board and room
    Nursing services
    Ancillary services
    Drugs, medications, supplies (pharmacy)
    Miscellaneous

Expenses:
    Payroll (may be allocated to departments)
    Administrative department

       Nursing department
       Housekeeping department
       Dietary department
       Maintenance and upkeep
       Laundry
       Ancillary services
       Depreciation
       Interest
       Taxes
    Net income

An alternative type of profit and loss statement showing a nondepartmental recording of expenses may be made. Since this is optional (except that Medicare requires the departmental allocation of expenses to verify costs), we list the following statement:

Income and revenue:
    Room and board
    Nursing services
    Ancillary services
    Drugs, medications, supplies (pharmacy)
    Miscellaneous

Expenses:
    Payroll
    Food
    Laundry
    Utilities and telephone
    Insurance
    Miscellaneous supplies
    Linens and bedding
    Hospital supplies and pharmaceuticals
    Payroll tax
    Kitchen supplies
    Grounds upkeep
    Maintenance
    Equipment and construction
    Office supplies and stationery
    Travel expenses
    Interest
    Depreciation
    Property taxes
  Net income

The distribution of the net income also could be stated so as to indicate whether it was surplus, allocated to amortize the mortgage, or taken as profits.

In order to indicate the distribution of net earnings that are being retained in the flow of cash, the additional information may be added to the financial statement:

Receipts:
Disbursements:
Excess of receipts over disbursements:
Fund balance at beginning of period:
Fund balance at end of period:
    Operating fund:
    Reserve fund #1:
    Reserve fund #2:
    Petty cash:

The owner may wish to include a statement to indicate his proprietorship, to show its increase and his withdrawals. Such a statement may be:

Receipts:
Disbursements:
Excess of receipts over disbursements:
Owner's capital at start of accounting period:
Total of net income and capital:
Less owner's withdrawal during accounting period:
Balance, owner's capital, at close of accounting period:

The businessman may wish a statement of his proprietorship or net worth. While any number of methods could be used, it is customary to divide the statement into four general categories: current assets, fixed assets, current liabilities, and fixed liabilities. Subtopics of this statement will be equivalent to the number and type of accounts the administrator wishes to establish. The accepted accounts that are set up in any business are optional. Bookkeeping and accounting are highly individual, and are fashioned according to the type of nursing home operation. We suggest these:

Current assets:
    Cash
    Accounts receivable
    Prepaid expenses

Inventory
Miscellaneous
Fixed assets:
    Real estate
    Less depreciation
    Fixtures and machinery
        Less depreciation
    Reserves
Current liabilities:
    Notes payable
    Accounts payable
    Wages due
    Taxes due
Fixed liabilities:
    Mortgage and accrued interest
    Long-term notes
Net worth or equity

The sole owner may wish to return to the original accounting formula to show: Assets equal liabilities plus proprietorship. His statement will in this case be arranged as follows:

Current assets
Fixed assets (less depreciation)
    Grand total assets
Current liabilities
Fixed liabilities
    Grand total liabilities
    Owner's capital
        Total (liabilities plus capital)

In this formula the grand total assets should equal the total liabilities plus capital. This will indicate that the statement is in balance.

The partnership statement divides the item, "Owner's capital," between the two or more partners, thus:

First partner, capital
Second partner, capital
Etc.

The corporation statement will usually show "Owner's capital" in two parts:

Capital stock
Retained earnings
   Total stockholders' equity

It is suggested that the administrator consult with his accountant to establish the type of accounts he will need. The sole proprietor will likely set his accounts to match closely the annual income tax statement for profit and loss of a business. The corporation, on the other hand, will have a detailed accounting system. The guiding principle is to decide how much definition is needed in the accounting system, then establish those accounts.

Balancing the Accounts

Determination of the various accounts to be kept indicates their logical arrangement, or the order in which they would appear in the financial statement. Widely used is a numerical system of identifying and efficiently locating accounts in the bookkeeping procedures. However, some accountants use functional or alphabetical classifications and some have devised mnemonic or code designations.

Once established, the accounts should be periodically posted and then periodically cleared. This clearing process is known as balancing the accounts. Thus, when all items are posted pertaining to the accounting period, it will be necessary to accumulate these and clear the account for the next accounting period.

The trial balance is to prove the equality of the debits and credits. The sum of debits and credits should always equal zero, or the books are out of balance. The trial balance is to detect errors in achieving this balance. It also summarizes the various accounts.

The administrator should practice balancing accounts in order to familiarize himself with the accounting process. While it is not within the scope of this text to qualify the administrator to be a bookkeeper, he must, nevertheless, become familiar with the accounting procedure. Detection of errors in accounting is a skill in itself. Normally, errors result from incorrect additions and subtractions, wrong postings, incorrect numbers, and omissions. Mistakes in the accounting procedure are often traced to the posting of accounts, such as posting to the wrong account, the wrong classification of a posting, or failure to post a transaction at all.

It is sometimes necessary to make adjustments in the balance for an accrued item, deferred income, and deferred expense. Some typical adjustments might be depreciation, bad debts, and correcting entries. The trial balance is normally prepared at the end of the month and may be done by listing both debits and credits of each account.

Accounting for Cash and Receipts

Like any business, the nursing home will need a systematic method of accounting for cash and receipts. The flow of cash in the operation is directly related to the solvency of the business. A patient may pay for services in as many as a half-dozen ways. She may pay a portion in cash, a portion from a Social Security check, or the state may make, in her behalf, a Medicaid payment. Her relatives may supplement the nursing service with their check, leave a deposit for her petty cash, and pay for ancillary services. The actual receipts may be in the form of a draft, certified check, postal or bank money order, cashier's check, personal check, or cash.

Bank deposits are a method of safeguarding income; their management includes documentation, making deposits, and withdrawals. The nursing home should establish a bank deposit system in keeping with good business practices. Each deposit should be identified and posted in a deposit journal. Cash can be identified or posted separately in a cash journal, using a receipt system for all income. It is normal practice to make different persons responsible for handling cash, making deposits, and recording receipts.

The monthly bank statement should be checked and reconciled monthly. With the use of modern computers, it will give a total of the deposits and disbursals and show the balance in the account. This statement also serves as a cross-check on outstanding checks and nonrecorded checks. Nonrecorded checks are quite typical when the owner serves as his own administrator. The bank statement will alert the administrator to noncollectable items.

Reconciling the bank statement with the accounts of the nursing home should be done monthly. The first step is to verify and note errors in the statement. Next, arrange the checks in the order written and compare with the check journal to determine which checks are outstanding. Then, compare deposits and record any additional deposits made during the accounting period. Now complete the reconciliation:

Bank balance
Add additional deposits not listed
Subtract outstanding checks
    Balance should equal accounts balance

The petty cash fund in the nursing home is for small miscellaneous items, and may be established by the system known as the "imprest" system. First determine the amount needed in the fund, cash a check for this amount and place it in the petty cash drawer. Thereafter, the cash on hand, plus vouchers for purchases, should equal the fund total. The fund may be replenished by writing a cash check equal to the vouchers on hand. The vouchers are posted to the respective accounts.

Notes and Drafts

Borrowing money is an accepted practice in business. Normally, there are several considerations concerning business borrowing: the cost of borrowing, the time allowed for repayment, the security or collateral, the amount available, and the resultant effect on the balance statement. Borrowing is usually necessary to make purchases, to maintain the flow of cash, to settle or extend accounts, and to achieve a balance of cash.

Notes may be classified as to interest-bearing, discount, receivables, and payables. The difference between discount and interest-bearing notes is whether the lender collects the interest in advance (discount) or on maturity (interest-bearing).

Computation of interest can be done easily with the use of a book of interest tables or by the use of the formula:

Principal × rate × time = interest

In the past, the use of the 360-day year and the 30-, 60-, 90-, and 120-day note period was popular. With the advent of the computer, notes of any length and the fraction of a percent of interest are now becoming common.

Discount or discounted notes are sometimes used in business. For example, the nursing home purchases a fixture to be paid for in equal monthly payments. The vendor may discount the note, that is, sell it for less than the amount of the principal. The nursing home will then pay the financial institution which purchased the note. Since the monthly payments include both principal and interest and the nursing home pays back all of the original amount of the note, the purchaser of the note earns both interest and the discount.

The accounting procedure for notes is usually one of allocating the amount of principal to the proper account and the amount of interest to an expense account. The practice of some mortgage holders of collecting escrow payments for taxes and insurance should also be considered in posting of accounts.

Occasionally, a note may not be paid at maturity. If it carries an endorsement, a certificate of protest is sent to each endorser who is then liable for payment plus the protest fee.

Notes are negotiable instruments with the holder having certain legal rights. The fact that he holds the note gives him the right to collect without proving the existence of the debt. The note is his proof. Therefore, when collection out of town is necessary, the holder may secure the services of a bank to make the collection and transfer on the note.

Sometimes, a firm will issue what is called a sight draft or a time draft for the purpose of collecting an account. More recently, laws pertaining to maximum rates and disclosure of interest have been passed. The administrator should be fully acquainted with these laws.

Accounts Receivable

Typically, nursing homes receive their income from several sources. When services are rendered, and until reimbursement is made for these services, they are known as accounts receivable. In a nursing home, this includes payments due from private patients, reimbursement due from Medicare, payment due from Medicaid vendor, and miscellaneous receivables. The home may have rendered ancillary services, the pharmacy dispensed drugs, provided medical supplies, rented special equipment, or provided laundry services. For accounts receivable, a billing procedure is established.

Normal billing procedures require that certain things be done periodically. The procedure should include:

Establish the billing cycle, e.g., monthly
    For charges for nursing services
    For charges for purchases
    For charges for ancillary services
Prepare the monthly statement
    Mail the monthly statement
Post the receipts to the individual account
Deposit the receipts

Billing procedures vary widely; but the basic elements of charging, billing, and posting receipts will occur in any system, whether it is computerized or hand written.

The recent enactment of the Fair Credit Reporting Act of 1971 protects the consumer. The act specifically says that you must tell why credit is refused a customer. If you obtain information from a credit bureau and use the information as the basis for refusal of credit, you must give the bureau's name and location. The act further specifies that the bureau must then tell the customer the basis for the report resulting in loss of credit.

Credit is related to accounts receivable, since credit is extended anytime collection for services is not made in advance. Many nursing homes belong to credit bureaus which, for a small fee, will provide a credit search on a prospective account. In any event, a statement of credit will be a necessary item to be secured at the time business arrangements are concluded.

Occasionally, collection problems will arise. The older an account becomes, the more unlikely it is that recovery will be made. Because the patient will run up a sizable bill in any given month, an effort should be made to collect it regularly. As a last resort, an attorney or collection agency could be used. As in every business, some bad debts will arise.

Finally, some special problems of accounting arise when goods or services are sold to employees or to stockholders. Accounting for overpayment or the recovery of a bad debt already written off requires special handling.

Assets and Depreciation

It is a normal practice in business to classify assets through evaluation as either short-term or long-term. However, all items except land will depreciate in value. Of course, some things may inflate in value; but inflation is not entered in normal bookkeeping, only depreciation. *Depreciation is the allocation of cost over the useful life of an asset to determine the true cost of operation.* Depreciation is caused by the deterioration or depletion in value of an asset over a period of time. Some items may be considered to have some salvage value at the end of the depreciation period. Depreciation does not mean an item becomes worthless; it merely means the item's cost has been allocated to its estimated useful life.

Accounting for depreciation is usually on the basis of cost, or the "book" value. *Normally, cost is the purchase price, plus any additional expense required for getting the asset ready for use.* The Internal Revenue Service publishes *Tax Information on Depreciation,* Publication 534, which outlines two systems, Class Life (ADR) System and Guideline Class Life System, for determining the life of an asset for depreciation purposes. IRS normally will expect that salvage value to be deducted before taking depreciation. It should also be pointed out that the use of Internal Revenue methods of determining depreciation are for the benefit of the taxpayer in determining his fair tax on earnings. Another schedule of depreciation may be used that is more reasonable for other accounting purposes than paying taxes. In borrowing money, for example, one will be seeking to show the fair market value, which may be quite different from the depreciated value.

Accounting methods have been adopted for allocation of depreciation. These are:

The straight-line method. The cost, less the salvage value, is divided by the years of useful life.

Production-units method. An estimate of the total productive units of the item is made and then divided by the useful life of the asset.

Declining-balance method. By doubling the rate that is used to compute the remaining balance, greater depreciation is allocated during the first years and less during the last. You may use different percentages, e.g., 125%, 150%, 200%.

Sum-of-years-digits method. Example (using an estimated three years): one plus two plus three (years) equals six, so that the first year depreciation would be 3/6, the second year, 2/6, and the third year, 1/6

Payroll Accounting

Accurate payroll accounting is a must for several good reasons. Perhaps the best reason is to maintain good employer-employee relationships by the elimination of errors in computing the paycheck. The nursing home is primarily engaged in the sale of service. This means that good control over the payroll will ensure good financial control. Of course, tax requirements make it imperative that accurate records are kept. If a wage dispute should arise or an audit by the Wage and Hour Division of the U.S. Department of Labor should be made, records will need to be absolutely accurate.

There are several payroll records that are needed: some type of timecard or timebook; a payroll register, which helps in accumulating the periodic payroll; notice of earnings with each employee's check;

an individual employee's register; finally, a sickpay register. Of course, if another basis for paying such as bonuses, piecework, etc., is used, records by hours still have to be kept to determine if minimum wage and overtime requirements are met. The payroll register summarizes a periodic payroll and should contain:

Employee's name and identification data
Hours worked
Overtime
Pay rate
Total earnings
Deductions
    F.I.C.A. (Federal Insurance Contributions Act)
    Federal withholding taxes
    State withholding taxes
    Miscellaneous
Net pay
Pay period
Check number
Date issued

In addition to the payroll register, which should be completed for each pay period, the administrator will need to record each recipient's record separately so as to be able to compile a summary of individual data for tax purposes. The individual employee record should contain:

Employee's name and identification data
Summary of earnings from payroll register
Basis for preparing W-2
Totals to show when the employee reaches
    F.I.C.A. maximum earnings
    State unemployment tax maximum

Normally, the payroll check is drawn on a special account. It should include a statement of earnings with:

Hours worked
Overtime
Total wages
Deductions
Net pay

Some nursing homes find a special check, printed for the payroll only, to be advantageous. It is well to have the employee's name on his check, the same as that listed on his Social Security card and the permanent records. This is particularly true for female employees.

Corporations, Proprietorship, Nonprofit Organizations

The organization of the business is peculiar to the owner or owners. American businesses have adopted several forms of ownership, including the corporation, proprietorship, partnership, and the non-profit organization.

The legal status of the corporation is that of a separate entity, which limits the liability of the stockholders to the extent of their ownership. The ease of transferring ownership by the mere sale of stock, while not disrupting the control or management of the concern, is one of its advantages. Its ability to raise capital by the sale of stock issues more than offsets the limitations on its borrowing capacity.

The legal status of the proprietorship is vested in the owner, who is said to be "doing business as_____Nursing Home." The single proprietor is liable to the full extent of any obligation his business may incur, which could exceed his total ownership, e.g., a liability incurred for negligence. The sole owner is usually limited by the amount of capital he can raise, or allow to remain, in the business.

The partnership is treated like the sole owner for all legal purposes. Each owner is normally liable for the acts of the partner or partners. Some states allow a limited partnership to exist when at least one partner assumes unlimited liability.

The voluntary nonprofit organization exists by charter—issued by the Secretary of State of the incorporating state—and must function within the stated purpose of its original charter. Profits are usually returned to the business or used for charitable purposes. Otherwise, the nonprofit institution functions like any corporation, except for tax requirements which may be eliminated.

Accounting procedures for the corporation and the proprietorship are similar, except for the equity accounts. The sole owner will have a proprietor or equity account. Each partner will have an equity account. With the stock corporation, equity is divided into common or preferred stock, retained earnings, and stockholders' equity accounts. Profits may be distributed as dividends for the corporation and as withdrawals for the sole owner or partnership. The charter requires the corporation to keep accurate records of all stock and to issue certificates promptly in the transfer or sale of stock. Licensing agencies are now requiring affidavits of ownership which must be filed when ownership of a nursing home is transferred.

Long-Term Liabilities

Long-term liabilities are directly related to long-term assets, which we previously discussed, i.e., fixed assets as real estate. Normally, a long-term liability is classified thus because it requires more than one year to be amortized. It is related to long-term assets because these are usually the security for the liability. We commonly call such liabilities, mortgages; however, it may be in the form of a promissory note or a bond issue.

There are several requirements for long-term liabilities. There must be a schedule for repayment. The terms, including interest, discounts, etc., must be stated. When secured by a mortgage, adequate insurance shall be provided, an escrow amount may be established, and the mortgaged property must be maintained in good repair. A foreclosure clause may be included and conditions for early payment may be agreed upon. It is sometimes a practice to include either a penalty or a minimum amount for prepayment.

Lending institutions vary widely, from the Savings and Loan Association, which specializes in real estate, to an individual or a bank dealing in commercial loans. When the mortgage is guaranteed by the Federal Housing Administration, it is said to be an "FHA mortgage"; such mortgages, however, are made by commercial lenders. Should the loan be from a commercial bank, it is called a "commercial mortgage." Banks may give interest rates equivalent to the Savings and Loan Association, but the length of time for repayment is likely to be less.

The use of bonds is usually limited to corporations and is normally issued by an underwriter. The underwriter may use a bank as trustee. The trustee normally holds the mortgage, holds the sinking fund for payments, acts as payee to retire the bonds, and may, in the event of default, foreclose.

Bonds are issued by several methods. The serial bond is popular, having a definite date to retire each bond of a particular issue. They are also known as sinking fund bonds. Another type is a coupon bond, which is much like serial bonds, except that coupons are used to make payment of the interest. Registered bonds are similar to stock in that the ownership is registered. When an unsecured bond is issued, it is called a debenture. When the bond is secured by collateral, it becomes a trust bond. The administrator will need to seek legal counsel, since the sale of stocks and bonds is a highly technical aspect of the operation of a business. Much of this activity is regulated by the Securities and Exchange Commission.

Electronic Data Processing and Machine Bookkeeping

Computers have come into the business field since World War II (the first electronic computer was perfected in the 1930s). Mechanical computers can be traced to the eighteenth century. Computers are related to mathematics and are based on Boolean algebra, binary notation, and differential equations. The first generation of computers were mechanical; the second, electronic tubes; the third, solid-state transistors. More recently, the integrated circuit has brought a vast reduction in the size of the unit. A desk-top computer is now practical when constructed with three-dimensional integrated circuits that put hundreds of electronic circuits into a small cube, the size of the head of a pin.

Machine bookkeeping is sometimes known as keypunch posting machine bookkeeping. The machine is set for multiple accounts and gives instant updating; but it does require a trained operator. However, the skilled secretary can acquire the skill to operate one in a minimum of time.

The first step in electronic data processing is usually the use of punched-card accounting. While most of the bookkeeping may be done mechanically with punched-card collators, some calculation, e.g., payroll, will require a computing section. Data from business transactions can be punched on cards and then sorted, tabulated, posted, and, when a computer is connected, calculated. Information may be in either letter or digital form.

Punched-tape accounting is similar, except that the data are punched on a tape in a chronological order. Sometimes this can be done automatically as on a cash register, and then the processing is done by an electronic computer.

Pure electronic data processing requires an input source, a processing or computational unit, storage units, and a method of output. Input of data may be done by the use of punched cards, punched tape, magnetic tape, or optical scanning. The nursing home can install a special adding machine which prints letters capable of being fed into a computer by optical means. Processing is sorting, tabulation, or computation. Output is in the form of statements for billing, checks, journalizing for financial records, summaries, and analyses.

Taxes

The administrator must be sure that he operates his business in compliance with all tax laws. These laws apply to levies by municipals, state, and federal government.

The sole owner is taxed as an individual, while normally the corporation is assessed a tax on its profits, and then the individual is taxed on his wages and dividends from the corporation. It is possible, however, for the small incorporated nursing home to be taxed as a partnership or proprietorship by agreement with the Internal Revenue Service. Considerations that influence the tax picture of a business are: whether equipment is leased or purchased, depreciation schedules, profits taken as dividends, methods of accounting, and net income as related to taxable income.

Penalty for income tax evasion is a danger to be realized and avoided. The ethical administrator would not knowingly evade payment of taxes. *In simple terms, concealment of income to avoid payment of taxes is illegal. Any unreported income and any illegal deductions taken may be counted as evasion.* The government does not expect the businessman to pay more than he rightly owes; therefore, the administrator can rightly take every deduction that is a true business expense.

State taxes, for which the businessman is responsible, include unemployment taxes, corporation franchise tax, and income tax. Municipal taxes include a sales tax on the sale of certain items, and, in some cities, income tax. Municipal sales taxes, when assessed, are levied whether or not there also exists a state sales tax, as is the case in practically all the states.

Federal taxes include income tax from the owner and withholding tax for the employees, a corporation tax, estate or trust tax, federal unemployment tax, F.I.C.A. (employer's part, Medicare and Social Security).

Certain taxes are required to be deposited regularly in a bank designated as a depository. These include Social Security (OASDHI) and Medicare, with both the employee's and the employer's contribution; income tax withheld for employees; federal unemployment tax; and, in some states, the municipal or state sales tax. It is advisable for the administrator to consult with the Internal Revenue Service to determine his liability, since it will vary with the amount of withholding.

Flow of Cash

Perhaps the single most important thing the administrator does as a businessman is to maintain an adequate flow of cash to enable him to pay his obligations promptly, to meet long-term payments at maturity, and to maintain solvency. The flow of cash is related to the immediate cash available, i.e., the bank balance, or readily available convertibles to cash. We say we apply an acid test to our business when we compare all readily available convertible assets to our current liabilities.

Working capital is another term for flow of cash. Normally, *current assets less current liabilities equal working capital*. The source of working capital varies with the business, but may be supplied from various sources. Cash on hand may accrue from surpluses or be contributed by the proprietor. Accounts receivable is related to working capital, since most banks will lend against it as collateral. Inventory or merchandise is sometimes thought of as working capital since it may be sold or mortgaged. When the flow of cash is not great enough for the businessman to meet promptly his obligations, he may need to convert some assets to cash, such as the sale of surplus inventory, or securing a short-term or long-term financing. In the case of the sole owner, he may increase his investment; but the corporation may sell a new issue of stock. It should be noted that most financiers consider this working capital as the owner's "risk money" and expect him to raise it rather than borrow it.

The preparation of the statement of working capital is based on an accounting period and a specified date. If the administrator wishes to know his status at a specific time, he lists assets and liabilities at that time as in his balance sheet. *However, for the analysis of working capital, he should compare the change between two or more statements to note the trend toward improvement or deterioration of his financial status.*

An administrator will need to analyze closely his financial statements to note trends that may be developing. Information he may desire is:

The amount and the change in the amount of cash balance.
The change in assets.

Additional liabilities, accounts, mortgages, etc.
The source of funds, i.e., sales, income, etc.
The application of funds.

The statement will be compiled from information recorded in the ledger account, the current income statement, and the latest net worth statement. He will note trends, the application of funds, and the changes in his source of capital.

Methods of Bookkeeping

Selecting the best method of bookkeeping will depend upon many factors. The size of the nursing home and, whether it is under sole ownership, a partnership, a corporation, or a nonprofit organization, may dictate the type of system. Outside help is always valuable to any type of business, whether it is only an annual audit, a quarterly preparation of reports, or a full accounting service.

Some businesses choose to do their own accounting. When this is done, some provision must be made for maintaining the system. Office space and equipment will vary; however, the basic elements are always present. An accounting desk, chair, filing cabinet, and storage for accounting material will be needed. A vault or small safe should be acquired as security for key records. The correct style of books, binders, and holders needs to be selected. Some calculating machinery will also be needed. The simplest is a calculator-adding machine. One may add a posting machine, an electronic-posting-computing machine, or a complete electronic data-processing system. Normally, however, when electronic data processing is used in the nursing home, only punch card, punch tape, or optical scanning input equipment is installed. Information is sent to a data center for processing. It is now possible for the nursing home to secure a remote input-output machine to address a computer, for which time has been purchased.

Employees needed for an accounting system may be a bookkeeper, a billing or statements clerk, or an accountant. Most nursing homes employ office personnel who are assigned these duties.

Some nursing homes find the use of a bookkeeping or accounting service adequate. If no employee has the skill to oversee the bookkeeping system or prepare the payroll, the administrator should contract for this service. Certain data are prepared in the office by a secretary and then sent to the accountant or central accounting center.

Affiliates use this system extensively. An outside accountant could, theoretically, keep accounts from either a purchase order system or from the deposit book and the canceled checks. However, he will need full details on each check as to the nature of the expenditure. It is also necessary for the administrator to be prepared to document expenditures.

Trends in accounting, in recent years, require the increased use of data, i.e., accrual accounting for Medicare, the increased cycling of data, such as costs vs. budgeting, the allocation of reasonable costs, etc. Electronic aids are the only answer to meeting these demands.

Chapter **26**

Classification of

Revenue and Expense

Income: Basic Maintenance and Nursing Care

The administrator, as a businessman, needs to determine the basic charge for services in order that he may be competitive. *The charge is usually based on the actual cost, or expenses actually incurred, and allowance for loss or risk, and a fair return on the investment.*

Charges are affected by several factors. Competition between nursing homes will affect the price, because people have learned to shop for nursing care. Contracted services, such as with Medicaid, may establish maximum prices allowable. Inflation in the economy, variations of locale and section of the country, the demand for space, and the volume of business will affect charges.

Methods of pricing vary somewhat: however, the monthly or daily charge seems to be most popular. Charging a monthly rate simplifies bookkeeping; but it is inflexible for the short-term patient. Also, it is difficult to correlate with some payment plans of third-party payers. On the other hand, the daily charge may be difficult to correlate with Medicaid when fees are paid in several ways.

Problems of pricing can be traced to several sources. One is in public relations, when the general public fails to understand the high cost of services, the ever increasing wage spiral, and inflationary costs. Another problem is the failure of many nursing homes to use true cost accounting to verify charges. The administrator must bear the responsibility of communicating the true cost of providing services to the public, the patient, and to contractual agencies.

There are a number of costs that relate to the basic maintenance of the patient, which is usually thought to be room, board, and laundry, direct and indirect costs, i.e., food, utilities, supplies, repair, janitorial expenses, etc. For a realistic appraisal, all costs are apportioned or allocated. Only then can the administrator set a fair charge for services.

Income: Ancillary and Miscellaneous Services

Perhaps the most abused and misunderstood area of charges is in ancillary and miscellaneous services. In the absence of true cost accounting, both on an accrual and a departmental basis, the nursing home administrator has little to base a charge on, except an approximation.

When informing a prospective patient of the additional charges, first the administrator should explain the basic service being offered, what it does and does not include. It is best that a clear understanding of additional charges be determined at the time of entry. A full review of the charges should be made, and then an agreement in writing, stating all charges, should be given the prospective patient. This statement of charges will vary from nursing home to nursing home. It should be noted that contractual agencies, such as Medicaid, specifically designate what is to be considered a part of the basic maintenance charge, nursing care, and what may be charged in addition. Medicare has also adopted a conservative attitude, choosing to limit the charges to what is considered reasonable.

In determining the cost of additional charges, the administrator allocates all true cost, or percentage of cost, to a particular service; to this is added risk, return on investment, and profit. A true-cost method of dividing labor should be adopted, as should a percentage method of allocating space and maintenance. Finally, a fair allocation of administrative costs is made.

Some of the areas in which additional charges are usually made are: drugs and medical supplies (pharmacy), beauty and barber care, laundry and cleaning, laboratory, speech therapy, physical therapy, occupational therapy, inhalation therapy, oxygen, equipment rental, and x-ray.

Operational Expenses Classified

To give the administrator some basic knowledge as to how to classify operational expenditures, listed below are some of the more common expenses in the operation of the nursing home. These data have been selected from a state department of public welfare report, for which the administrator is now responsible if he has the Medicaid contract.

Administration
    Administrator's salary
    Assistant administrator
    Receptionist
    Clerk-typist
    Bookkeeper
    Accountant
    Owner
    Other
        Total administration salaries
Office supplies and expenses
    Office supplies
    Telephone
    Travel
    Advertising
    Licenses and fees
    Professional services
    Legal services
    Employee benefits—payroll
    Employee benefits—nonpayroll
    Interest (other than buildings and equipment)
    Accounting and auditing
    Insurance
        Buildings
        Equipment
        Vehicles
        Other
            Total office supplies and expense
Property expense
    Real estate taxes
    Interest on mortgages
    Rent
        Total property expense
Motor vehicle expense
    Taxes
    Interest on auto note
    Rent
    Other expense
        Total motor vehicle expense

Depreciation
    Buildings
    Equipment
    Vehicles
        Total depreciation
Plant operation and maintenance
    Salaries
        Maintenance engineer
        Janitor
        Gardener
        Other
    Fuel (Gas, electricity, water)
    Supplies
    Repairs
        Total plant operation
Dietary department
    Salaries
        Dietitian
        Food service manager
        Cook
        Assistant cook
        Kitchen helpers or aides
        Other
    Raw food
    Supplies
        Total dietary department expense
Laundry and Linen
    Salaries
    Linens and bedding
    Contracted services
    Laundry supplies
        Total laundry and linen expense
Housekeeping department
    Salaries
        Executive housekeeper
        Maids
        Janitor (when not carried under maintenance)
    Housekeeping supplies
        Total housekeeping department
Nursing department
    Salaries

      Director of nurses
      Registered nurses
      Licensed vocational nurses
      Nurse's aide
      Orderlies
      Other
    Supplies (medical)
    Total nursing department
Consultants and other services
    Physician and utilization review
    Pharmacist
    Clergy
    Records librarian
    Total consultants and other services
Recreation and Rehabilitation
    Salaries
      Physical therapist
      Physical therapist aide
      Occupational therapist
      Occupational therapist aide
        Recreational activities director
      Social director
    Supplies
    Total recreation and rehabilitation
Other expenses
    Bad accounts write-off
    Miscellaneous taxes
    Refunds and allowances
    Total other expenses
    GRAND TOTAL ALL OPERATIONAL EXPENSE

The classification of each expense will be determined by the administrator. There is one area, however, that proves to be a chief concern to the accounting system. Some items are classified as nonoperating expenses; that is, they are expenses that cannot be charged against the operating accounts. Some are capital expenses and others are accrued liabilities. Perhaps it is difficult to make sizable payments to defray certain nonoperating items and to have these payments come from the profit of the enterprise. It is necessary to understand the nature of the business statement before being fully aware of the cause. Some things are expenses simply because they are the cost of making money. Others are considered as a part of the capital equity of the owner. Nonoperating expense is charged against the capital account. Some of the items, e.g., accrued taxes withheld are carried in the capital account, although the money belongs to the employees. It is simply money withheld from the employee's check. Other items, e.g., notes payable may be funds borrowed against accounts receivable; it will be replaced when the patients pay their accounts. The following items may be classified as nonoperating liabilities:

> Notes payable
> Taxes withheld
> Accrued expenses
> Accrued interest
> Accrued insurance
> Dividends payable
> Bonds payable
> Mortgage principal

Profit and Loss: Analysis of the Financial Statement

Every business will wish to keep a balance sheet on the state of the business. This is simply a financial statement balancing the assets against the liabilities to give the net worth or equity in the business. However, this is often not sufficient, since other ratios or percentages may be necessary to show a trend in the business. There are several types of ratios that may be beneficial. A partial list of ratios that may pertain to the operation of the nursing home is:

> Current assets to current liabilities
> Total assets to total liabilities
> Current assets to total assets
> Fixed assets to fixed liabilities
> Surplus to net worth
> Net worth to total assets
> Net profit to income
> Accounts receivable to income
> Income to fixed assets
> Income to net worth
> Profit to net worth
> Profit to total assets

Learning to use the information as given in the ratios is a complete study for the administrator. However, there are certain obvious uses for the information. *The primary use of statements is for the management to determine efficiency and to predict future trends.* Since a ratio is based on past operation, it can be useful in establishing future business policy. Of course, every businessman is interested in his equity and the return on his investment. Ratios reveal this information. A secondary reason for financial statements is in obtaining credit. A statement will reveal the nursing home's ability to repay a liability, should it be necessary to secure additional credit. It is normal procedure for the loan department of a bank to ask for an annual financial statement.

Government agencies, such as the licensing agency, may ask for a statement, since it is useful for them to predict financial trends in health care costs. Taxation is also based on that statement. It is deemed wise for the small businessman to correlate closely his expense accounts to conform somewhat to the annual tax return.

Analysis of Profit

Every business must make a profit to remain in operation. The nursing home is no exception. However, it is possible to operate for a period of time without making a profit, because of assets and credit. It is also possible for the administrator to be unaware of the state of the business and suddenly find himself in financial difficulty. However, wise management and financial forecasting will often reveal such a tendency before it becomes a reality. It is therefore necessary that the businessman know constantly whether the business is making a profit.

Profit means a net or surplus remaining after the expenses of the operation have been defrayed. However, this profit margin is dependent upon several things. In its simplest terms, it is the net return on sales.

Profit is affected by price level trends and the occupancy of the nursing home. Volume also determines the ability of the nursing home to compete. The expense of borrowing money for long-term investments or short-term flow of cash definitely affects profit. The turnover of capital in order to meet expenses, which may also vary greatly, will affect the profit margin.

Businessmen have learned to look for certain healthy business signs; the two best indicators are a steady increase in net worth and an increase in working capital after profit taking. Working capital is determined by the difference between current assets and current liabilities.

The amount of profit a person desires to make may be related to his debt-paying ability. Should the administrator not have sufficient working capital to make prompt payment of obligations, it may be desirable to increase profits to gain capital. It is theoretically possible to reduce expenses in order for the working capital to be replenished. It is possible for a business to be making a "paper profit" and not have ready cash to meet obligations. It is also possible to operate for some time on investor's capital or on "the depreciation."

Where profit should go is always a question. The stockholder wants dividends; the worker wants better wages; the owner wants withdrawals or equity. Normally, profits can be channeled into three areas; paying for assets, increasing working capital, and withdrawals or dividends. Every business needs a balance of these. Until enough working capital is created, profits should stay in the business. One danger a business may face is inflation and rising price trends in the economy. For example, the businessman may purchase a business that requires a certain amount of operating capital, but because of inflation and rising prices the need for operating capital may double within a short period of time. In effect, his profits remain in the business to gain additional operating capital. Often, a businessman may discover he has bought too large a capital-investment mortgage, or sudden remodeling demands must be financed with immediate working cash.

Analysis of Loss

In the simplest of terms, loss is sustained when expenses exceed income. However, there are other indicators that signal a loss within certain areas of the operation. The business may lose its working capital or the capital investment may diminish. Normally, excessive operating costs, wages, or unusual expenditures will bring about a loss. Lower gross revenue because of low occupancy may be the cause. Sometimes excessive capital investment for nonproductive assets may cause a loss. While there may be a net gain in net worth, a loss may be sustained in the working capital.

The administrator should be wary of certain indicators that signal a loss in the operation. The first and foremost is failure to meet promptly current obligations. A low amount of working capital, such as a poor bank balance, indicates danger, although it may be only temporary. An unfavorable financial statement of current assets and current liabilities may indicate a difficulty. If ready cash reserves or convertible reserves are exhausted, it may indicate a trend. Sometimes an increase in accounts receivable collection or noncollection could indicate a trend.

The administrator should rely on periodic statements to indicate profit or loss. His analysis may give the first indication of danger. In making an analysis he will look for specific indicators such as the following:

Note the current ratio for trends from one quarter to the next. Some say that a two to one ratio—twice the current assets as to the current liabilities—is necessary; however, each administrator will decide on the best ratio for his nursing home.

The "acid test" is a good indicator, since it shows how much ready cash is available. In the application of this test, the administrator notes only the actual ready cash available to meet current day-to-day operational expense.

Other indicators are: the increase or decrease in working capital, the ratio of net profit to working capital, a rise in noncurrent assets, or a decrease in net income and net profit.

How does one determine the "right" indicator of profit or loss? It is possible to compare a single nursing home with the nursing home industry, to use Dun & Bradstreet ratios, to compare competitive prices, or to use a simple *rule-of-thumb: patient services are more than adequate, indicating efficiency, the mortgage is being paid, the working capital is adequate, the employees feel well remunerated, and the proprietor is pleased.*

Chapter *27*

Medicare Cost Reimbursement

Health Insurance Reimbursement Principles

Medicare has adopted reasonable cost as the basis for reimbursing the providers of the services under Health Insurance. It should be noted again that *Health Insurance contains two parts: Part A, which is Hospital Insurance, and Part B, which is Medical Insurance.* Part A includes such providers of services as: hospitals, skilled nursing facilities, extended care benefits, and home health agencies. This discussion is primarily applicable to reimbursement procedures for nursing homes as skilled nursing facilities offering extended care benefits. The administrator should remember that constant changes are taking place in reimbursement practices. It is strongly advised that he discuss reimbursement, in detail, with his Medicare representative of the Social Security Administration.

Congress originally intended Medicare to be paid for at cost, since most of the providers were thought to be nonprofit organizations. However, because of the contention that even a nonprofit organization needs to amortize its investment (capital assets), and that the long-term elderly patient is more costly to care for than the short-term young patient, some concessions were made in allowances. First, depreciation was allowed, even though some nonprofit facilities may have been built with federally assisted, long-term, low-interest loans.

Hospitals were granted an 8½% excess nursing cost if they were nonprofit, and 1½% times the trust-fund interest rate, if proprietary. Payment was to be on an interim basis. Carriers were appointed to serve as the fiscal intermediaries to determine reasonable costs and to make payments, e.g., the Blue Cross Association and the Mutual of Omaha Insurance Company.

Because monthly payments were to be allowed, the average daily cost reimbursement method or the percentages of charges reimbursement method may be adopted by the provider of services. Payment made by either of the two methods is then adjusted annually to conform to "reasonable cost" and to conform to an annual audit.

The responsibility rests with the provider to develop an accounting system that will show the reasonable cost. Medicare, however, strongly believes that only an accrual accounting system which will show departmental costs is needed. In addition, it is the responsibility of the nursing home to collect the deductible from the patient or to apply for co-insurance.

Reasonable Cost As Basis for Reimbursement

The principle of reasonable cost originated with the Blue Cross-Blue Shield Insurance Association, a nationally known hospital-medical insurance firm that grew from the idea of group insurance to spread the risk over prepaid groups. Employees of Baylor Hospital, Dallas, Texas, were the first to be covered. Reasonable cost was adopted by Congress for the reimbursement of Medicare. The idea is advanced that *the fair and average cost of a service or medical need within a locale is the allowable reasonable charge.*

To discover the actual cost, no more and no less, requires accurate accounting, such as the uniform accounting of all homes within a locale, and accrual accounting within each home. One problem of reasonable cost is determining what is reasonable for the depreciation of a facility. Another is the question of the imputed value of donated services and goods.

A number of questions may be raised in adding up the cost of giving a service. Who funds research within a home? What about nursing schools and their costs? What about bad debts? What are the differences in cost for various age patients? How do you fund an increase in working capital? What about improvements to the capital asset?

The use of reasonable cost demands a uniform application of several principles. The cost must be a true cost, no more and no less than actual cost. All true costs must be applied and they must be properly apportioned to the department or unit utilizing the service. It must be a fair apportionment. Costs must be the actual accrued cost within the period of the service; they must not be abnormal for a given locality.

There are certain costs that Medicare will not recognize. Some system of keeping these costs separately must be developed within the accounting procedure. Some costs not recognized are: personal comfort items, convenience items, noncovered level of care, non-certified care. Medicare further insists that the nursing home care be for the same illness for which the patient was admitted to the hospital, or for an illness contracted during confinement.

There are certain other excluded services for which Medicare will not pay, such as when the provider fails to supply information to substantiate its charges or when the service was not incurred during a patient's coverage period. The administrator may consult the *Social Security Handbook* or go to the local office of the Social Security Administration for further information.

Depreciation and Imputed Interest

The nursing home is allowed to recover its capital investment at a depreciated rate under the provision of Medicare. Normally, depreciation is computed by one of three methods: straight-line method, the sum-of-the-digits method, and the double-declining-balance method.

Many businessmen use depreciation as a customary operational expense and do not fund it for future replacement of the capital investment. They argue that it is an expense of doing business and that the theoretical funding is the same as the mortgage principal payment. On the other hand, some businessmen consider the capital asset as the "untouchable" of business. They fund their depreciation in order to replace equipment or facilities. It should be pointed out that with inflation soaring higher each year, an asset will not be fully funded at the end of its expected life. Also, at accelerated depreciation, one will have some advantage over straight-line depreciation funding.

When the depreciation is funded, it is contended, capital is not available for operation, nor will it be, theoretically, available for other capital needs. The businessman who does not fund depreciation will usually argue that capital used as operational capital is more productive for profits than that invested in capital funds for depreciation. He will also maintain that replacement is almost always more complex, owing to advancement in technology. Thus a piece of equipment, when it is to be replaced, will always cost more. On the other hand, when income is considered, it will be distorted when a fund for depreciation is not set aside. The businessman may also be encouraged into overexpansion because of an apparent abundance of cash.

The question of imputed interest caused considerable discussion when the Medicare program was in its infancy. The question came about because of the apparent differences between the nonprofit organization and the proprietary institution. The question concerns the imputed interest in the capital investment and a reasonable reimbursement for benefits that may be derived by the Medicare patient from its use. The government contends that many hospitals have been financed by Hill-Burton funds and philanthropic gifts which do not merit reimbursement. The administrator holds, however, that depreciation is the method of replacing depleted capital assets and should be reimbursed.

The Reimbursement Procedure

The administrator should have no difficulty establishing a reimbursement procedure with Medicare. Their method is two-fold: the extended care billing, and the adjusted annual audit. The implications, however, are serious when the procedure is abused, making it imperative that the administrator adhere rigidly to the true-cost principle.

There are two methods of interim reimbursement which work well with the nursing home accounting system. The extended care facility will choose one and develop a good accounting system to ascertain the interim charge.

The *average-daily-cost method* uses the principle that the extended care facility accounting methods can adequately establish the true cost of patient care, which may be reduced to an average daily cost. The billing for interim reimbursement will then be for each patient-day, less deductibles.

The *percentage-of-charge method* is sometimes used. In this, the administrator will assume a percentage, perhaps 80% to 90% of the customary charge, and then bill for reimbursement, less deductibles, of course. In both cases, it is understood that this is merely a formula for interim finances only. The actual amount of reimbursement will be determined and adjusted at the annual audit.

It should be pointed out that precise methods of accounting will be required to substantiate the amount of reimbursement. The actual billing procedure for interim reimbursement will be made each 30 days. The appropriate form is so designed that it serves as the basis for admission:

> *Identifying information* to be provided: Name, address, hospital insurance number, physician, provider, provider number, co-insurance information, the signature of patient and/or representative, admitting diagnosis, surgical, and current diagnosis.
>
> *Statement of services:* Itemize services rendered, charges for accommodations, and ancillary charges.
>
> *Period of services rendered:* dates of services, date of guarantee, date of utilization review, date active care ended, date benefits exhausted.
>
> *Physician's certification:* Must be signed and on file.

The Annual Audit

The annual audit will document and give an impartial accounting of the actual cost of patient care. It will serve as the Medicare basis for making the final reimbursement for services rendered for the year less the interim reimbursement taken. It could mean that the extended care facility will receive additional payment, or it could mean refunding to Medicare for overpayment.

There are customarily two bases for accounting: cash accounting and accrual accounting. While cash accounting is widely used, Medicare expects the skilled nursing facility providing extended care benefits to convert to accrual accounting. At the beginning of the program, the cash basis was acceptable. Now it is not, and a method of departmental allocating of costs is necessary.

The annual audit will require specific information for which established methods of verification will be required. The participating facility will be automatically sent a set of audit forms and given 90 days to complete and submit them. Failure to submit them may be the basis for denial of payment or the assessment of a 2% penalty. The above submission is subject to spot-checking by Medicare auditors who make a random audit and verification of items submitted. In some extreme cases, a full verification of transactions will be made.

The impact of the annual audit is obvious. It will prove up the accounting system or it will bring some difficulty and perhaps embarrassment. Some considerations of interest to the administrator are listed below.

Denial of a portion of interim financing may be made when expenditures are rejected as applying to the true cost of providing care.

Substantial payment may be made at the end of the year in cases where adequate records have been kept and interim reimbursement was set low.

A professional accountant will be needed to supervise the submission of the final audit forms. He should be secured at the beginning of the contract in order that he can recommend accounting procedures to meet the new demands for departmental allocation of expenditures.

The true cost of doing business will be given the administrator. He may choose to make some adjustments in his charges.

Utilization Review and Patient Termination

When Congress established the Medicare program, it was concerned that the facilities should provide the level of care needed by the patient and that this care be rendered by means of certain specific services. It was recognized that a method of reviewing the utilization of essential medical facilities and health care personnel was necessary. Thus, a utilization review committee is established by the skilled nursing facility as a provision of participation in Medicare. This requirement now covers the Medicaid skilled nursing facility.

Utilization review, of course, has a direct effect on the financing of patient care. It may abruptly terminate the reimbursement of cost on behalf of the patient who is no longer certified as needing skilled nursing care. When the skilled nursing facility is found to be not fully accredited to qualify for assurance of payments, this has been deemed retroactive, requiring reimbursement to Medicare. In such cases, the administrator then bills the patient. Because of these rigid requirements and the likelihood of imposing undue financial burden on the patient, he should review his patient care practices to ensure that he is providing only the skilled nursing care which is required under his Medicare contract.

When utilization review terminates reimbursement of cost, the administrator will need to have made an agreement with the patient or his representative for alternative financing. It is well that an agreement be made to this effect at the time of admission. The home may also face a reduction in reimbursement when a dual agreement with the state assistance program is held by the home and a patient no longer eligible for Medicare becomes a recipient of Medicaid.

The utilization review plan is a basic requirement of each skilled nursing facility and hospital; each establishes its own unique plan within the guidelines established by the conditions for participation in Medicare. Each patient is to be reviewed periodically once they become a long-term case. Short-term cases are reviewed on a sample basis. The review will determine the quality of care, professional services included, the effective utilization of services, and the medical necessity for continuing skilled nursing care.

The requirement for certification includes the initial certification by the physician, which must be on file for the period for which reimbursement is claimed, a recertification by the 12th day and recurrent reviews, not to exceed one in each 30 days.

In order to maintain good financial management of the nursing home, all admissions must be deemed fully proper and necessary and therefore eligible for Medicare payment, and there must be an agreement by the patient arranging for other means of support—such as personal responsibility, co-insurance, or Medicaid—in case of a termination of Medicare coverage.

Assurance of payment may be assumed in all cases until disapproved. However, to be eligible for assurance of payment, the skilled nursing facility must: be fully accredited to participate in the Medicare program, must actively evaluate cases, and have a functioning utilization review team. Recent changes in evaluation procedures require the submission of criteria in the form of a medical information summary. The information required includes: diagnosis, primary and secondary, hospital diagnosis, the specific degree of the patient's physical limitations, the physical therapy required, medications, physician's orders, and the skilled nursing care required.

Chapter 28

Comparative and Analytical

Cost Finding

Methods of Cost Accounting

Cost accounting is determining unit costs for purposes of distribution and control. Nursing home costs may be best controlled when they are properly allocated to the cost units through proper accounting methods.

Allocation of costs depends on fully determining the expenses of providing a particular service. There are administrative costs to be divided among all services. The question of how much depreciation is allocated or how much of the overhead should be allocated, as well as other indirect costs, is the basic problem of cost accounting.

Job-accounting, as for example, figuring the cost of making an x-ray, or providing a meal, is one method. *Process accounting* is sometimes used, which may also include the cost of board per month, or laundry service. Other methods include *cost units or centers,* the use of *percentage of costs,* or simply the *average cost* over a period of time. In the nursing home, the primary cost accounting method is computing *cost per patient-day.*

For true cost accounting, there are several requirements. The administrator adopts a base period in which costs will be compared; this may be a month, a quarter, a day, or a year. Secondly, accounting is then done regularly to establish the base cost and to establish the trends in cost.

349

The adoption of a basic unit is required. It may be per patient, per item, or per service. It may be a combination of more than one unit. One may choose to account for ancillary services per item or per service. Thus, the billing may read "nursing service," at a certain price, and "extra charges," at a charge per service.

Once the units are established, allocating costs is made according to comparable units. Thus, nursing services will be allocated a percentage of the administrative cost, a percentage of the depreciation, etc. The decision as to what percentage to use will be a matter of determining a fair allocation of the use for that service. To illustrate, a 10,000 square-foot building may have 4000 square feet in bedrooms, 1000 square feet in the dining room and kitchen, 250 square feet in a therapy room, and the remainder in service and recreation areas. Using such figures, the accountant could reasonably allocate costs for depreciation to each of these units on a percentage basis.

Cost as Related to Patient-Day

The use of the cost of providing services on a daily basis is valuable to the administrator for several reasons. It may indicate efficiency when the determination is made periodically. The administrator certainly needs this information to establish his charges. Medicare will expect an interim financing charge based on related patient-day costs. The administrator will find that the periodically computed patient-day costs are effective indicators of trends in the business. Finally, knowing the patient-day cost helps him determine his profits.

In determining the cost per patient-day, the administrator first establishes a procedure for accounting for all costs. He should select an accounting period that can produce an average cost. The period must not be so long as to fail to average certain types of expenses; for example, the second quarter of the year fails to reflect the same high utility cost as the winter quarter; thus a truer average could be noted between costs of the two accounting periods. Also, variations in occupancy may cause a variation of cost because of the allocation of fixed expenses. Normally, a financial period is adopted for cost accounting.

Because the occupancy of the home will cause some variation in the per-day cost, it is essential that the administrator spread his cost over as broad a base as possible. However, with high inflation, too broad a base is not always recommended. One may use either the average occupancy of the accounting period or the occupied bed-days.

The method of determining occupancy may be by a percentage of the total number of beds, e.g., 80% for January, 90% for February, and 100% for March, for an average of 90% for the quarter. However, this is not absolutely accurate because of the variation in the days of the month. The administrator may prefer to count the actual days and thus obtain an absolutely accurate figure, e.g., January 1, 50 patients; January 2, 49 patients; January 3, 51 patients, etc.

Another factor concerning the number of patient-days is the fact that the nursing home may care for more than one level-of-care, i.e., both skilled and custodial patients. In this case, the accounting will be for those costs specific to each type of care and the occupancy counted accordingly.

The determination of the cost per patient-day can best be shown by this example:

Total costs for the month:	$28,440.00
Total occupied bed-days for month:	2,370.00

Then: $\dfrac{\$28,440.}{2,370} = \$12.00$ per patient-day

The administrator should set up his accounting procedures to supply this information periodically. It is possible to refine the information even further to reveal costs in certain areas. For example, the administrator could substitute any specific cost, such as food, utilities, supplies, etc., in place of a total cost. The result would be the cost per patient-day for the specific item.

Cost as Related to Departmentalization

The administrator will need more specific costs than the total cost per patient-day. He may wish to group certain specific costs on a departmental basis. All direct and indirect costs should be allocated by department before he can efficiently measure the true cost for each working unit. Suppose the administrator wished an apportionment of the cost of the wages of the dietary department. He would compile his costs thus:

Salaries:
    Dietitian
    Food service manager
    Cooks, helpers

Administrative, allocated at 21%
Maintenance and janitorial, allocated at 25%
Total dietary wage cost

With such information, the cost of wages per patient-meal could be computed. All that would be necessary is to select the base period, accumulate the costs as indicated, and count the meals served during the period. Thus all costs divided by the number of meals yields the cost of wages per patient-meal.

To keep the account of costs of a department more nearly shows the administrator the true cost of each unit of work. He may find it necessary to initiate efficiency measures to improve the financial return of certain units. Because he knows which units are not productive in relation to costs, he can more easily set up control measures. Each department cost may be established as it relates to the total cost. In this manner, the administrator may establish, over a period of time, what he considers to be a reasonable cost for each unit.

It is also possible to compute the cost of improvement by entering the anticipated cost into the formula. He may start with an estimated increase in cost to the individual patient, e.g., supplying each patient with a specific item daily at a known cost. Thus this may be added into the total monthly cost for a particular cost center.

Before cost-finding data can be effectively utilized, a systematic system of recording and accounting will need to be established. It can then be analyzed periodically for trends in the business costs.

Chapter *29*

Purchasing, Inventory Control, and Budgeting

Methods of Controlling Purchases

There is perhaps a greater need for controlling the purchases of nursing home supplies and goods than for any other measure of management efficiency. Because of the illusive nature of purchasing, its ability to deceive, the lag in accounting and the close relationship to solvency in business, the administrator will need to institute means of control. Essentially, control measures require a standard, a system of feedback of information for comparison, and corrective action. Thus, to control purchasing will maintain a balance in the operational expense, ensure proper accounting, and aid in budgeting for future needs.

The elements of a control system include: requisition of purchase, placement of orders, delivery, invoicing, payment, and accounting for money used. A purchase order system comprises a method of receiving requests or requisitions for purchases, approval by an authorized person, the issuance of a purchase order, and the placement of the order with the vendor.

Authority to place orders is given to a purchasing agent, who also has to approve purchase orders. Some nursing homes may choose to place the purchasing agent under bond. Normally, the department supervisors will only requisition supplies from stock that has been purchased. The administrator will also reserve the right to make purchases, but he should coordinate them with those of his purchasing agent.

The third part of the system is a central place for receiving deliveries of purchases. This may be a single department or the responsibility of one person. Several functions are performed by the receiving department, including

Receiving deliveries
Checking deliveries against invoices
Checking deliveries against purchase orders
Signing for deliveries on bill of lading (delivery ticket)
Returning unordered goods
Noting shortages
Noting damages on invoice and bill of lading
Storing goods until distributed
Notifying proper department of arrival
Certifying receipt to accounting department

The final step in the system is payment for goods. When the invoice and purchase order have been checked against delivery, and it is ascertained that they were ordered and that they arrived in good condition, the receiving agent authorizes payment.

Methods of Controlling Inventory

The administrator needs to control the size of the inventory of materials and supplies for several reasons. He will wish to limit the size to an efficient level in order to ensure enough supplies to meet demand, but not to waste purchasing power by an oversupply. Too little an inventory means waste of time, poor service, and perhaps danger to the patient. Too large an inventory means too much space in storage, too much capital in inventory, and an additional tax burden at the end of the year. The control method gives the administrator a check on the availability of supplies, serves as a system of accounting, and helps to guard against loss. There are two methods of inventory control: a periodic count and a perpetual inventory balance.

Smaller businesses generally use a periodic inventory. The count of all items in supply may be taken monthly, quarterly, and yearly. For accounting purposes the taking of the inventory will usually coincide with the accounting period. An inventory should be taken at the beginning and at the end of the accounting period. Thus, when one considers the number of a particular item purchased during a particular period, it is possible to determine the cost vs. usage of the item. Note the following:

Beginning inventory
Add purchases made during accounting period
Subtract ending inventory
Remainder is total used during accounting period

The beginning and ending inventories will also give an accurate check on the increase or decrease of the capital account.

For purchasing purposes, a system of storage of supplies that will readily indicate the inventory will be needed. Some items like fixtures and furnishings may need an identification system.

The perpetual inventory has all the elements of the periodic inventory, except that a separate record is kept for each item. It is updated at the time of the use of any item. It is absolutely necessary that supplies be checked in and out systematically, and that the records be constantly updated. This method works best with data processing; however, even the smallest nursing home may utilize it effectively.

Certain additional controls of inventory include secure storage rooms, a periodic check of supplies, supervision of the use of supplies, and adequate maintenance.

Control as Related to Departmentalization

The administrator will perhaps have the most problems with inventory and purchasing control because of departmentalization. The responsibility for supplies is a matter of assignment and supervision. The administrator should assign to a person within each department the responsibility for making requisitions, for receiving supplies, and accounting for their use.

Supervision of the inventory when a departmental distribution system is used functions along the same lines as the central system. A purchasing agent authorizes and makes purchases when they are requisitioned by the heads of departments. The distribution system extends from central receiving and holding to departmental receiving and storage. Each department is then organized to distribute supplies. For example, the dietary department has storage for food staples, perishables, frozen foods, liquids, etc. These are distributed daily, of course, by an authorized person who will requisition replacements and be responsible for accounting for supplies on hand.

Some supplies lend themselves to distribution through a central supply. Normally, medical supplies, furnishings, bedrails, wheelchairs, or emergency equipment can be handled centrally. Again, receiving, stocking, and distribution can be systematized by assigning responsibility: each department will assign one person to requisition and receive supplies. When multiple storerooms are used, there is the same routine of requisition and receiving, but the matter of distribution is more difficult to control. Stocking, maintenance, and security are harder to control, and distribution is more difficult to supervise.

Several problems related to departmental control arise. Correlation of purchasing is difficult, since a delay in ordering, either by the purchasing agent or the one making the requisition, means that the order does not go out in time to secure delivery, and therefore may make it necessary to maintain a large inventory. A system, such as setting a minimum number or amount to be kept on hand, will facilitate the necessary lead time for ordering. Lead time is calculated to include: time to make the requisition, time to approve a purchase order, time to place the order, time to take delivery, time to restock storerooms, and an estimated time to allow for a margin of safety. The safety margin will consider errors in ordering, problems of prompt delivery, delivery of damaged goods, the working hours of the receiving personnel, and the critical nature of the item being ordered. Once the amount of lead time is known, and cost accounting has determined normal usage, it is a simple matter to calculate the minimum to be kept on hand.

Some difficulty may arise from distribution, methods of transport, prompt storage, proper receiving, loss or damage while awaiting storage, etc. However, without the proper feedback of control data, it may be difficult to reduce to a minimum the misuse or loss of supplies In fact, pilfering by employees may occur over a period of years without a supervisor's suspecting theft. Inventory control may eliminate it.

Budgeting Objectives

Budgeting makes use of past experience to forecast future expenditures. Since one would also forecast expected revenue, he will utilize a budget to see that his costs stay within his expected income.

There are a number of budget objectives. The administrator will wish to forecast future business operations. Using experiential data accumulated through good accounting procedures, the administrator is able to forecast his expected expenses and to anticipate income and thus determine his expected profit.

Anticipated expansion may be included in the budget objectives. By controlling operations and improving efficiency according to budget objectives, the administrator may work for an expansion program.

Anticipated changes in operation may be predicted from studies of budgetary feasibility. Ultimately, budgets are guides for controlling expenses. This is done through budget coordination or budgetary restrictions. The requirements of budgeting are: to establish the budget period; to collect budgetary data; to correlate the data; and to project the data to future periods.

Assembling a budget is perhaps the most valuable function of the administrator. Ultimately, it is the administrator who is responsible to see that the mechanics of budgeting are established and adhered to. A procedure for budgeting includes the steps given below.

First, instruct the various departments to furnish requests. These will include improvements, machinery, equipment, routine supplies, and staffing needs.

Request accounting to furnish expense data from previous accounting periods. The profit and loss statement will yield the most information; however, income statements, capital accounts statements, and cost studies will be needed.

Carefully analyze such items as growth in services, income, and other needs. Consider future improvements and new expenses.

Finally, project the budget, using data collected, budget objectives, growth potential, and future needs.

The Budget Period

The selection of a budget period may seem relatively simple; yet there are problems related to establishing uniform periods of budgeting. Areas of difficulty may be noted. The length of the budget period should be established to cover all expected trends in expenses and income. There is a definite relationship with the past experience. For example, one may have had abnormal remodeling needs owing to change in the requirements of the licensing agency. To project the same remodeling costs into a future budget may be unwise, unless it can be shown that the unusual costs were absorbed by diverting regular remodeling funds to this requirement. Outdated data from a past budget period may make the information useless. For example, wages progressively increase because of minimum wage regulation or labor demands for higher wages. FICA contributions are also on a rising scale. Some data are not available and may cause some difficulty. Taxes on property are revised yearly by the various tax districts and may not be available at the time the budget is established.

The administrator may make some assumptions concerning the budget period. First, the future period should relate to the previous period. A low-occupancy period of the past may be adjusted to fit the anticipated occupancy of the future. Second, the period should be long enough to be practical. One month's experience is of little value to projecting for a year ahead. Third, it should not be so long as to restrict growth. The rigid adherence to a five-year budget would certainly be foolish. Finally, the budget period should be broken into workable units.

The most common budget is for a year, with, perhaps, some modification for each quarter. This normally corresponds to accounting periods. Accounting data are usually accumulated by months, quarters, and then by the year, making a yearly budget more or less universally accepted. It is wise to project past a year, perhaps to a fifteen or eighteen months' total, to allow for the time the budget is in preparation.

Once the budget period is decided, it should remain for a number of years or until some good reason is presented to change it. The comparison between several years will be valuable; also, personnel will begin to expect a revision on a yearly basis.

Budget Data

The administrator needs to establish routine methods of accumulating the budget data which will be coordinated with his accounting procedures and will probably be equivalent to his monthly ledger accounts. Administrators have found that accounts may be assembled in the order of the financial statement and that the budget may be assembled in the same order.

Identifying budget data is equivalent to identifying the various ledger accounts of business expense, business income, and capital expenditures. The revenue account will serve as the source for projecting future revenues. The operational accounts or business expense accounts will need to be divided into fixed expense items and variable expense items. The capital accounts may be a part of the budget, since working capital, additional investment, and future profit may be forecast.

The sources of budget data are the accumulated accounting procedures of the past accounting periods. Some data will be drawn from the full previous period, while other data may be for only a portion of the period. They are adjusted, of course, to comparative values for equal time periods.

Revenue and income data sources are from only those periods or portions of periods that reflect true past experience projected into the future. It is the norm that is to be achieved. Should the normal occupancy be 90%, it would be unwise to project the 95% occupancy that may have been enjoyed for a short period. Revenue data also need to be adjusted to take into account future growth and improvement. Such adjustment may reflect a new procedure inaugurated midway during the previous accounting period. When savings accrue for efficiency measures or changes in the operation, the adjustment will be considered in the projection. Occasionally, accounting procedures may change during a period, making it imperative that these changes be recognized as related to past data.

The capital account may have to be increased owing to increased capital needs. On the other hand, a surplus from the previous budget period may reduce budgetary needs. This may be true for reasons of anticipated stock sales, or the sale of surplus assets. Occasionally, profit taking, enlargements, remodeling, or paying off a mortgage may be considered in budgeting.

Fixed-Cost Items

There are a number of fixed-cost items in any budget that influence the preparation and projection of future needs. Because such items may dictate other budget allowances, it is well for the administrator to identify and assess their affect.

Identifying fixed-cost items is to assume that any item of expense, either capital or operational, is fixed for budgetary purposes, regardless of other needs. It may be noted that no item is absolutely fixed, because sooner or later it may vary or be paid off. Long-range items, such as mortgage payments, permanent improvements, such as buildings, real estate and/or land, and any item that may remain stable for the entire budget period may be considered as fixed costs. However, some accountants consider only capital improvements in this category. For budgeting purposes, however, it is well to differentiate between those specific items that are variable, and those that may be considered constant. Some specific items that are usually considered fixed in cost are listed here.

Depreciation, which is determined for the period and then divided into equal monthly amounts.

Insurance, which is usually by contract (normally to cover three years), may be funded monthly to cover the expected premiums.

Professional expense, such as legal retainers, licenses, dues.

Consultant fees for which contracts are issued.

Contracted services, such as termite and pest control.

Mortgage payments, which are adjusted each year, if an escrow amount is included to cover the payment of taxes and insurance.

Interest payments are considered to be constant for budgetary purposes.

Principal payments are also considered to be constant.

The administrator will soon note the effect on his budget if he is committed to paying too many fixed costs, with payment schedules set too often, and principal payments too large. *The amortization of capital improvements must be spread over the most optimum period, the pay-out soon enough to make way for more improvement, but not so soon that cash is drained from the business operation.* Learning to assess what fixed items are necessary, contracting for them wisely is a fundamental responsibility of the businessman/administrator.

Variable-Cost Items

The effect of variable-cost items on the budget is not easy to determine. The basic idea is to obtain all the data possible and then make the wisest assessment of the anticipated expenses. When the total cost is an accumulation of many different costs, it is difficult to project future expenditures.

Identifying variable-cost items is relatively simple, since costs in these categories tend to vary because of price, quantity, number, and usage. Normally, we say that when the accumulated cost of purchases within a budgeted period for specific business expense is not constant, it can only be variable. Some accountants do not make any distinction, except to say that fixed assets are nonvariable. However, this does not help the administrator to assemble his budget costs. Predicting the costs of variable-cost items may be done by one of the following methods of projection: from the price data of the vendor; from average use data; from per-unit cost times demand; or from an assumed base.

The administrator needs some specific basis for projecting costs. It is not enough to say, for example, that the nursing department spent x dollars last year. The careful analyst will determine all the specific costs, i.e., supplies, wages, etc., which when totaled equal x dollars. Such data may then be projected to reflect the anticipated usage.

Probably the most useful method of projection is the use of per patient-day costs. This permits a variety of combinations of past data. For example, if the cost of an item increased during the past period and the average use per patient is known, the formula is:

$$\text{unit cost} \times \text{number units} \times \text{time factor}.$$

Another item may be a relatively stable-use item and its entire cost may be projected with minor correction for an anticipated change in occupancy.

If the operation of a specific unit or department is relatively stable, accumulated cost totals for previous periods may be assumed as adequate. However, when the administrator has reason to believe some change is necessary in the cost data, he will analyze specified items, in order to make predictions. Other areas that present difficulty in predicting costs are repairs and maintenance, foodstuff and dietary supplies, janitorial supplies, medical supplies, utilities and telephone (long distance), and auto or transportation.

Coordinating and Communicating the Budget

The administrator will find his budget of great benefit in comparing the state of the business at given times. He will want to know whether expenses are staying within predictions, and whether the profit margin is being maintained. If either is not, he must seek to remedy the situation. His best method is to establish a way of communicating the limitations of the budget to his employees.

Coordination of the budget starts in the assembling of it. *The administrator needs to set up a system for the methodical evaluation of requests, an accurate appraisal of data, and a fair hearing of each need presented.*

Coordinating the use of the budget will ensure the equal application of it. When a proper control system is established, the administrator will have the necessary feedback of data to make a periodic comparison of the actual spending by the various departments. Measures of correction can then be applied in those areas needing restraint.

Coordination of the cost of unbudgeted items can be expedited, if the administrator makes some allowance for them in his budget. New items are accepted only afterward: evaluation as to need, effect on the budget, and effect on related departments. Friction and ill will between the personnel of the various departments may be kept to a minimum, when they are treated impartially in budget allocations.

Communicating budget information, so as to encourage the cooperation of personnel, may be accomplished in several ways. The budget may be presented with a challenge. Departmental heads should know what they have to spend; they usually can be counted upon to improve efficiency and increase productivity, when they receive a fair budget to meet the needs of their several departments.

The administrator may publish the budget in order to notify personnel and coordinate efforts. Certainly, the budget should be reviewed at intervals within the budget period. Accounting can supply the necessary data. Such information can be used at staff meetings, in private, or as published.

In formulating cost control and budget data, the administrator may wish to correlate projections with his profit and loss statement. By first counting the occupancy for each period of the profit and loss statement, he can resolve each budget item to per patient-day cost, monthly total, or yearly grand total. He should take care that specific levels of care are counted and compared with only related accounts applicable.

First, count the bed-days; this should be a regular part of the accounting system. Counting the patients each day can be accomplished thus:

Patient count for the month of:_____

Day:	Personal care:	Intermediate care:	Skilled care:	Daily total
1	_____	_____	_____	_____
2	_____	_____	_____	_____
3rd through 31st day				
Totals:	_____	_____	_____	_____

By accomplishing this census count daily and accumulating monthly, the necessary data is available for budget projections.

The second step is to formulate a regular summary of the monthly accounts in such a fashion that budget analysis can be accomplished easily. Not only can you summarize expenses for the given month, but by using the census information you can also calculate cost per patient-day for each account. An appropriate form could be developed like the one included here as the Summary of Accounts.

SUMMARY OF ACCOUNTS.

Type of expense	Patient-day	Monthly total	Yearly total
Administrative	_____	_____	_____
*Utilization review	_____	_____	_____
Maintenance	_____	_____	_____
*Skilled services	_____	_____	_____
*Intermediate services	_____	_____	_____
*Custodial services	_____	_____	_____
Dietary expense	_____	_____	_____
Housekeeping expense	_____	_____	_____
Laundry expense	_____	_____	_____
Consultants	_____	_____	_____
Recreational expense	_____	_____	_____
Restorative expense	_____	_____	_____
TOTAL EXPENSES	_____	_____	_____

The administrator will use the data in the Summary of Accounts to project the budget. In this case, he will need to make some adjustment for anticipated changes in occupancy. Thus he can multiply the per patient-day cost by anticipated daily occupancy and by 30 to get the monthly budget total, or by 365 to get the yearly budget total.

Income may be dealt with in the same manner. By substituting income for expense in the form, we may project income data as in the form for Summary of Income Data.

SUMMARY OF INCOME DATA

Type of income	Patient Day	Monthly total	Yearly total
Skilled nursing care:	_____	_____	_____
Intermediate care:	_____	_____	_____
Personal care:	_____	_____	_____
Ancillary:	_____	_____	_____
TOTAL INCOME	_____	_____	_____

Using this form and accurate census information, and inserting previous patient-day costs, monthly totals, or yearly totals, you can calculate the remaining columns. Thus, if you received accounting data concerning monthly income or expenditures for a specific count, you could calculate the per patient-day cost and project the information into the future budget period by calculating the anticipated yearly total. It is also possible for accounting data to be cumulative, that is, the

*These items are compared with specific occupancies. All others may be considered community services, computed with the total occupancy, unless the administrator is charged with keeping separate books on each distinct service offered.

yearly total accumulated from the beginning of the budget period to the date of the report. Another variation is to replace the yearly total with the actual budget allowances changed to patient-day cost. This way, you can compare the patient-day cost with the budgeted cost.

Anticipated Enlargement of the Facility

Frequently, the administrator is called upon to compile data to substantiate an anticipated building program. The Summary of Income Data form should be completed, especially the income and expense items resolved to per patient-day costs. Then using this data with the anticipated occupancy of the new facility, a projection of income and expense may be completed (see the sample form headed "Projection of Income and Expense"). This information, when compared with the payout of the anticipated debt computed at the anticipated rate of interest for the expected time, will reveal whether it is practical to undertake the enlargement program. One may compute a number of probable debt-retirement plans before finding which will be satisfactory with the anticipated net-before-debt retirement. You may need to decide whether you should include depreciation in the costs or leave it out to show a larger net.

PROJECTION OF INCOME AND EXPENSE
Projection of income:

No.: Type of beds:	Patient-day:	Total daily:	Total monthly:	Total yearly:
_____Skilled	× $ _____	= $ _____	× 30 = $ _____	× 12 = $ _____
_____Intermediate	_____	_____	_____	_____
_____Custodial	_____	_____	_____	_____
Total income @ 100% occupancy:	_____	_____	_____	
@ 80% occupancy:	_____	_____	_____	
@ 60% occupancy:	_____	_____	_____	

Projection of costs:

_____Skilled	_____	_____	_____	_____
_____Intermediate	_____	_____	_____	_____
_____Custodial	_____	_____	_____	_____
Total costs @ 100% occupancy:	_____	_____	_____	
@ 80% occupancy:	_____	_____	_____	
@ 60% occupancy:	_____	_____	_____	

Anticipated net before debt retirement: (income less cost)

Net profit @ 100% occupancy:	_____	_____	_____	
@ 80% occupancy:	_____	_____	_____	
@ 60% occupancy:	_____	_____	_____	

For Further Study

Selected Readings in Financial Management of the Nursing Home

Meyers, Robert J./ McCahan Foundation (Bryn Mawr, Penna.), *Medicare.* Homewood, Ill.: Richard D. Irwin, Inc., 1970.

Myer, John N., *What the Executive Should Know About the Accountant's Statements.* American Research Council, Inc., 1964.

Pyle, William W., and White, John Arch, *Fundamental Accounting Principles.* Homewood, Ill.: Richard D. Irwin, Inc., 1968.

Social Security Handbook. Washington, D.C.: U.S. Department of Health, Education, and Welfare.

Appendix: Official Terminology

The American College of Nursing Home Administrators has adopted the following definition to be used as "a base line from which to work with some degree of uniformity." These definitions are also recommended by the American Nursing Home Association. (Used by permission.)

A NURSING HOME or its equivalent is a facility, institution, or an identifiable unit of an acute hospital or other care facility licensed for:

1. Care for persons who because of physical or mental conditions, or both, require or desire living accommodations and care which as a practical matter can best be made available to them through institutional facilities, or other acute care units of hospitals, providing a protective and/or supervised environment, and

2. Care of persons and patients who require a combination of health care services and personal care services which are in addition to the above and may include, but are not necessarily restricted to, one or more of the following care services:
   a. Therapeutic diets.
   b. Regular observations of patient's physical and mental condition.
   c. Personal assistance including bathing, dressing, grooming, ambulation, transportation, housekeeping (such as bedmaking, dusting, etc.) of living quarters.
   d. A program of social and recreational activities.
   e. Assistance with self-administered medications.
   f. Emergency-medical care including bedside nursing during temporary periods of illness.

g. Professional nursing supervision.
h. Skilled nursing care.
i. Medical care and services by a licensed practitioner.
j. Other special medical and social care services for diagnostic and treatment purposes of rehabilitative, restorative, or maintenance nature, designed to restore and/or maintain the person in the most normal physical and social condition attainable.

A NURSING HOME ADMINISTRATOR means any individual who by training and experience is qualified to assume the responsibility for planning, organizing, directing, and/or controlling the operation of a nursing home or its equivalent.

The PRACTICE OF NURSING HOME ADMINISTRATION means the performance of any act or the making of any decision involved in the planning, organizing, directing, and/or control of the operation of a nursing home or its equivalent.

Bibliography

Recommended books, journals, and selected association and government agencies to be used as references for the Associate of Applied Science Degree in Long Term Health Care. Prepared by the Program Director for Nursing Home Administration, McLennan Community College, Waco, Texas 76708.

Books

American Hospital Association. *Food Service Manual.* Chicago: American Hospital Association.

American Medical Records Association. *Organizing Health Records.* Chicago: American Medical Records Association.

American Safety Council. *Safety Guide for Health Care Institutions.* Chicago: American Safety Council.

Anderson, Ronald A., and Kumpf, Walter A. *Business Law.* Cincinnati: South-Western Publishing Co., 1972.

Anthony, Catherine Parker. *Structure and Function of the Body.* 4th ed. St. Louis: C. V. Mosby Co., 1972.

Bainum, Robert. *Getting Approved for Medicare: A Guide for Nursing Homes.* Silver Springs, Md.: Cathry Cash, Agent , 1966.

Berlo, David K. *The Process of Communication.* New York: Holt, Rinehart and Winston, Inc., 1960.

Bonner, Hubert. *Group Dynamics.* New York: The Ronald Press, 1959.

Bredow, Miriam. *Medical Secretarial Procedures.* 5th ed. New York: McGraw-Hill, 1959.

Brown, Forest. *Social Work Training Manual for Nursing Home Personnel.* Oklahoma City: State Department of Health.

Bryant, Donald C., and Wallace, Karl R. *Oral Communication.* New York: Appleton-Century-Crofts, Inc., 1954.

Chruden, Herbert J., and Sherman, Arthur W. *Personnel Management.* 4th ed. Cincinnati: South-Western Publishing Co., 1972.

Cloyd, Frances. *Guide to Food Service Management.* Boston: Cahners Books, 1972.

Cole, Jonathan O., and Wittenborn, J. R. *Drug Abuse: Social and Psychopharmacological Aspects.* Springfield, Ill.: Charles C. Thomas, 1969.

Committee, T. C. *Managerial Finance for the Seventies.* New York: McGraw-Hill, 1972.

Crooks, Lois A. *Long Term Care Facility Administration.* Washington, D.C.: U.S. Department of Health, Education & Welfare; HE 20:2558:L86.

Dean, W. B., et al. *Basic Concepts of Anatomy and Physiology.* 3rd ed. Philadelphia: J. B. Lippincott Co., 1966.

Department of Health, Education, and Welfare. *Working with Older People.* Washington, D.C.: Government Printing Office.

Diamond, Jay, and Pintel, Gerald. *Mathematics of Business.* Englewood Cliffs, N.J.: Prentice-Hall, Inc., 1970.

Downs, James C. *Principles of Real Estate Management.* Chicago: Institute of Real Estate Management, 1970.

Drucker, Peter F. *The Practice of Management.* New York: Harper & Row, 1954.

Feingold, Carl. *Introduction to Data Processing.* Dubuque, Iowa: Wm. C. Brown Co., Publishers, 1971.

Felice, Joseph P., and Carolan, Patrick J. *Tune in to Health.* New York: Standard Publishing Co., 1973.

Field, Minna. *Aging with Honor and Dignity.* Springfield, Illinois: Charles C. Thomas, 1968.

Finney, Harry A., and Miller, Herbert E. *Principles of Accounting: Intermediate.* Englewood Cliffs, N.J.: Prentice-Hall, Inc., 1965.

Fish, Harriet U. *Activities Program for Senior Citizens.* West Nyack, N.Y.: Parker Publishing Co., Inc., 1971.

Frobisher, Martin. *Microbiology in Health and Disease.* 13th ed. Philadelphia: W. B. Saunders Company, 1973.

Gruner, Charles R., et al. *Speech Communication in Society.* Boston: Allyn & Bacon, Inc., 1972.

Hall, Edward T. *The Silent Language.* Garden City, N.Y.: Doubleday, 1973.

Heckman, I. L., and Huneryager, S. G. *Human Relations in Management.* 2nd ed. Cincinnati: South-Western Publishing Co., 1967.

Hoagland, Henry E. *Real Estate Finance.* 5th ed. Homewood, Ill.: Richard D. Irwin, Inc., 1973.

Hoffman, Adeline M. *The Daily Needs and Interests of Older People.* Springfield, Ill.: Charles C. Thomas, 1970.

Hospital Research and Educational Trust. *Being a Nursing Aide.* Chicago: Hospital Research and Educational Trust.

Hospital Research and Educational Trust. *Being a Ward Clerk.* Chicago: Hospital Research and Educational Trust.

Howe, Phyllis Sullivan. *Basic Nutrition in Health and Disease.* 5th ed. Philadelphia: W. B. Saunders Co., 1971.

Huffman, Edna K. *Medical Records Management.* Berwyn, Ill.: Physicians Record Company, 1961.

Huffman, Edna K. *Medical Records Management.* 6th ed. Berwyn, Ill.: Physicians Record Company, 1972.

Jacobs, H. Lee, and Morris, Woodrow W. *Nursing and Retirement Home Administration.* Ames, Iowa: The Iowa State University Press, 1967.

Johnston, Dorothy F. *Medical Surgical Nursing: Workbook for Practical Nurses.* 3rd ed. St. Louis: C. V. Mosby Company, 1972.

Johnston, Dorothy F. *Total Patient Care.* 3rd ed. St. Louis: C. V. Mosby Company, 1972.

Joint Commission on Accreditation of Hospitals and Nursing Homes. *Standards for Accreditation of Extended Care Facilities.* Chicago: Joint Commission, 1966.

Kazmier, Leonard J. *Principles of Management.* New York: McGraw-Hill, 1974.

Kotschevar, Lendal. *Food Service for the Extended Care Facility.* Boston: Cahners Books, 1973.

Krech, David, and Crutchfield, Richard S. *Elements of Psychology.* 2nd ed. New York: Alfred A. Knopf, 1969.

Kutscher, Austin H. *Death and Bereavement.* Springfield, Ill.: Charles C. Thomas.

Laird, Donald A., and Laird, Eleanor. *Psychology, Human Relations and Motivation.* 4th ed. New York: McGraw-Hill Book Co., 1967.

Levey, Samuel, and Loomba, N. Paul. *Health Care Administration: A Managerial Perspective.* Philadelphia: J. B. Lippincott Company, 1973.

McCarthy, E. Jerome. *Basic Marketing.* 4th ed. Homewood, Ill.: Richard D. Irwin, Inc., 1971.

McQuillan, Florence L. *Fundamentals of Nursing Home Administration.* 2nd ed. Philadelphia: W. B. Saunders Co., 1974.

Manfreds, Marguerite Lucy. *Psychiatric Nursing.* 9th ed. Philadelphia: F. A. Davis Co., 1973.

Massie, Joseph L. *Essentials of Management.* 2nd ed. Englewood Cliffs, N.J.: Prentice-Hall, Inc., 1970.

Mauser, Ferdinand F., and Schwartz, David J. *American Business.* 3rd ed. New York: Harcourt Brace Jovanovich, 1974.

Mayakawa, S. I. *Use and Misuse of Language.* Greenwich, Conn.: Fawcett Publications, Inc., 1973.

Mayo Clinic Committee on Dietetics. *Mayo Clinic Diet Manual.* Philadelphia, Pa.: W. B. Saunders Co., 1971.

Medical Economics, Inc. *Physicians' Desk Reference.* Oradell, N.J.: Medical Economics, Inc.

Meldman, Monte J., et al. *Occupational Therapy Manual.* Springfield, Ill.: Charles C. Thomas, 1969.

Memmler, Ruth Lundeen. *Human Body in Health and Disease.* 3rd ed. Philadelphia: J. B. Lippincott Co., 1970.

Merrill, Toni. *Activities for the Aged and Infirm.* Springfield, Ill.: Charles C. Thomas, 1972.

Merton, Robert K., and Nisbet, Robert. *Contemporary Social Problems.* 3rd ed. New York: Harcourt Brace Jovanovich, 1973.

Miller, Benjam F., and Keane, Claire Brachen. *Encyclopedia and Dictionary of Medicine and Nursing.* Philadelphia: W. B. Saunders Co., 1972.

Miller, Dulcy B. *Extended Care Facility: A Guide to Organization and Operation.* New York: McGraw-Hill Book Co., 1969.

Musselman, Vernon A., and Hughes, Eugene H. *Introduction to Modern Business.* 6th ed. Englewood Cliffs, N.J.: Prentice-Hall, Inc., 1973.

Myer, John N. *Understanding Financial Statements.* New York: The New American Library, 1968.

Myers, Robert J. *Medicare.* Bryn Mawr, Pa.: McCahan Foundation, 1970.

National Fire Protection Association. *Life Safety Code.* 21st ed. Boston: National Fire Protection Association, 1967.

Naylor, Harriet H. *Volunteers Today.* New York: Association Press, 1967.

New York Times. *Social Profile: USA Today.* New York: Van Nostrand Reinhold Co., 1970.

Niswonger, C. Rollin. *Accounting Principles.* 11th ed. Cincinnati: South-Western Publishing Co., 1973.

Odiorno, George S. *Management by Objectives.* New York: Pitman Publishing Corp., 1970.

Ohio Trade and Industrial Education Service. *Nursing Procedures for* the *Practical Nurse.* Columbus: Ohio Trade and Industrial Education Service, 1972.

Pinkert, Michael S. *The Ready Foods System for Health Care Facilities.* Boston: Cahners Books, 1973.

Popenoe, David. *Sociology.* New York: Appleton-Century Crofts, 1974.

Public Health Service. *A Guide to Nutrition and Food Service for Nursing Homes and Homes for the Aged.* FSA2.6/2/N95. Washington, D.C.: Government Printing Office, 1971.

Pyle, William W. and White, John Arch. *Fundamental Accounting Principles.* 6th ed. Homewood, Ill.: Richard D. Irwin, Inc., 1972.

Rilh, Thomas A., and Gilmore, Alden S. *Basic Concepts of Aging.* Washington, D.C.: Government Printing Office.

Ring, Alfred A. *Real Estate Principles and Practices.* 7th ed. Englewood Cliffs, N.J.: Prentice-Hall, Inc., 1972.

Rogers, Wesley W. *A Teaching Plan and Outline for General Administration in the Nursing Home.* 2nd ed. Austin, Texas: National Association of Boards of Examiners for Nursing Home Administrators, 1974.

Rogers, Wesley W. *Testing and Review for the NAB Exam.* 2nd Ed. Austin, Texas: National Association of Boards of Examiners for Nursing Home Administrators, 1973.

Root, Kathleen Berger. *The Medical Secretary: Terminology and Transcription.* 3rd ed. New York: McGraw-Hill Book Co., 1972.

Ross, Carmen F. *Personal and Vocational Relationships in Practical Nursing.* 3rd ed. Philadelphia: J. B. Lippincott, 1969.

Routh, Thomas A. *Choosing a Nursing Home.* Springfield, Ill.: Charles C. Thomas, 1970.

Rudd, Jacob L., and Margolin, Reuben J. *Maintenance Therapy for the Geriatric Patient.* Springfield, Ill.: Charles C. Thomas, 1968.

Saxton, Lloyd. *The Individual, Marriage, and the Family.* 2nd ed. Belmont, Calif.: Wadsworth Publishing Co., 1972.

Shafer, Kathleen, et al. *Medical Surgical Nursing.* 5th ed. St. Louis: C. V. Mosby Co., 1971.

Shapiro, David S. *The Mental Health Counselor in the Community.* 2nd ed. Springfield, Ill.: Charles C. Thomas, 1968.

Shrope, Wayne Austin. *Speaking and Listening.* New York: Harcourt, Brace, and World, Inc., 1970.

Smith, Huston. *The Religions of Man.* New York: Harper, Colophon Books, 1958.

Smith, Nila Banton. *Read Faster and Get More from Your Reading.* Englewood Cliffs, N.J.: Prentice-Hall, Inc., 1958.

Social Security Administration. *Social Security Handbook*. Washington, D.C. Government Printing Office.
Stewart, Marie M. *Business English and Communication*. 4th ed. New York: McGraw-Hill, Inc., 1972.
Stroman, J. H. *The Secretary's Manual*. New York: New American Library. 1968.
Texas Association of Homes for the Aging. *Manual on Volunteer Services*. Austin, Tex.: Texas Association of Homes for the Aging.
Thomas, Clayton L. *Tabors Cyclopedic Medical Dictionary*. 12th ed. Philadelphia: F. A. Davis Co., 1973.
Yoder, Dale. *Personnel Management and Industrial Relations*. 6th ed. Englewood Cliffs, N.J.: Prentice-Hall, Inc., 1970.
Zaccarelli, Herman E., and Maggiore, Josephine. *Nursing Home Menu Planning—Food Purchasing, Management*. Boston: Cahners Books, 1972.
Zelko, Harold P. *Successful Conference and Discussion Techniques*. New York: McGraw-Hill, Inc., 1957.

Journals

Accent on Living. P.O. Box 726, Bloomington, Illinois 61701.
Administrative Management. 51 Madison Avenue, New York, N.Y. 10010.
Better Nutrition. 25 West 45th Street, New York, N.Y. 10036.
Dynamic Maturity. 1225 Connecticut Ave., N.W., Washington, D.C. 20036.
Family Health. 1271 Avenue of the Americas, New York, N.Y. 10020.
Food Management. 757 Third Avenue, New York, N.Y. 10017.
Harvest Years. 104 East 40th Street, New York, N.Y. 10016.
Job Safety & Health. Supt. of Documents, Attn.: "S.L." Mail List, Washington, D.C. 20402.
Journal of the American Geriatrics Society. Williams & Wilkins Co., Baltimore, Md. 21202.
Mature Years. 201 8th Avenue So., Nashville, Tennessee 37202.
Modern Maturity. 215 Long Beach Blvd., Long Beach, Ca. 90801.
Modern Nursing Home. 230 West Monroe Street, Chicago, Illinois 60606.
Nursing Homes. 222 Wisconsin Avenue, Lake Forest, Illinois 60045.
Nursing Outlook. 10 Columbus Circle, New York, N.Y. 10019.
Psychology Today. 1330 Camino Del Mar, Del Mar, Ca. 92014.
R.N.: National Magazine for Nurses. Oradell, N.J. 07649.
Today's Health. 535 North Dearborn Ave., Chicago, Illinois 60610.

Associations, Societies, Institutions

American Association of Homes for the Aging. 315 Park Avenue South, New York, N.Y. 10010.

American Association of Retired Persons. 1225 Connecticut Avenue, N.W., Washington, D.C. 20036.

American College of Nursing Home Administrators. 8641 Colesville Road, Suite 409, Silver Spring, Md. 20910.

American Foundation for the Blind. 15 W. 16th Street, New York, N.Y. 10011.

American Health Care Association. 1200 15th Street, N.W., Washington, D.C. 20005.

American Heart Association. 44 East 23rd Street, New York, N.Y. 10010.

American Hospital Association. 840 North Lake Shore Drive, Chicago, Ill. 60611.

American Medical Association. 535 North Dearborn Street, Chicago, Ill. 60610.

American Nurses' Association, 10 Columbus Circle, New York, N.Y. 10019.

American Registry for Physical Therapists. 30 North Michigan Avenue, Chicago, Ill. 60602.

American Rehabilitation Foundation. 1800 Chicago Avenue, Minneapolis, Minn. 55404.

American Speech and Hearing Association, 1001 Connecticut Ave. N.W., Washington, D.C. 20036.

Center for Health Administration Studies. 5555 South Ellis Ave., Chicago, Illinois 60637.

Center for Studies in Aging. North Texas State University, Denton, Tex. 76203.

Gerontological Society. Suite 520, One Dupont Circle, Washington, D.C. 20036.

International Food Research and Educational Center. North Easton, Mass. 02356.

Joint Commission on Accreditation of Hospitals and Nursing Homes. 200 East Ohio, Chicago, Ill. 60611.

National Association of Boards of Examiners for Nursing Home Administrators. P.O. Box 9706, Austin, Tex. 78766.

National Council on Aging. 44 West 45th Street, New York, N.Y. 10036.

National Council of Senior Citizens, Inc. 1627 K Street N.W., Washington, D.C. 20006.

National Geriatrics Society. 11 East 48th Street, New York, N.Y. 10017.

National Fire Protection Association. 470 Atlantic Avenue, Boston, Mass. 02110.

National Health Council. 1790 Broadway, New York, N.Y. 10019.

National Recreation Association. 8 West 8th Street, New York, N.Y. 10011.

National Rehabilitation Association. 1029 Vermont Avenue, N.W. Washington, D.C. 20005.

National Society for Crippled Children and Adults. 2023 Ogden Avenue, Chicago, Illinois 60614.

National Society for the Prevention of Blindness. 16 East 40th Street, New York, N.Y. 10016.

Governmental Agencies

Administration on Aging. Dept. of Health, Education, and Welfare, 330 Independence Ave., S.W., Washington, D.C. 20201.

Bureau of Census. Department of Commerce, Washington, D.C. 20233.

Bureau of Outdoor Recreation. Room 2024, Interior Building, Washington, D.C. 20240.

Department of Health, Education, and Welfare. 330 Independence Ave. S.W., Washington, D.C. 20201.

Department of the Interior. Interior Building, Washington, D.C. 20240.

Department of Labor. 14th and Constitution Ave. N.W., Washington, D.C. 20240.

Environmental Protection Agency. Washington, D.C. 20242.

Food and Drug Administration. 200 C Street. S.W., Washington, D.C. 20204.

General Services Administration. 19th and F Street, N.W., Washington, D.C. 20405.

Government Printing Office. Public Documents Department, Washington, D.C. 20402.

Interstate Commerce Commission. 12th and Constitution Ave., Washington, D.C. 20230.

Small Business Administration. 1441 L Street N.W., Washington, D.C. 20416.

Social Security Administration. 6401 Security Blvd., Baltimore, Md. 21235.

Veterans Administration. 810 Vermont Ave., N.W., Washington, D.C. 20420.

Index

376